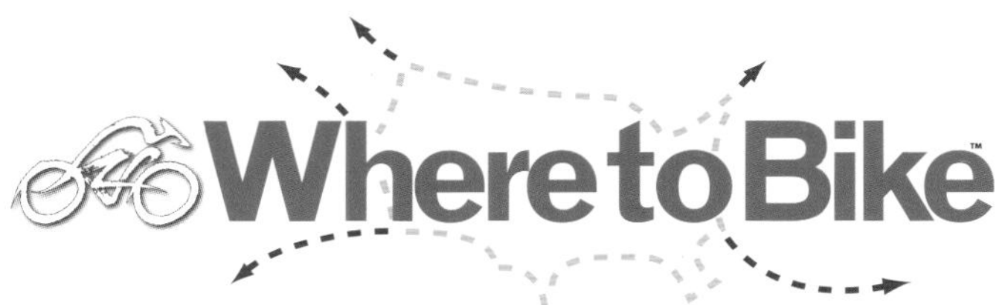

Orange County

- North Inland
- North Coast
- Central Inland
- Central Coast
- South
- Kids' Rides

By Peter Dopulos

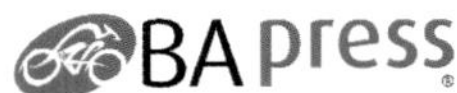

Where to Bike LLC

Email: mail@wheretobikeguides.com
Tel: +61 2 4274 4884 - Fax: +61 2 4274 0988
www.wheretobikeguides.com

First published in the USA in 2012 by Where to Bike LLC.

Design and Layout - Justine Powell
Advertising - Phil Latz
Photography - Peter Dopulos unless otherwise specified
Mapping - Justine Powell, Bicycling Australia
Printed in China by RR Donnelley
Cover - Photo by Peter Dopulos

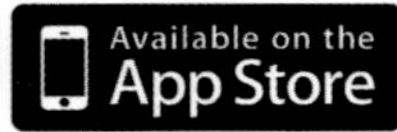

Library of Congress Control Number: 2012938394
Author: Peter Dopulos
Title: Where to Bike Orange County
ISBN: 978-0-9871686-8-9
978-0-9871851-1-2

The Cycling Kangaroo logo is a trademark of Lake Wangary Publishing Company Pty Ltd.

Where to Bike is a proud sponsor of World Bicycle Relief.

Where to Bike is a proud member of the Bikes Belong Coalition, organizers of the People for Bikes campaign; and the League of American Bicyclists.

peopleforbikes.org

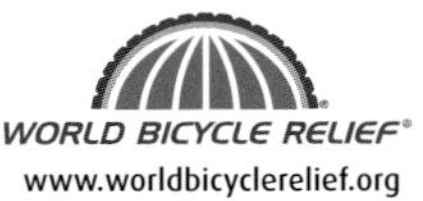

www.worldbicyclerelief.org

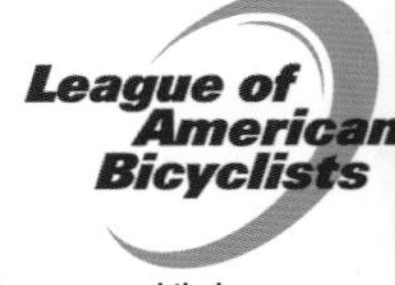

www.bikeleague.org

Also in this series:

Where to Ride Melbourne
Where to Ride Adelaide
Where to Ride Perth
Where to Ride Sydney
Where to Ride Canberra
Where to Ride South East Queensland
Where to Ride Tasmania
Where to Ride Western & Northern Victoria
Where to Ride Eastern Victoria
Where to Ride Sydney MTB
Where to Ride London
Where to Bike Chicago
Where to Bike Washington, D.C.
Where to Bike Philadelphia
Where to Bike Los Angeles
Where to Bike New York City
Where to Bike Portland
Where to Bike Los Angeles Mountain Biking

Coming soon:

Where to Ride Auckland
Where to Ride Melbourne Mountain Biking
Where to Bike Orange County Mountain Biking

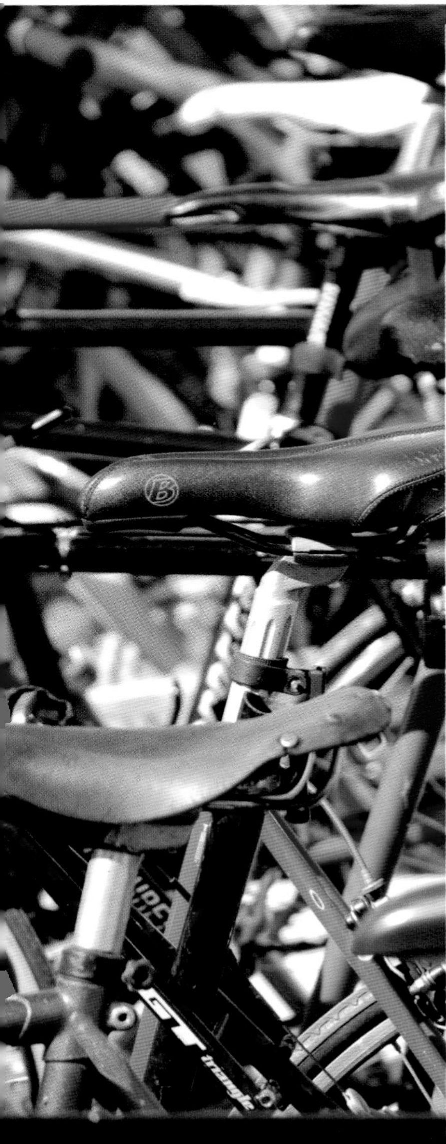

About us...

Cycling has many health and environmental benefits, but in addition to these it's a fun leisure time activity for all ages. Bike touring is also a great way to get up close and personal with a new destination. Where to Bike guides provide locals and tourists alike with advice on the best ride options for fun, exploration and relaxation on two wheels.

Most of our team are active cyclists; we love to ride and hope that we can inspire and motivate readers to join us on two wheels. We're committed to our vision of enhancing all aspects of cycling through these Where to Bike guides and our other publications.

Available in printed hard copy through bike shops and book stores, Where to Bike publications are also offered in digital format online. Check the iTunes store for an eBook version if you prefer a soft copy, or download the IOS App and we'll guide you along the route of each ride as you go!

Look out for other Where to Bike titles and the 'cycling kangaroo' logo in news stands and bookstores; it's your key to quality cycling publications.

We have made every effort to ensure the accuracy of the content of this book, but please feel free to contact us at feedback@wheretobikeguides.com to report any changes to routes or inconsistencies you may find.

For more information about *Where to Bike Orange County* and other books in this series, visit **www.wheretobikeguides.com.**

Image Matt Wittmer

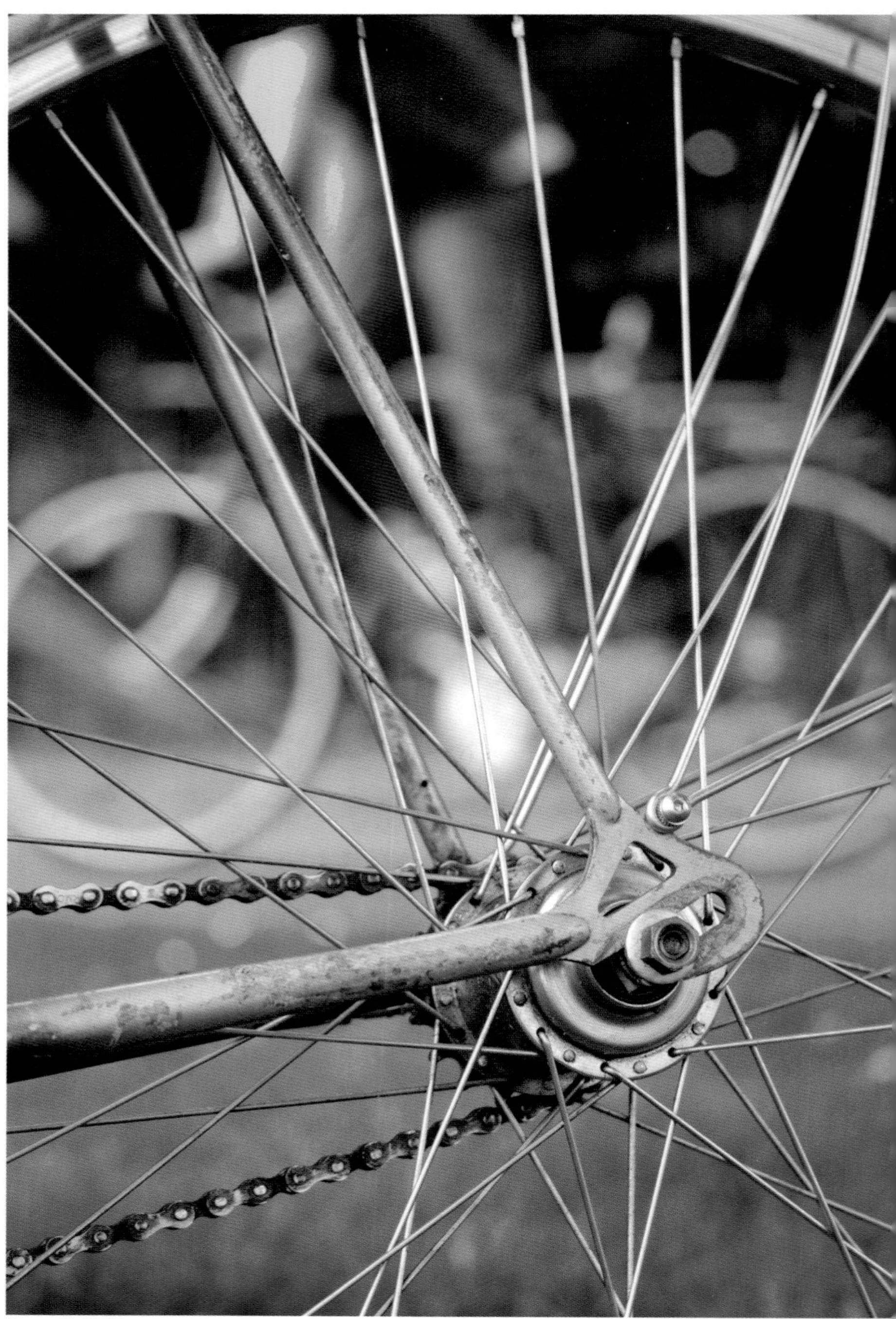

Image Matt Wittmer

Foreword by Garry Brown

Executive Director, Orange County Coastkeeper

An Insiders Guide to Orange County Bikeways

With perfect weather, and over 1,000 miles of bike trails, Orange County is a cycling paradise. Thirty-four cities along with the County of Orange have dedicated bike lanes and trails to cycling. Cycling is not just a form of transportation and recreation – in Orange County it is a way of life. Along with the miles of bike trails and dedicated bike lanes, Orange County is also home to an extensive network of roadways and traffic. Knowing where to go, and how to get there is an important part of enjoying the bikeways that make Orange County a singular and an exceptional place to live and visit.

here to Bike Orange County is a treasure trove of formation that will guide the reader throughout rious destinations in Orange County. From hilly rba Linda in the north to central, historical wntown Santa Ana, to the beaches of San Clemente d beyond, this guide can literally direct the cyclist on ites from the inland areas to the beach and back. The ites are linked together, allowing for full day rides as ll as short family friendly jaunts. Cyclists can begin ir day in the foothills and follow a freshwater river the waves of the Pacific Ocean. A day of surfing can n into cycling-surfing safari! My wife and I enjoy weekly ride that takes us from the front door of home, past the Bolsa Chica wetlands and ends at surf mecca of Huntington Beach. *Where to Bike ange County* also introduces the reader to different ts of Orange County and the unique restaurants and utiful parks and attractions that even some natives e yet to discover.

Orange County has worked to balance the many nsportation options available to those who live, rk, and play here. Part of this balance comes in form of bicycling, and areas designed for safe enjoyable riding. In 2009, the Orange County nsportation Authority (OCTA) adopted the 2009 nmuter Bikeways Strategic Plan (CBSP). The SP is a plan of the existing bikeways in the county, well as a proposal for new bikeways. Where to e Orange County is a user friendly translation of this regional planning document and takes the concept of the CBSP to the next level by providing maps and step by step guidelines for enjoying the bikeways of the county.

Since I founded it in 1999, Orange County Coastkeeper has grown to become the leading environmental organization working to preserve the waterways and coastline of Orange County. With millions of residents and visitors every year, Orange County's breath-taking beaches are world-renowned. The county also has miles of fresh water rivers that course from the inland areas and drain at the beaches. What I find most appealing about *Where to Bike Orange County* is that cyclists can use it to experience the beautiful natural resources of Orange County through its extensive network of bike routes along Orange County waterways. Whether you are a casual weekend rider or more serious with your commitment to cycling, this book is a treat. The bikeways in Orange County increase appreciation and awareness of our environment. Users of Orange County bike trails and bike lanes can enjoy what Orange County Coastkeeper has worked to keep clean – our water. Grab your bike, leaf through the pages of *Where to Bike Orange County* for a new part of Orange County to discover, and enjoy the ride!

Garry Brown

Executive Director, Orange County Coastkeeper

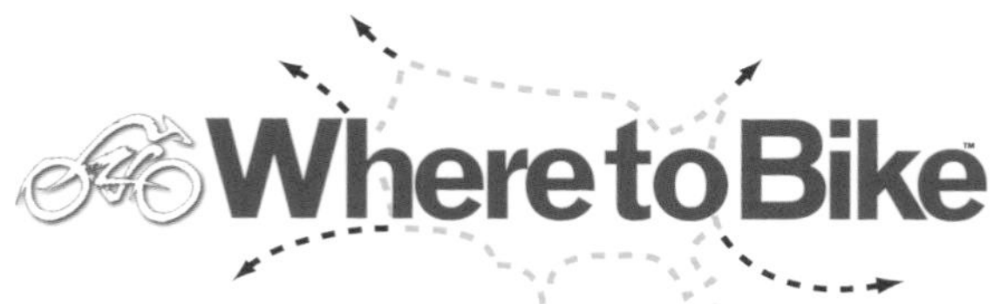

Orange County

Contents

North Inland

North Coast

entral Inland

entral Coast

uth

Kids' Rides

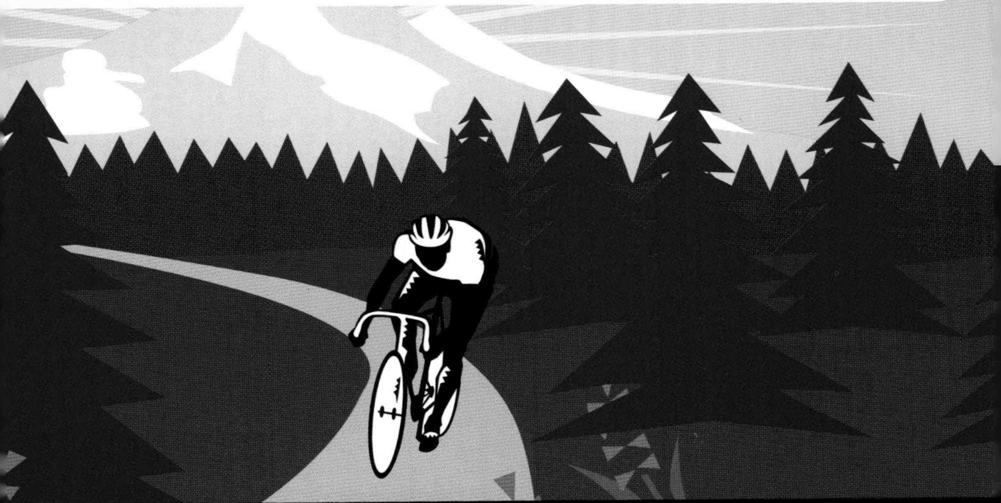

Author's Note

In writing this book I spent a year of my life riding thousands of miles, exploring parts of Orange County I hadn't known existed, and re-visiting old haunts with fresh eyes. Along the way I enjoyed the company of dear friends and made new ones, while riding with strangers and family alike. I exuberantly set out on this journey which was a good thing, because if I had paused for too long to think about the task and the amount of work that lay ahead, I might have had second thoughts. Now with most of the pages completed and put to print, I look back and marvel at the effort it took and all the help I received along the way.

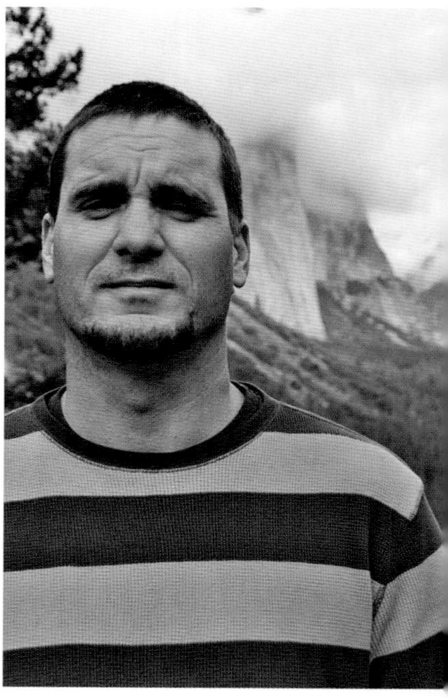

Orange County is a decentralized patchwork of suburbs, usually with one municipality bleeding seamlessly into the next. As I developed these routes, my overall vision was to connect the entire county through a web of bike rides that would allow cyclists to ride from the most northerly section to the most southerly part of the county. For most people this would mean simply following Pacific Coast Highway from Seal Beach to San Clemente, and while this route would run through the county, it would leave out most of the county as well. Think of these rides as a network of interconnected bikeways and paths that would allow any cyclist to navigate the entire county by bike.

From a cyclist's point of view, Orange County is as close to bicycle nirvana as I have experienced. Although not every city is crisscrossed by bike lanes, there are still literally thousands of miles of bike lanes and paths. The cities of Irvine, Fullerton, Huntington Beach, Dana Point and San Clemente, to name a few, have invested considerable resources to developing comprehensive transportation plans that include cycling infrastructure. Combine this with the incredibly diverse terrain these routes pass and you will find a ride for everyone. There are long, car-free river rides, flat coastal routes, and inland challenging climbs through steep foothills. And while Orange County often gets painted as bland and cookie cutter, for those willir ride these routes you will find a great deal of va and diversity, not just in the rides themselves, but i cities and the people who live here as well.

But it's not just the paint on the road or a bike signs thrown up that make this county su pleasant place to ride. In the thousands of miles I throughout the county, I did not have a single nega confrontation with a motorist. Orange County, w the car still reigns supreme, seems to provide proof cars and bikes can peacefully coexist.

As you ride these routes I would welc comments and questions, discoveries or concerns email at wheretobikeOC@gmail.com, Facebook c wheretobikeOC.com.

Be safe, ride on.

Peter Dopulos
Author & Photographer

bout the Author

eter Dopulos discovered his passion for cycling at age five when he borrowed a neighbor's shiny red e and took it for a joy-ride. Despite the punishment received thereafter, a life-long obsession of all gs bicycling was born. As an adult he became a sically-trained chef, spending two decades running hens and ultimately building a catering business. ay he shares cycling with his wife, two kids and one willing to listen to him talk about bikes.

knowledgements

t and foremost, I need to thank my wife, Tracy, and kids, Max and Bella. Their schedules were juggled quite a few Sunday brunches were missed in order me to do those longer rides, or re-take photos that n't turn out right. But most of all, I want to thank n for all the miles we rode together and the patience y had when this year-long project took my attention y from them. The family rides were the sweetest es of this book.

To Sharon and Paul, aka Mom and Dad, the family es we did when I was a child inspired me to make ain my own kids had as many wonderful bicycling mories as I have.

To Keith Lewis of Swoop's World Radio, who e some of those miles as well and who has been constant supporter and cheerleader, thank you. Barbara Holbrook, without whom I would have sed this wonderful opportunity altogether, I offer sincere gratitude. A thank you goes also to Garry wn of Orange County Coastkeeper, for his support wonderfully penned foreword.

Producing a book of this size and detail requires a numental effort by many, and the hard working group Bicycling Australia rose to the challenge. Justine and y were invaluable in their careful criticisms and ting and without them this endeavor would not have n possible. To Phil, thanks for the opportunity to nd over a year working at something I love.

Finally, a special thanks to all the friendly cyclists I met along the way that let me take their pictures and helped me with suggestions of their favorite rides or their favorite place to eat. Happy trails to you all – keep on rolling.

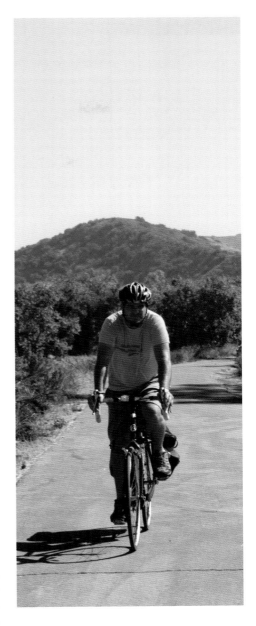

Introduction

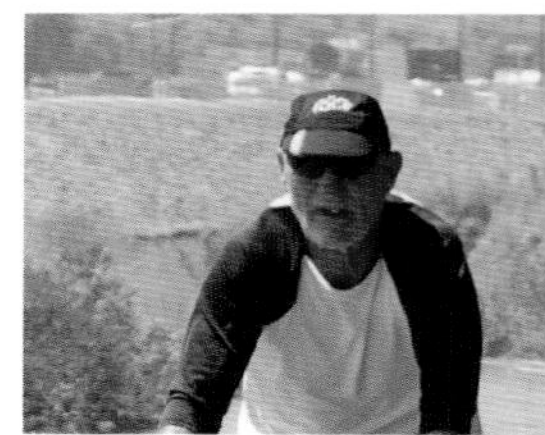
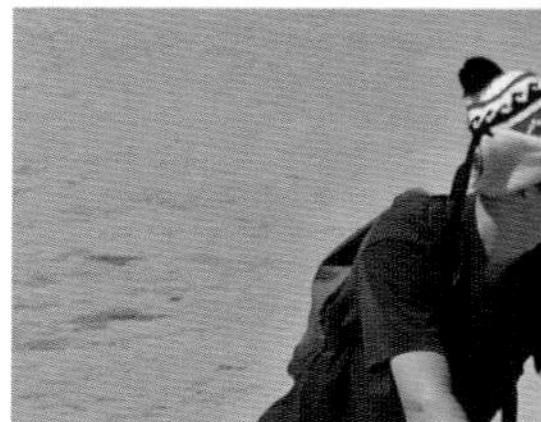
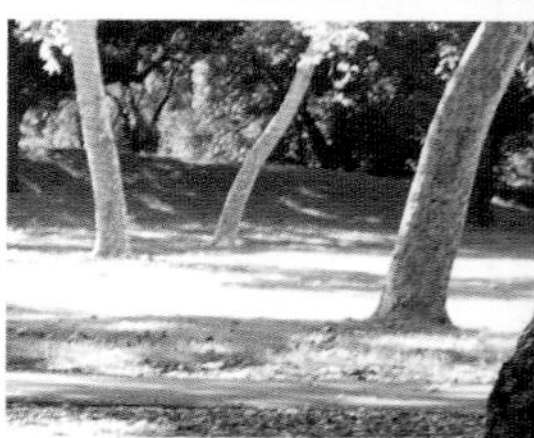
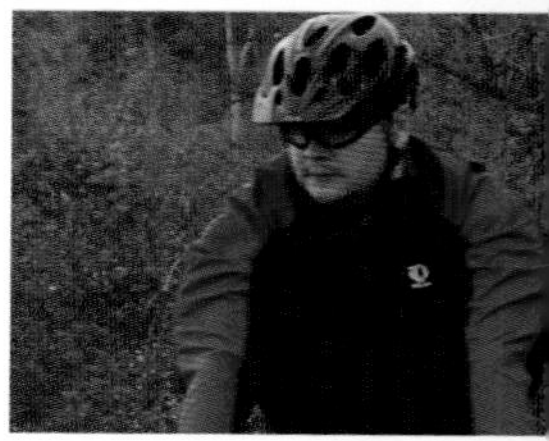
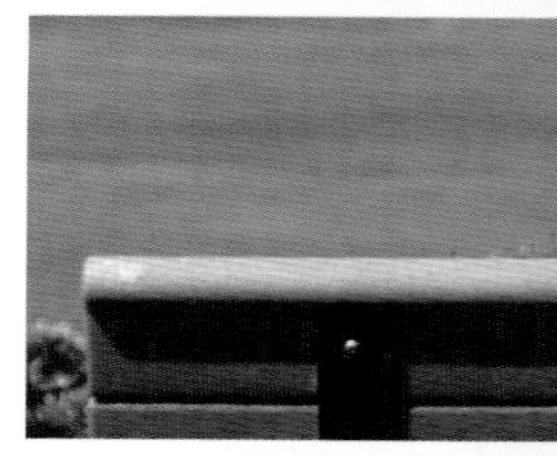
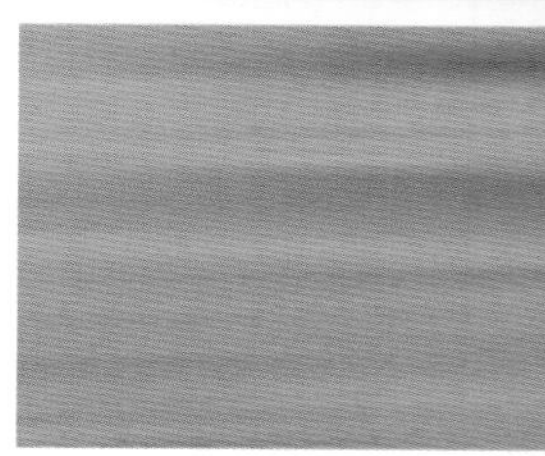

Once an agricultural center, Orange County has grown from a suburb of Los Angeles into its own metropolitan entity. Although the smallest county in California by land area, it's the third largest in population behind Los Angeles and San Diego counties. In this small space with lots of people, bikes have become an increasingly important and efficient mode of transportation. Not surprisingly, many of Orange County's 34 cities have realized that alternatives to car travel are more important than ever and are adopting transportation models that include bus, rail and bicycles. In the famously master planned communities of the central and southern parts of the county, bicycle routes have been designed into the very fabric of the communities and as a result the bike culture has taken root and blossomed.

Cycling in the county is booming with more routes and lanes than ever before. Whether you are interested in commuting, training or casual recreation, in the 53 rides that follow there is a little something for everyone. The first section of the book is the North Inland where you will find an interesting mix of hilly and flat rides through older cities such as Fullerton and La Habra as well as spins through newer parts of the county such as Yorba Linda and Placentia. The North Coast section features mostly flat, coastal and river rides through Seal Beach, Sunset Beach and Huntington Beach.

Moving further south takes you to the Central Inland section where the county pushes up against the Santa Ana Mountains. Rides through here often involve climbs and in a few instances take you through rugged wilderness. The Central Coast is probably the most bike-friendly section of the county with nearly every major thoroughfare here boasting a bike lane. The South section rides are primarily coastal with a few rare flat rides, and miles of hills to climb.

If you are traveling with young riders, as I often am, you will find plenty of kids' rides in the final section that are scattered across the county, often near one of the longer adult rides. Here you will find a range of outings from the safe, flat loops that are ideal for the beginners to longer rides for those kids ready to increase mileage. Also, look for the family-friendly icon among the adult rides for routes that more experienced families can explore.

Unfortunately, due to its decentralized, suburban nature, the car is still king in Orange County. Each city retains autonomy regarding its transportation efforts and some have been quicker to incorporate cycling than others. So until the time arrives when the entire county is connected by a web of bike lanes and paths, use those freeways for what they were meant for; to carry your bike to the part of the county you want to ride.

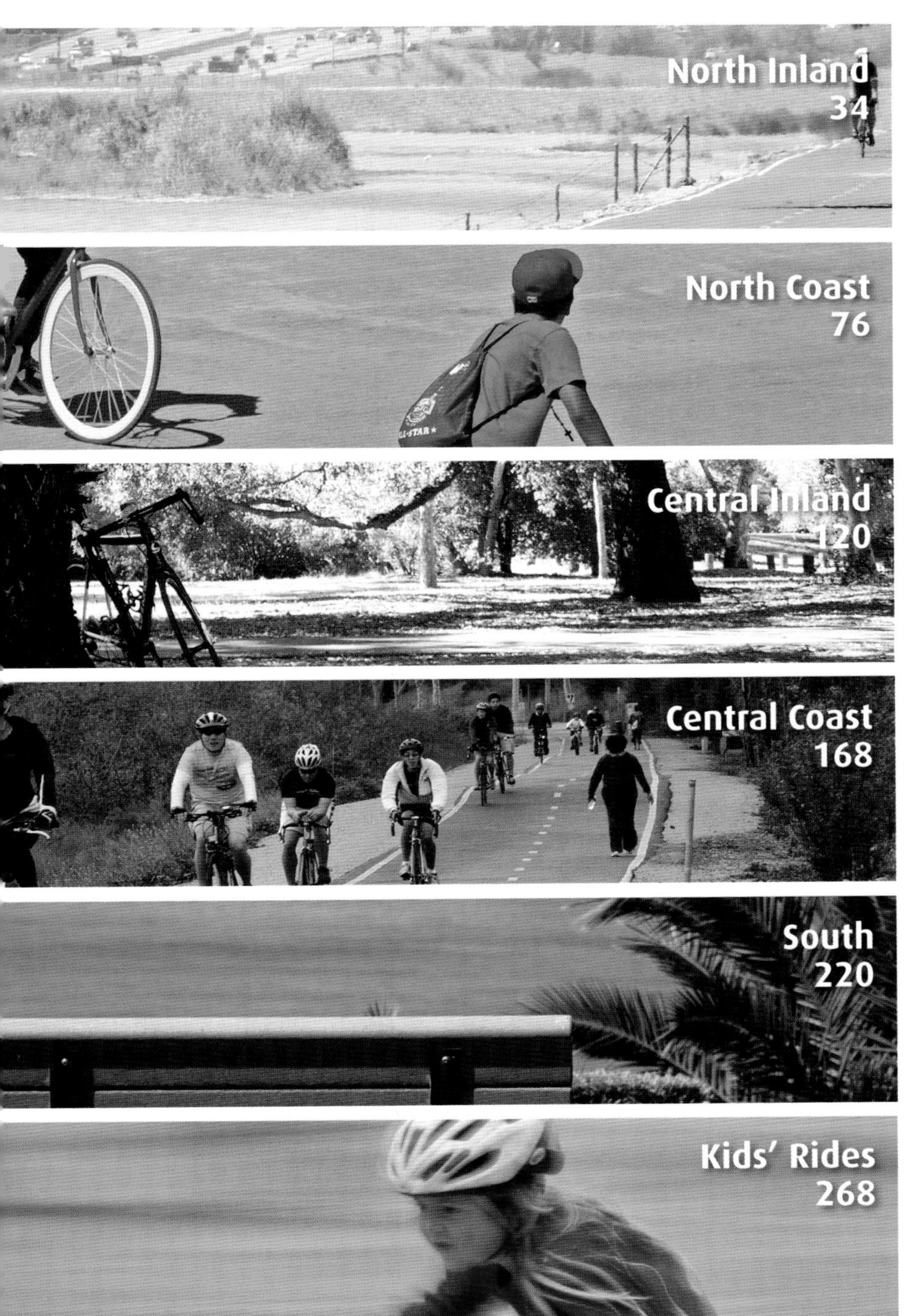
North Inland
34
North Coast
76
Central Inland
120
Central Coast
168
South
220
Kids' Rides
268

How to Use This Book

Although Orange County is often divided simply as north and south, for the purpose of this book the 53 adult rides have been divided into five color-coded regions, with a sixth section dedicated to 32 kids' rides. From flat coastal outings in the North Coast section, to the hilly routes of the South, browse these chapters to find the right ride for your skill level and riding style.

Locating a ride is simple and often the best place to start is the Ride Overview section. Here rides are listed by section along with pertinent data including length and elevation as well as icons that indicate the overall feel of the ride. The overview also provides the ride's start location, ride number and page number, as well as the ride scale.

The rides themselves are made up of four parts. "At a Glance" will provide quick details that include directions to the start, side trips, dining opportunities, links to other rides and what sort of traffic to expect. Icons located near the bottom of the page will indicate whether this ride travels on bike paths, on-road or along on-road lanes while icons along the top bar indicate the overall nature of the ride.

The "About" page is a detailed account of the ride and includes a bit of history about the area, information on points of interest and notes about the landscape ride traverses. Following this page is the Ride I and map which used together will guide you thro the ride. Maps were produced using a GPS unit make them as accurate as possible and include ic for points of interest, dining, water, restrooms shopping opportunities. Links to other rides a appear as they intersect the route.

Ride Scale

Each ride is assigned a Where to Bike rating wh provides a standard scale for all our guidebooks. Y will find these on the "At a Glance" page of each r as well as the Ride Overview section. It looks like th

The number of cycling kangaroos on red ov indicates the ride difficulty based on distan elevation and surface conditions. All the rides in t book are suitable for recreational cyclists, but wit that category there can be a lot of difference. The sc goes from one to five, with one meant for those new cycling or returning after a long time away. A rating five indicates a ride for the most experienced cyclis You will find most of the rides in this book fall in middle of this scale.

	1 pt	2 pts	3 pts	4 pts	5 pts
Distance – Road (miles)	<12	12-19	19-25	25-37	>37
Distance – MTB (miles)	<6	6-9	9-16	16-25	>25
Climbing (feet)	<500	500 - 1,000	1,000 - 1,500	1,500 - 2,000	>2,000
Surface	Paved smooth	Paved rough	Unpaved smooth	Unpaved moderate	Unpaved rough

Accumulated Points	Riding Level/Grade	Suggested Suitability
3	1	Beginner
4-5	2	
6-7	3	Moderately fit
8-9	4	
10+	5	Experienced cyclist

de Classifications

de Classifications are used to represent the distinct aracter of the ride itself and are usually a reflection the environment or landscape the cyclist will enjoy they travel the route.

In *Where to Bike Orange County*, there are six ssifications to look for on the ride At a Glance page:

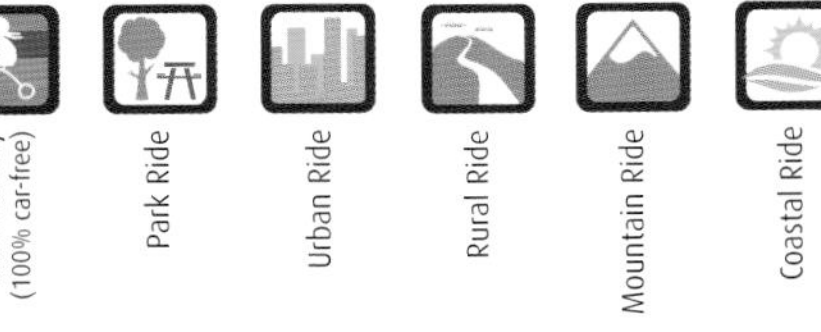

de Links

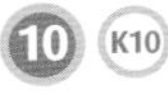

you're partial to adding to your ride, or simply erested in other routes nearby, information on ride ks can be found on both the ride At a Glance page, d on the maps.

At a Glance: Ride numbers included in the 'Links panel on the At a Glance page are considered direct ks—rides that intersect with, or can be accessed th ease from the current route.

Maps: Each map includes easy to identify ride link ons at either the location of junction, or at the closest int the linked ride can be accessed from the current e. The maps show all links, both direct and non-ect—and each link route is highlighted with an easy identify orange dashed line.

ke Shops and Rentals

ke shops and bike rental outlets are marked upon ch map with icons as above. Each icon carries a mber which correlates to a comprehensive store ting on page 306. Here you'll find the name, number d web details of the stores that are an easy pedal om all of the rides. No spares? No worries.

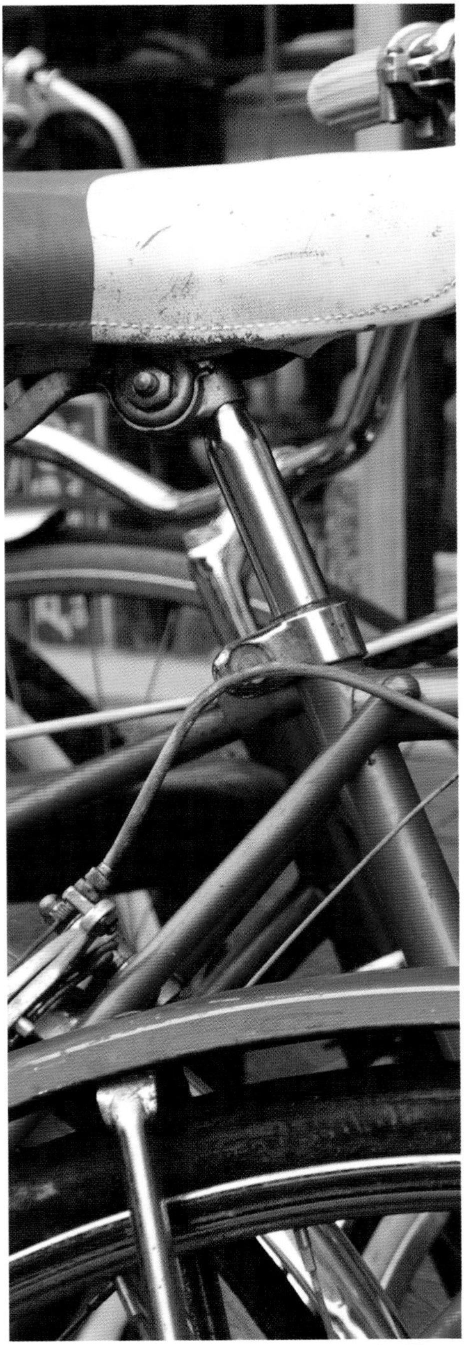

Image Matt Wittmer

Terrain Guide

To help you understand what to expect on the route, terrain types are described on both the At a Glance page, and directly on the maps with easy to follow colored ride lines, as follows:

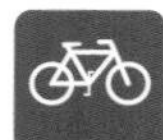

On-Road:

A *red ride line* depicts sections of the ride that are on-road. The cyclist shares the road with vehicular traffic, and is expected to abide by road rules and laws. These routes are either Class III Bike Routes, or are considered comparably safe for recommendation by the author.

On-Road Bike Lane:

A *green ride line* depicts sections of the ride where exclusive on-road bike lanes are provided. Here the cyclist is clearly separated from vehicular traffic by a traffic lane marked on an existing roadway that is restricted to cycle traffic. These routes are Class II Bike Routes, and are only indicated if such infrastructure is in place.

Protected On-Road Bike Lane:

A *blue ride line* depicts sections of the ride where exclusive, protected on-road bike lanes are provided. Here the cyclist is clearly separated from vehicular traffic by a physical barrier that is restricted to use by cycle traffic. Such barriers can consist of parked cars or painted curbs. These routes are also considered Class I Bike Routes, and are only indicated if such infrastructure is in place.

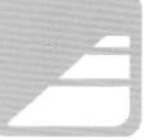

Designated Bike Path:

A *yellow ride line* depicts sections of the ride that are on smooth bike paths where the cyclist is completely separated from roads. The path can either be a sidepath (designated for use by cyclists) or a shared-use footway (for use by both cyclists and pedestrians). These routes are either Class I Bike Routes, or are considered comparably safe for recommendation by the author.

Off-Road:

A *brown ride line* depicts sections of the ric that are on wide, unpaved dirt trails, that a smooth enough for navigation by any ty of bike.

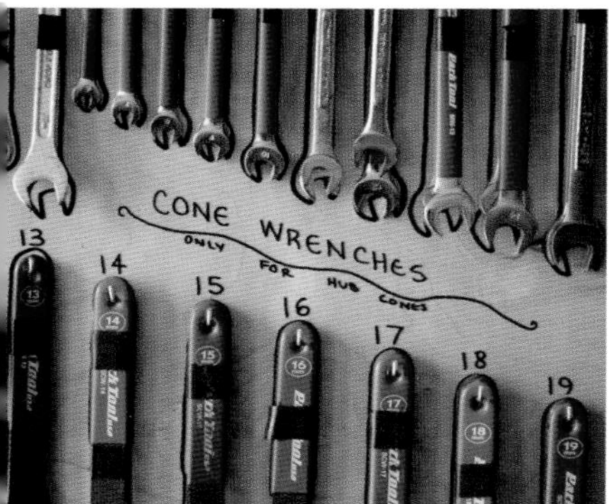

efore You Go

he benefits of an active lifestyle are beyond dispute and cycling can play a significant role getting fit and staying healthy. If you are new cycling or are returning after a lengthy hiatus, sult your doctor before hopping on a bike. It uld also be a good idea to make sure your bike equipment is in good working order. Nothing turn you off of cycling faster than getting nded miles away from home because your bike ke down.

fore you ride, some things to check:

- Inflate tires to proper pressure and check for damage.
- Check brake pads and cables work properly.
- Check gear cables and shifters work, allowing shifting to every gear.
- Clean and lubricate chain.

f your bike has been sitting in the garage uched, or worse, outside, for a considerable time sider taking it to your local shop for some TLC. es are simple machines that when well-maintained a pleasure to operate. Rusty, grinding, rubbing parts slate into a lot more energy spent by you to make simple machine move. And that can make even the rtest jaunt seem like the longest ride of your life.

What to Take

All of these rides, with a couple of exceptions, travel within easy reach of civilization and a nearby bike shop, meaning you don't need to carry much. But a few essentials will make your outings more enjoyable. Even if you don't enjoy repairing your bike, at the very least know how to change a flat.

- A helmet, properly fitted
- Gloves
- Water, plan to drink a quart per hour
- Snacks
- Cash, ID, medical info, credit card
- Cellphone
- Spare inner tube, tire levers, patch kit and pump/ CO2 cartridges and adapter
- First aid kit
- Wind breaker
- Bike lock
- Sunscreen

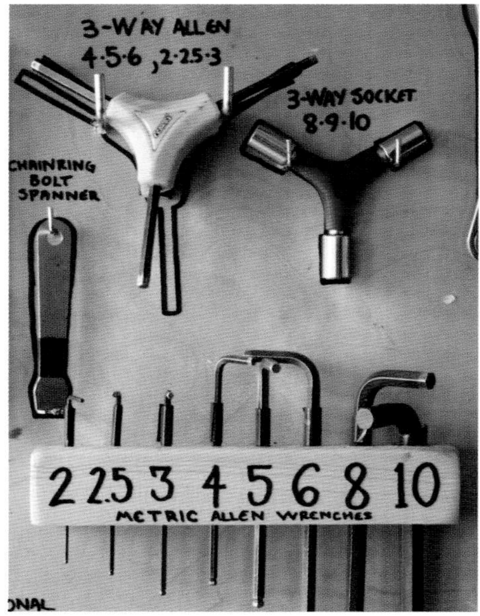

Ride Overview

North Inland

Page	Ride	Ride Name	Start Location
38	1	Anaheim Canyon Metrolink to Corona Metrolink	Anaheim Canyon Metrolink parking lot
42	2	La Habra/Whittier Loop	Portola Park, La Habra
46	3	La Habra Guadalupe Park/Loop to Children's Museum	Guadalupe Park, La Habra
50	4	Yorba Linda Recreational Trail	George Koch Park, Placentia
54	5	Placentia Loop	Tri-City Park, Placentia
58	6	Coyote Hills/West Fullerton Loop	Bastanchury Park, Fullerton
62	7	Laguna Lake Loop	Laguna Lake, Fullerton
66	8	Fullerton Loop	Berkeley Ave, near Fullerton College
70	9	Old Town Fullerton to Independence Park	Walnut Ave, next to Fullerton Station

North Coast

Page	Ride	Ride Name	Start Location
80	10	Cerritos Regional Park Up Coyote Creek Trail	Cerritos Regional Park
84	11	Cypress /La Palma Loop	El Rancho Verde bike path, La Palma
88	12	El Dorado Two Loop	Golden Grove in El Dorado Park
92	13	San Gabriel River Trail to Coyote Creek Trail and Back	In front of End of River Café, Seal Beach
96	14	Seal Beach Loop (Westminster)	In front of Out-spoken bike shop, Sunset Beach
100	15	Electric Avenue, Seal Beach	San Gabriel River Trail, Seal Beach
104	16	Tour of Huntington Beach	Yorktown Ave, across from City Hall
108	17	Fountain Valley Green Belt	Greenbelt in Fountain Valley
112	18	Bolsa Chica to Santa Ana River	Bolsa Chica State Beach, intersection with Warner A
116	19	The Big Loop	Intersection of Warner Ave and PCH, Huntington Be

Central Inland

Page	Ride	Ride Name	Start Location
124	20	Santa Ana Canyon Road	Eucalyptus Park, Anaheim Hills
128	21	City of Orange to Villa Park Loop	Historic Orange traffic circle
132	22	Santiago Canyon Road	Peter's Canyon Regional Park, Orange
136	23	Jamboree/North Tustin Loop	Centennial Park, Tustin
140	24	Irvine Regional Park	Orange County Zoo, Irvine
144	25	Peters Canyon Trail	Irvine Regional Park

Terrain	Kid-Friendly	Distance (miles)	Elev. Gain (feet)	WTB Rating
On Road / On Road Lane / Path	partial	42.55	2982	
On Road / On Road Lane / Path	no	21.53	984	
On Road / Path / Off Road	partial	1.81	85	
On Road / On Road Lane / Path	partial	18.55	563	
On Road Lane / Path	no	11.91	640	
On Road / On Road Lane / Path	no	8.94	1222	
On Road / On Road Lane / Off Road		3.26	240	
On Road / On Road Lane / Path	no	23.81	1715	
On Road / On Road Lane	partial	7.86	209	

Terrain	Kid-Friendly	Distance (miles)	Elev. Gain (feet)	WTB Rating
Path		11.29	240	
On Road / On Road Lane / Path	no	10.6	59	
On Road Lane / Path		7.66	91	
Path		17.3	244	
On Road / On Road Lane	no	13.0	132	
On Road / On Road Lane / Path	partial	2.49	43	
On Road / On Road Lane	no	22.67	247	
On Road / On Road Lane / Path	partial	7.24	226	
Path		16.85	185	
On Road / On Road Lane / Path	no	38.0	351	

Terrain	Kid-Friendly	Distance (miles)	Elev. Gain (feet)	WTB Rating
On Road / On Road Lane	no	16.96	1218	
On Road / On Road Lane / Path	partial	12.64	390	
On Road Lane / Path	no	32.55	1986	
On Road / On Road Lane	no	23.34	1294	
Path		2.95	85	
On Road Lane / Path / Off Road	partial	18.27	987	

Ride Overview continued

Page	Ride	Ride Name	Start Location
148	26	Santiago Creek Trail	Grijalva Park, Orange
152	27	Portola to Sand Canyon, Irvine	Portola Staging Area, Irvine
156	28	Hicks Trail/Peters East Branch Loop	Hicks Canyon Community Park, Irvine
160	29	Irvine Loop - Irvine Boulevard, Alton Parkway, Irvine Center Drive	Across from Northwood Park, Irvine
164	30	Rancho Margarita Loop	Trabuco Mesa Park

Central Coast

Page	Ride	Ride Name	Start Location
172	31	Santa Ana River Trail	Huntingon Beach State Beach
176	32	Pacific Electric Trail to SART	Corner of Maple St and Chestnut Ave, Santa Ana
180	33	Yale Loop	Across from Windrow Community Park, Irvine
184	34	Alton & Barranca Parkway Loop	Civic Center Park, Irvine
188	35	Walnut Bike Trail/Incredible Edible Park	Flagstone Park, Irvine
192	36	Shady Canyon Trail Loop	William R. Mason Regional Park, Irvine
196	37	Turtle Rock to UC Irvine Loop	Turtle Rock Community Park, Irvine
200	38	San Diego Creek Trail	Eastbluff Dr and Jamboree Rd, Newport Beach
204	39	Newport Beach/Back Bay Loop	Castaway Park, Newport Beach
208	40	Fairview Park/Mesa Verde Loop	Fairview Park, Costa Mesa
212	41	Balbo Peninsula	Newport Pier, Balboa Peninsula
216	42	Crystal Cove Park	Southern parking lot, Crystal Cove State Beach

East

Page	Ride	Ride Name	Start Location
224	43	Aliso Creek Bikeway	Sheep Hill Park, Laguna Hills
228	44	Live Oak Canyon Trail/O'Neill Regional Park	Trabuco Mesa Park, Rancho Santa Margarita
232	45	Irvine Metrolink to Mission Viejo via Muirlands	Irvine Metrolink station
236	46	Aliso Creek Trail to Aliso and Wood Canyons	Sheep Hill Park, Laguna Hills
240	47	Laguna Niguel Regional Park	Park entrance, Laguna Niguel
244	48	Salt Creek Trail	Salt Creek Beach parking lot, Dana Point
248	49	Dana Point Loop	Southern end Doheny State Beach, Dana Point
252	50	San Juan Creek to San Juan Capistrano	Dana Point Harbor, Ocean Institute
256	51	Dana Point to San Clemente and Back	Salt Creek Beach parking lot, Dana Point
260	52	Hilly San Clemente	Camino Capistrano, Pines Park, Dana Point
264	53	San Clemente Metro to Camp Pendelton	San Clemente Metrolink Station

Path		12.53	459	
On Road Lane / Path	no	15.85	762	
On Road Lane / Path		7.98	401	
On Road Lane	no	13.85	685	
On Road Lane	no	17.54	1033	

Terrain	Kid-Friendly	Distance (miles)	Elev. Gain (feet)	WTB Rating
Path		43.79	1118	
On Road Lane / Path	no	12.25	173	
On Road Lane	partial	4.88	50	
On Road Lane	no	17.57	529	
Path		8.27	147	
Path		13.78	612	
On Road Lane / Path	no	8.11	590	
Path		19.82	577	
On Road Lane / Path	partial	10.5	331	
On Road / On Road Lane / Path	partial	11.71	367	
On Road Lane / Path	partial	9.3	37	
Path		5.48	295	

Terrain	Kid-Friendly	Distance (miles)	Elev. Gain (feet)	WTB Rating
Path		18.86	1025	
On Road Lane / Path	partial	10.7	745	
On Road Lane	no	17.09	1174	
On Road / Path		11.31	329	
On Road / Path		4.44	194	
On Road / On Road Lane / Path	partial	11.3	884	
On Road / On Road Lane / Path	no	9.36	583	
On Road Lane / Path	partial	13.03	162	
On Road / On Road Lane / Protected On Road Lane / Path	partial	12.79	345	
On Road Lane / Path	no	16.03	1246	
On Road / On Road Lane / Path	no	29.01	1034	

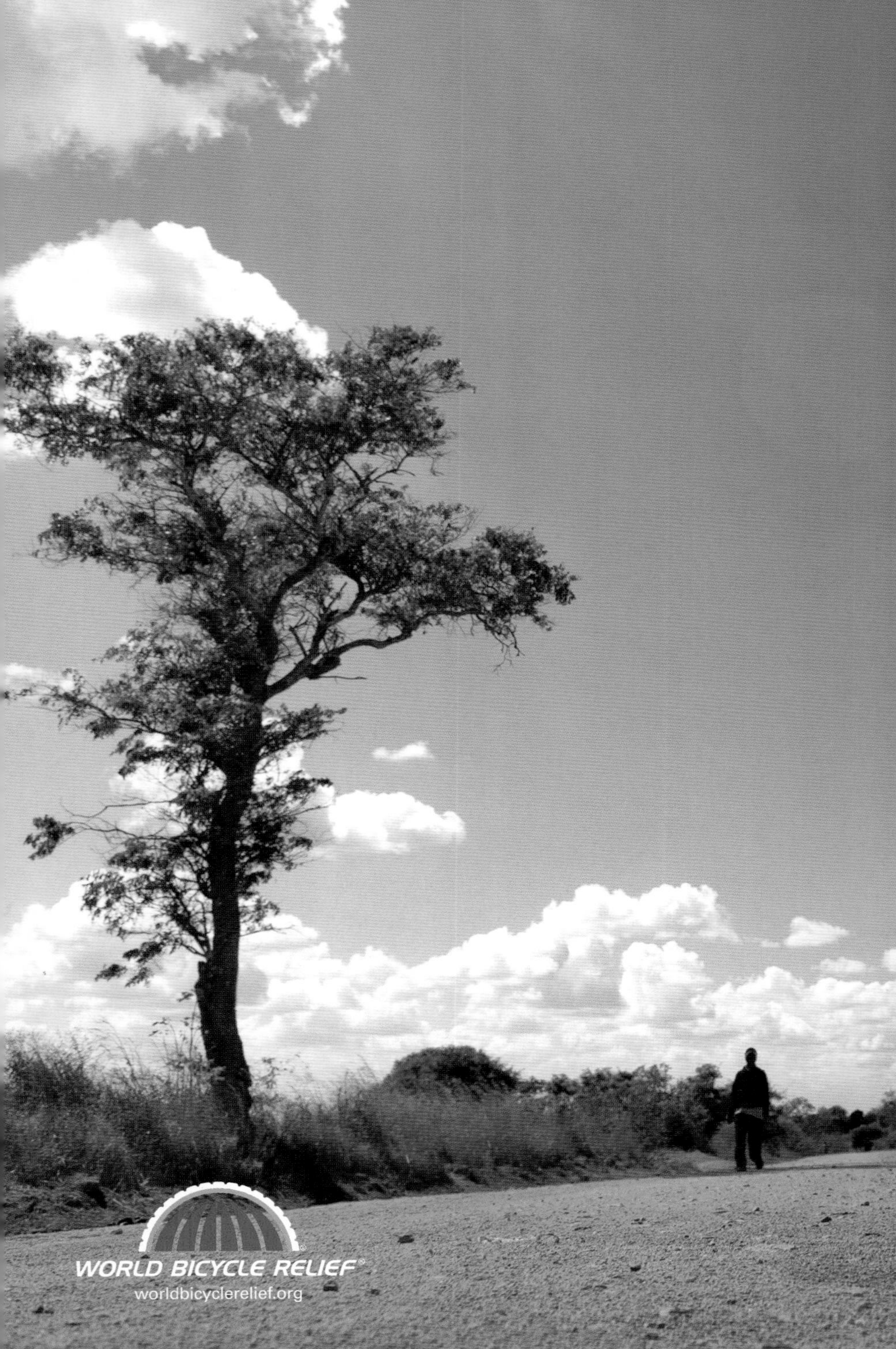
WORLD BICYCLE RELIEF®
worldbicyclerelief.org

On the Road

I have lived in a number of cities on both the west and east coast since I started cycling in my teens and I can honestly say that Orange County is one of the safest, friendliest places I have ever ridden my bike. That being said, riding your bike safely should always be your paramount goal as you explore these rides. And while accidents do happen, the good news is that you can do a great deal to prevent them altogether.

Without a doubt the single most important piece of equipment you can utilize is a helmet. They seem flimsy and insubstantial, but statistics support the argument that helmets save lives. The Insurance Institute for Highway Safety compiles data regarding cycling fatalities every year. According to their data, nationwide, 70 per cent of all cycling fatalities in 2010 occurred to those not wearing a helmet. In 2009, 91 per cent were not wearing helmets. The numbers speak for themselves, put on that helmet!

Cycling clothing is usually bright, garish almost, for a reason. You want to be seen. But that doesn't stop at what you wear. Make sure your bike has reflectors on the wheels as well as front and rear deflectors. If you ride at dawn or dusk, there are plenty of lighting systems out there to make yourself stand out.

When considering safety the best thing you can do to reduce accidents is ride predictably. Avoid erratic movements, ride in the direction of traffic, stay as far right as is safe. In California, cyclists are considered slow moving vehicles and are required by law to follow all traffic rules. That means you have both the right and responsibilities to travel on the road.

Cycling is a fast-paced, intensive activity that requires you to be constantly alert and actively evaluating your situation in a rapidly changing environment. Often the difference between an accident and safety is a split-second decision. Don't handicap yourself by wearing headphones. Plugged in, you won't hear other cyclist's communications and you

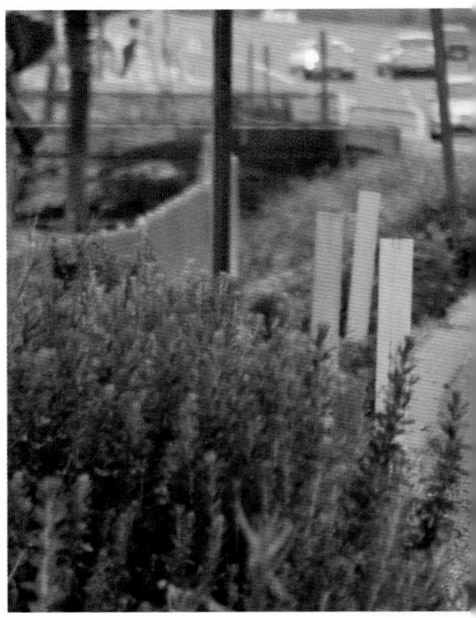

may miss that tiny cue that could have alerted yo danger.

Some Finer Points on Safe Riding

- Ride in the direction of traffic, whether on the r or the bike path.
- Stay in your lane.
- Pass only on the left and alert others of your in by calling out "on your left".
- Yield to pedestrians and equestrians.
- Use simple hand signals to indicate turns.
- When stopping, pull completely off the road o path.
- When approaching intersections, never assume motorists have seen you. Try to make eye cont and err on the side of caution.

Riding as a Family

Many of the rides in this book were ridden with wife and kids in tow. As a family we ride thousa of miles a year together and really enjoy this aspec cycling. While we have a great deal of fun doing family riding requires a bit more work and plann The first thing you need to consider when cyc

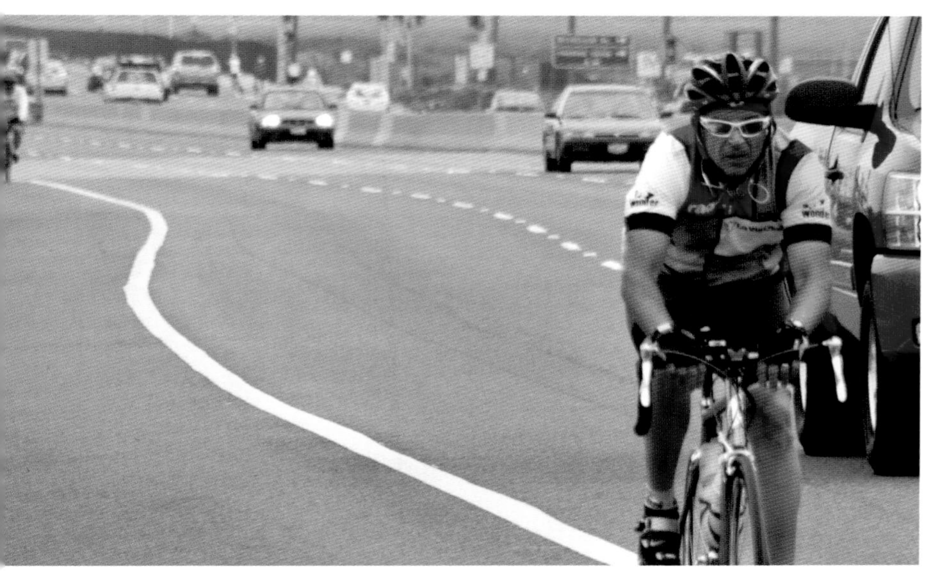

h kids is that you will need to ride to the level of least experienced rider. Pushing kids beyond their ity can have disastrous consequences so increase eage slowly. Riding with kids is not about getting where fast. Plan on making lots of stops on the way whenever possible have a fun destination as part of ride, something for them to look forward to.

Teaching kids to ride predictably is probably the gest challenge a family faces. Their attention nders, they will make sudden stops or turns and y often don't have enough experience to anticipate gers. To help with these factors, try to ride ngside your kids with them to the right. Before ing out make sure they know how to stop quickly can change gears if they are riding a multi-speed e. Don't assume they know how to do these things. raveling in pairs is unsafe, try to bracket the kids n one parent in front leading and the other behind kids. Rides in this book indicate whether a ride is nily-friendly, but if you decide to explore different is not covered by the book, ride the route first alone make sure your family has the necessary bike skills. st important of all, make sure your child's helmet is and properly fitted.

A Few Tips on Better Biking in General

Bicycling is becoming more popular every year and more companies are producing more styles all the time. Whether you buy new or used, find a bike that fits your size and riding style. The wrong bike is not only uncomfortable, it can be dangerous. Local shops survive on their service. Bring your bike in and ask them to look it over. A good shop can fit you for the bike, make repairs and help make sure you have the equipment you need.

A few simple things will make cycling more enjoyable. First make sure your saddle is the correct height. Your knee should only be slightly bent on the down stroke. Making sure your tires are inflated properly will reduce resistance, which in turn makes pedaling easier. Put the right tires on your bike. If you ride beach paths then you won't need those big knobby mountain bike tires. Clean and lubricate the chain regularly. If you learn nothing else about bicycle maintenance, know how to change a flat and always carry the tools you need with you. I can almost guarantee the moment you don't have a new inner tube, CO_2 or tire levers with you, will be the time you get a flat.

You, Your Bike and Transport in Orange County

Today's Orange County grew out of the need for affordable housing for those who had jobs in Los Angeles. When this boom occurred, tax dollars were thrown into the large scale construction of broad thoroughfares and freeways. There is no light rail or metro system in Orange County, nor are there any plans for such a system in the foreseeable future. That's the bad news. The good news is that the Orange County Transit Authority (OCTA) does an admirable job of connecting all 34 cities in the county by bus. Reliable, regular and cheap, nearly every ride in this book lies along an OCTA bus line. The other public transportation option is Metrolink which runs a number of commuter trains that cross through the central cities of Orange County.

OCTA

The Orange County Transportation Authority is a multi-modal transportation agency serving Orange County. This large agency is responsible for keeping the county moving by overseeing, Metrolink rail service, the 91 Express Lanes toll facility, freeway, street and road improvement projects, motorist aid services and by regulating taxi operations. Most importantly for cyclists, they run a countywide bus service.

OCTA operates in a 798 square-mile area serving more than 3 million residents in 34 cities and unincorporated areas. Its countywide system has 77 bus routes and 6,200 bus stops reaching nearly every corner of the county. Every OCTA bus is equipped to carry bicycles. For those who plan to take advantage of this convenient service, here are a few tips from OCTA on loading and unloading your bike.

Loading

- Be prepared to load your bike when the bus approaches. Remove water bottles, pumps and other loose items.
- Alert the coach operator that you are going to use the bike rack.
- Load your bike from curbside in front of the bu
- If the bike rack is up, release it by pulling dow with one hand.
- Lift your bike onto the bike rack and fit the whe into the proper slots.
- Raise the support arm over the front tire. A spr will pull the arm back securely latching your bi

Unloading

- Before the bus approaches your stop, tell the co operator that you will be removing your bike.
- From curbside in front of the bus, raise the sup arm off the tire.
- Lift your bike out of the rack.
- Fold up the rack if no one will be using it. The r will automatically lock in place.
- Step away from the bus with your bike.

Points to Remember

- The coach operator may not leave the bus to he load or unload bicycles.
- The bike racks are easy to use. You can load or unload your bike in less than 20 seconds.
- The bike nearest the bus can be unloaded with removing the front bike.
- The bike rack touches only the rubber tires and will not scratch or damage your bike.
- Bike racks are available on a first-come, first-served basis. Each bus is equipped with a rack which can hold two bicycles of any size or typ
- You may not bring bicycles onboard the bus un it is the last bus of the day on a particular route if the bike racks are full.

Visit OCTA's website at **www.octa.net** to numerous trip planning tools as well as an excell interactive map.

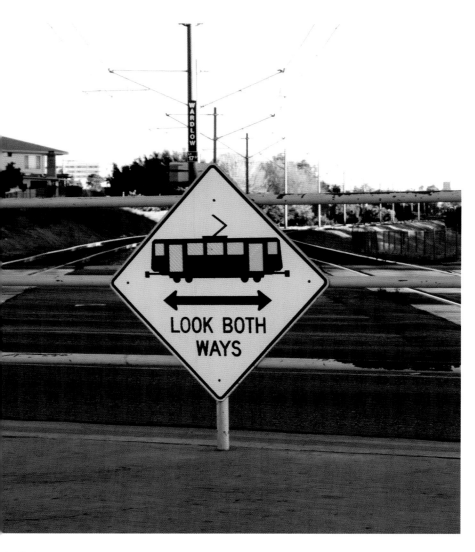

trolink

trolink is a commuter train system designed to cover entire region of Southern California. For the cyclist veling Orange County you will find the Orange unty Line most useful. This line makes 10 stops as uns through the central portion of the county. As a mmuter route expect more trains Monday through day, with the fewest number of options available on day, so plan appropriately. Bicycles are permitted on train cars and must be secured and stored in the designated storage area (each train car can hold up to two bicycles). The special Bike Car can hold up to 18 bicycles on the lower level.

For those looking for rides conveniently located near a Metrolink station, consider Rides 1, 8, 21, 29, 34, 45, 51, and 53.

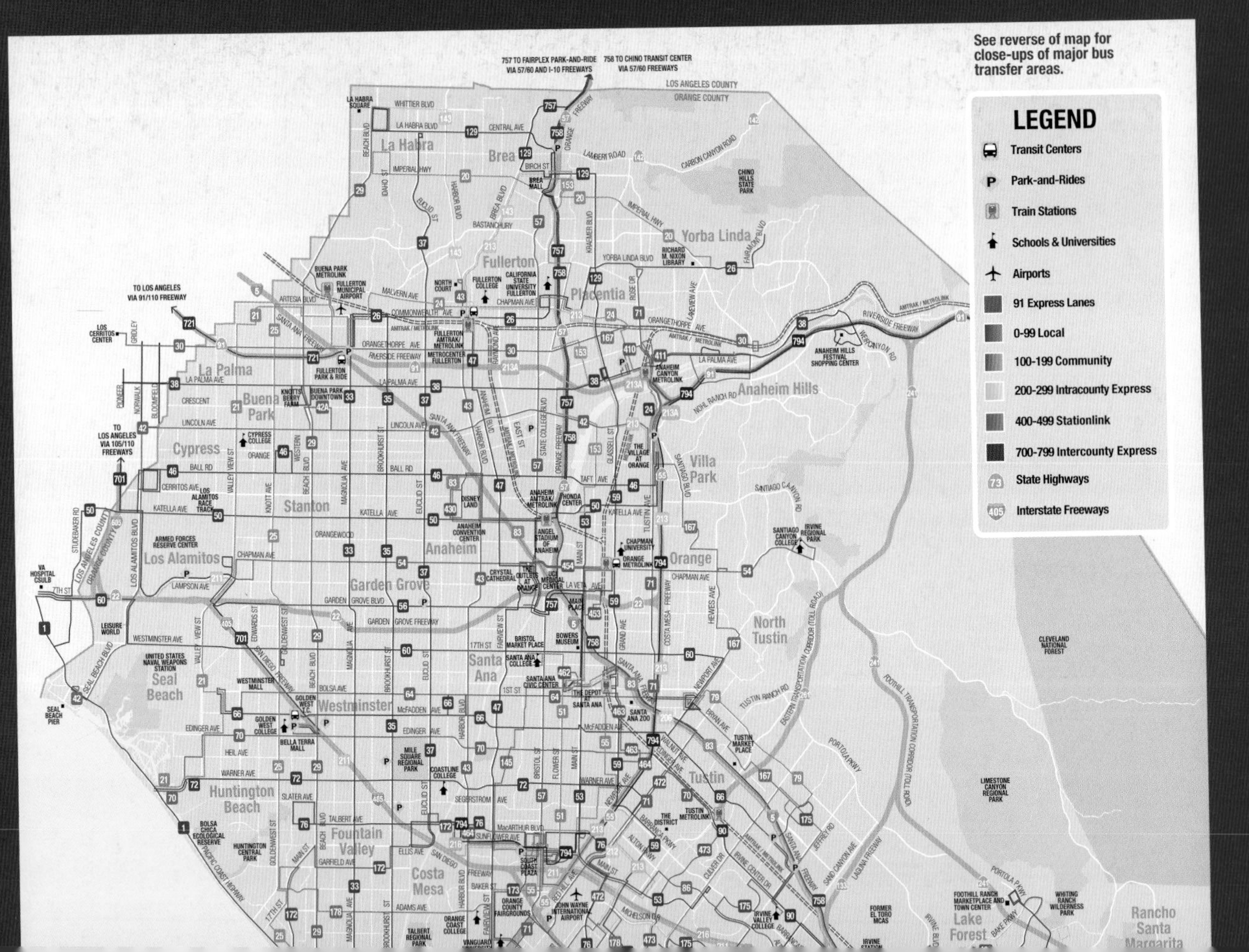

See reverse of map for close-ups of major bus transfer areas.
LEGEND
Transit Centers
Park-and-Rides
Train Stations
Schools & Universities
Airports
91 Express Lanes
0-99 Local
100-199 Community
200-299 Intracounty Express
400-499 Stationlink
700-799 Intercounty Express
State Highways
Interstate Freeways
757 TO FAIRPLEX PARK-AND-RIDE VIA 57/60 AND I-10 FREEWAYS
758 TO CHINO TRANSIT CENTER VIA 57/60 FREEWAYS
LOS ANGELES COUNTY
ORANGE COUNTY
TO LOS ANGELES VIA 91/110 FREEWAY
TO LOS ANGELES VIA 105/110 FREEWAYS
La Habra
Brea
Yorba Linda
Fullerton
Placentia
La Palma
Buena Park
Cypress
Stanton
Anaheim
Anaheim Hills
Villa Park
Orange
Los Alamitos
Garden Grove
North Tustin
Santa Ana
Seal Beach
Westminster
Tustin
Huntington Beach
Fountain Valley
Costa Mesa
Lake Forest
Rancho Santa Margarita
CHINO HILLS STATE PARK
CLEVELAND NATIONAL FOREST
LIMESTONE CANYON REGIONAL PARK
WHITING RANCH WILDERNESS PARK
IRVINE REGIONAL PARK
MILE SQUARE REGIONAL PARK
HUNTINGTON CENTRAL PARK
BOLSA CHICA ECOLOGICAL RESERVE
TALBERT REGIONAL PARK
UNITED STATES NAVAL WEAPONS STATION
ARMED FORCES RESERVE CENTER
LEISURE WORLD
SEAL BEACH PIER
VA HOSPITAL CSULB
LOS CERRITOS CENTER
LA HABRA SQUARE
BREA MALL
RICHARD M. NIXON LIBRARY
BUENA PARK METROLINK
FULLERTON MUNICIPAL AIRPORT
FULLERTON PARK & RIDE
BUENA PARK DOWNTOWN
KNOTT'S BERRY FARM
CYPRESS COLLEGE
LOS ALAMITOS RACE TRACK
FULLERTON COLLEGE
CALIFORNIA STATE UNIVERSITY FULLERTON
NORTH COURT
FULLERTON AMTRAK/ METROLINK
METROCENTER FULLERTON
ANAHEIM CANYON METROLINK
ANAHEIM HILLS FESTIVAL SHOPPING CENTER
THE VILLAGE AT ORANGE
DISNEY LAND
ANAHEIM CONVENTION CENTER
ANAHEIM AMTRAK/ METROLINK
HONDA CENTER
ANGEL STADIUM OF ANAHEIM
THE OUTLETS AT ORANGE
UCI MEDICAL CENTER
CRYSTAL CATHEDRAL
CHAPMAN UNIVERSITY
ORANGE METROLINK
SANTIAGO CANYON COLLEGE
MAIN PLACE
BOWERS MUSEUM
BRISTOL MARKET PLACE
SANTA ANA COLLEGE
SANTA ANA CIVIC CENTER
THE DEPOT AT SANTA ANA
SANTA ANA ZOO
WESTMINSTER MALL
GOLDEN WEST T.C.
GOLDEN WEST COLLEGE
BELLA TERRA MALL
COASTLINE COLLEGE
TUSTIN MARKET PLACE
TUSTIN METROLINK
THE DISTRICT
SOUTH COAST PLAZA
ORANGE COUNTY FAIRGROUNDS
ORANGE COAST COLLEGE
JOHN WAYNE INTERNATIONAL AIRPORT
IRVINE VALLEY COLLEGE
FORMER EL TORO MCAS
IRVINE STATION
FOOTHILL RANCH MARKETPLACE AND TOWN CENTER
FOOTHILL TRANSPORTATION CORRIDOR (TOLL ROAD)
EASTERN TRANSPORTATION CORRIDOR (TOLL ROAD)
RIVERSIDE FREEWAY
ORANGE FREEWAY
SANTA ANA FREEWAY
GARDEN GROVE FREEWAY
SAN DIEGO FREEWAY
COSTA MESA FREEWAY
LAGUNA FREEWAY
PACIFIC COAST HIGHWAY

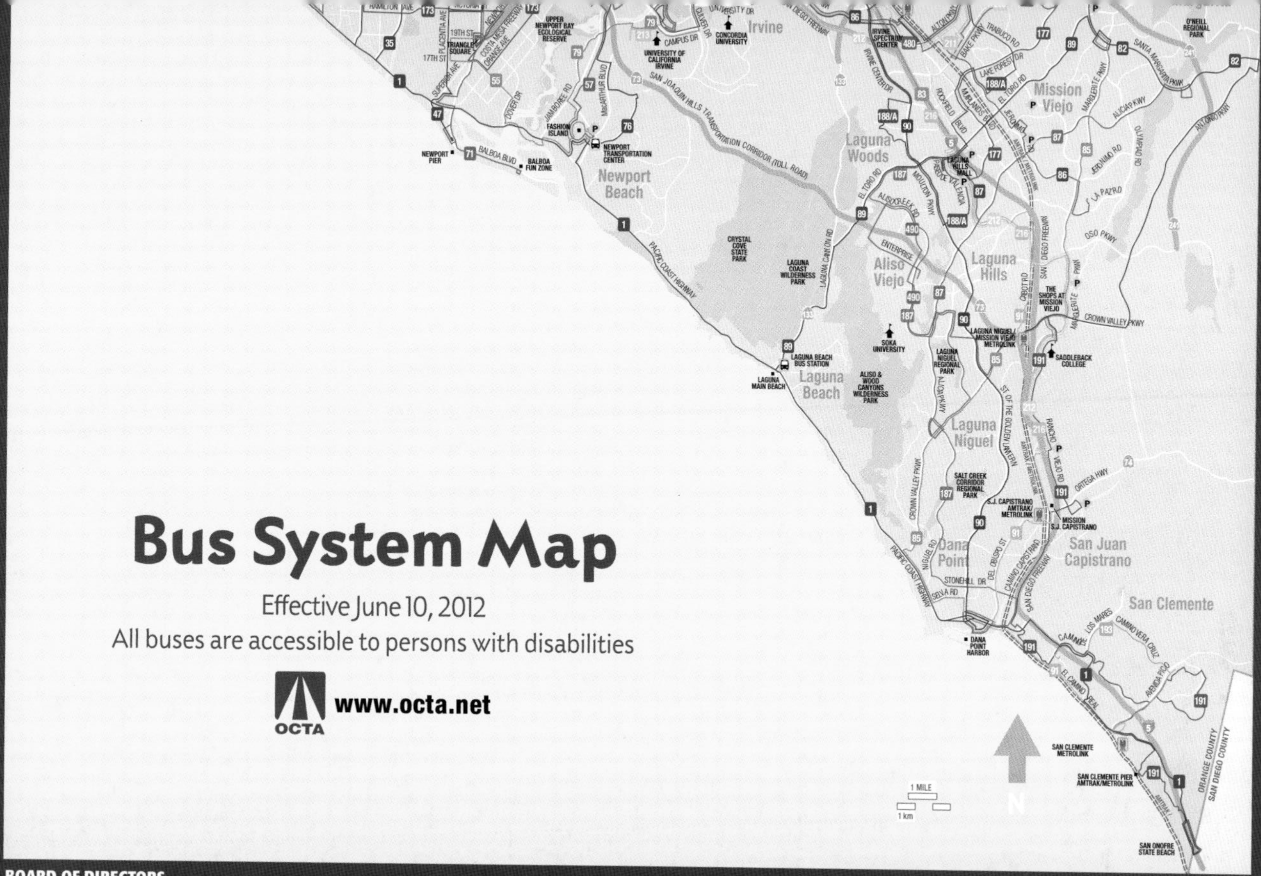

Bus System Map

Effective June 10, 2012

All buses are accessible to persons with disabilities

www.octa.net

Metro & Metrolink

metro.net
metrolinktrains.com

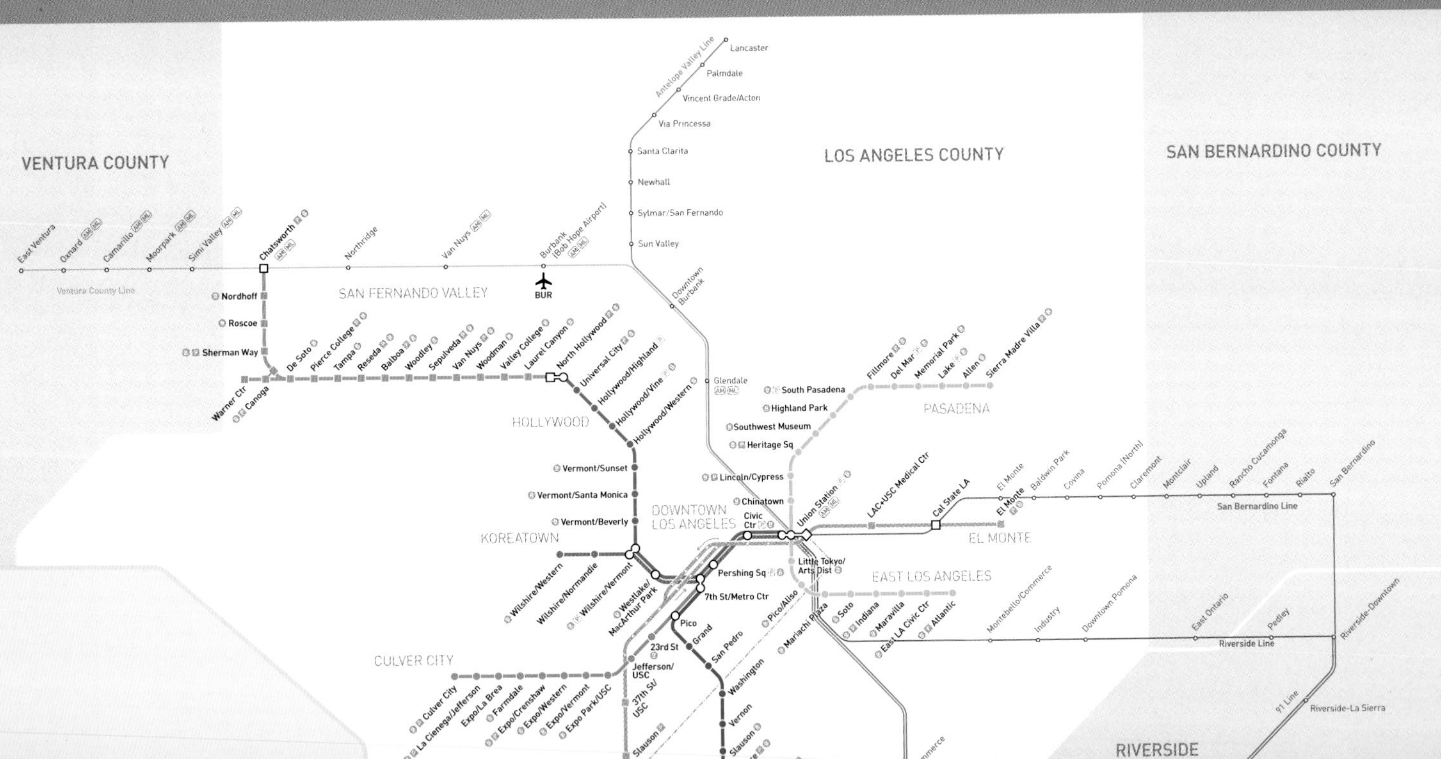

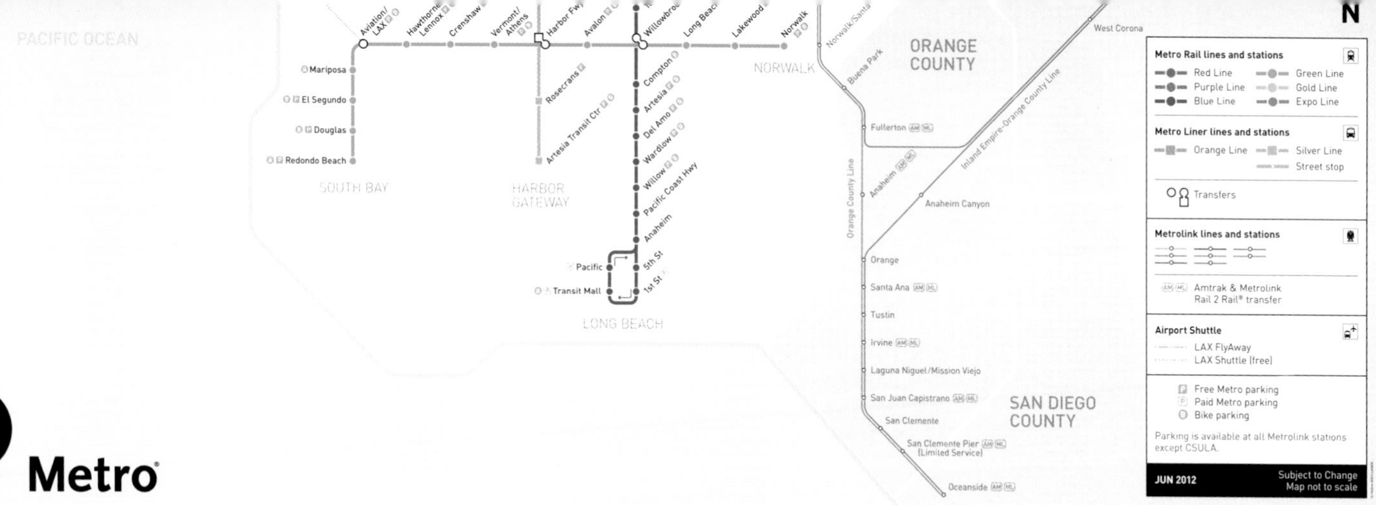

PACIFIC OCEAN

Aviation/ LAX
Hawthorne/ Lennox
Crenshaw
Vermont/ Athens
Harbor Fwy
Avalon
Willowbrook
Long Beach
Lakewood
Norwalk

Mariposa
El Segundo
Douglas
Redondo Beach
SOUTH BAY

Rosecrans
Artesia Transit Ctr
HARBOR GATEWAY

Compton
Artesia
Del Amo
Wardlow
Willow
Pacific Coast Hwy
Anaheim
5th St
1st St
Pacific
Transit Mall
LONG BEACH

NORWALK

Norwalk/Santa Fe Springs
Buena Park
Fullerton (AM) (ML)
Anaheim (AM) (ML)
Orange County Line
Inland Empire-Orange County Line
West Corona
Anaheim Canyon
ORANGE COUNTY
Orange
Santa Ana (AM) (ML)
Tustin
Irvine (AM) (ML)
Laguna Niguel/Mission Viejo
San Juan Capistrano (AM) (ML)
San Clemente
San Clemente Pier (AM) (ML) (Limited Service)
Oceanside (AM) (ML)
SAN DIEGO COUNTY

N

Metro Rail lines and stations
Red Line
Purple Line
Blue Line
Green Line
Gold Line
Expo Line

Metro Liner lines and stations
Orange Line
Silver Line
Street stop

Transfers

Metrolink lines and stations

(AM) (ML) Amtrak & Metrolink Rail 2 Rail® transfer

Airport Shuttle
LAX FlyAway
LAX Shuttle (free)

Free Metro parking
Paid Metro parking
Bike parking

Parking is available at all Metrolink stations except CSULA.

JUN 2012
Subject to Change
Map not to scale

Metro®

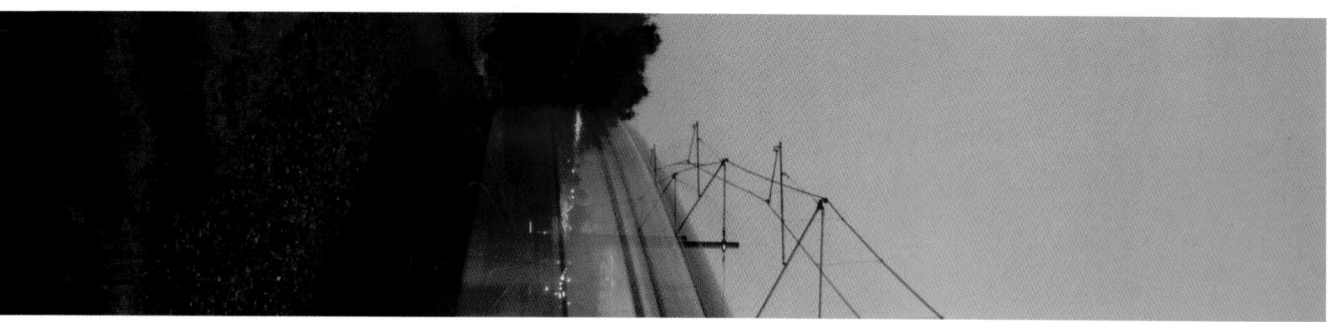

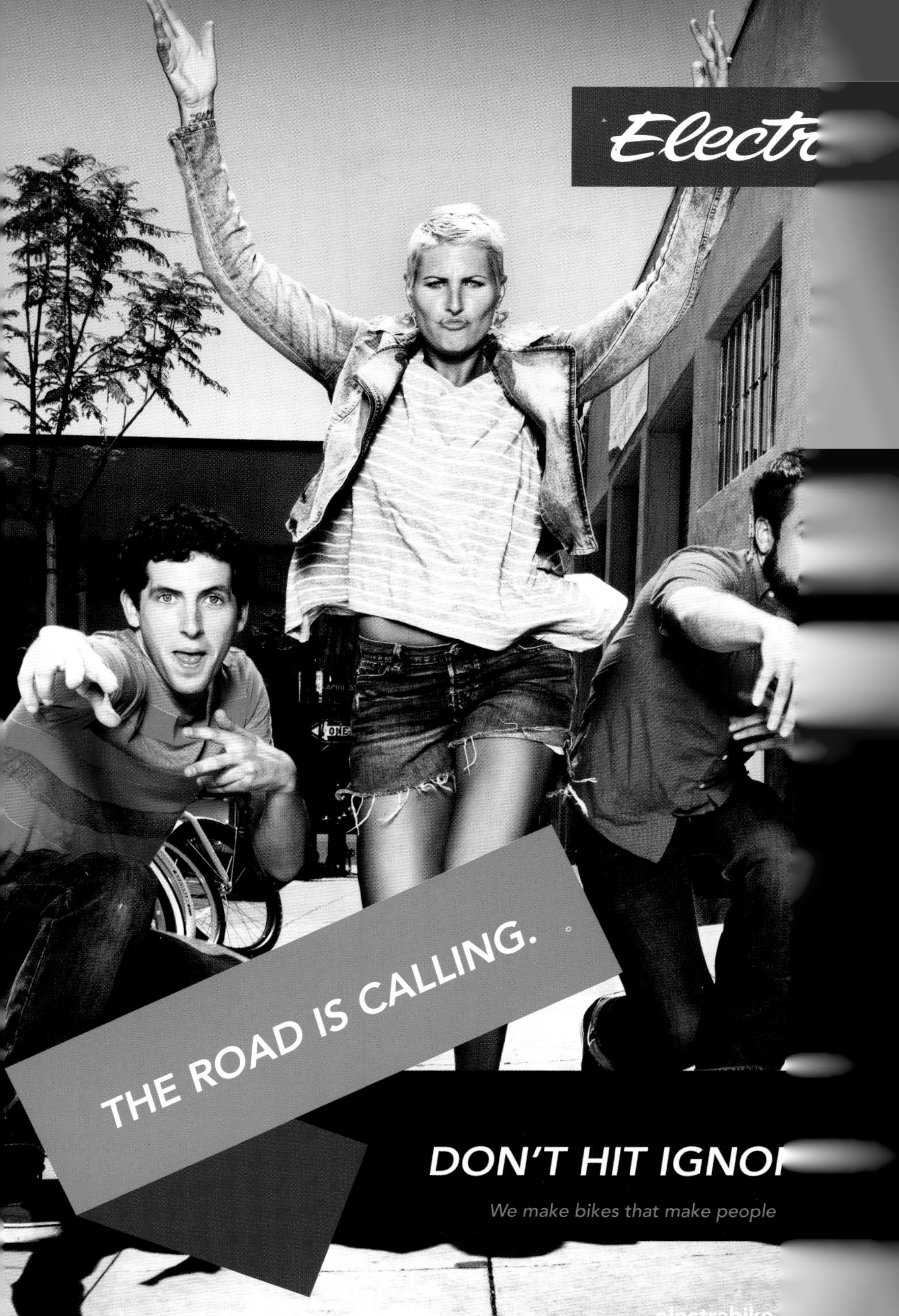
Electr
THE ROAD IS CALLING.
DON'T HIT IGNO
We make bikes that make people
electrabike.

North Inland

Bounded by Interstate 5, Los Angeles and San Bernadino counties and the Santa Ana River, this region presses up against the Santa Ana Mountains and includes the cities of Fullerton, La Habra, Yorba Linda, Brea and Placentia. This area once was coveted for its fertile soil, temperate weather and access to water that allowed it to become the center of an agricultural citrus boom that gave us the name Orange County. As Los Angeles' population grew, agriculture gave way to affordable housing and Orange County's suburbs were born.

Hilly, mountainous landscapes dominate much of this section and not surprisingly, you can expect to find plenty of climbs in many of the rides. For cyclists looking for flat rides, routes that travel alongside rivers and creeks are your best bet as elevation changes on these outings are mild. La Habra Guadalupe Park ride, a family-oriented ride, and the Santa Ana River Trail are two flatter rides worth exploring. And for those looking for climbing challenges, look no further that Coyote Hills with one of the steepest climbs in this section. Yorba Linda Recreational Trail and the Fullerton loop also offer climbs that are long and steady combined with challenging distances.

As cycling becomes more prominent in the county, many cities are working hard to incorporate bike paths and lanes into their transportation plans. Nowhere is this more evident than in Fullerton where the city has excelled in developing safe bike routes for both on and off-road cycling enthusiasts and this is reflected in the number of rides in and through Fullerton. As the oldest city in this section, Fullerton has a lively, pedestrian friendly downtown and well developed, integrated transportation system that includes miles of bike lanes. This town also boasts a vibrant, independent music scene and plenty of culinary diversions.

Two of the rides in this section actually travel into nearby counties demonstrating the opportunity bicycles offer as commuting and exploring vehicles. The La Habra/Whittier Loop crosses into Los Angeles County as it spins past charming, historic Whittier. And the longest, most challenging ride of the section travels along the Santa Ana River Trail, through the Santa Ana Mountains to Corona in San Bernardino County.

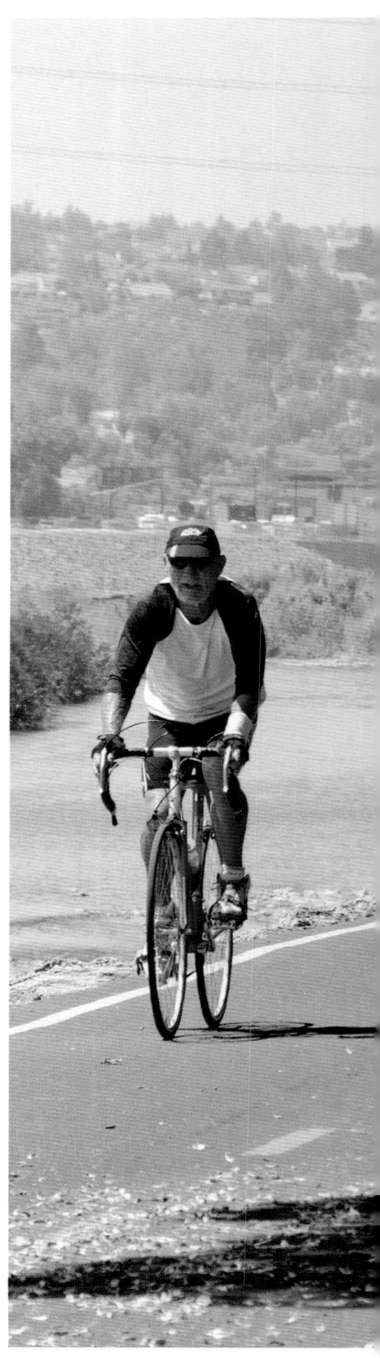

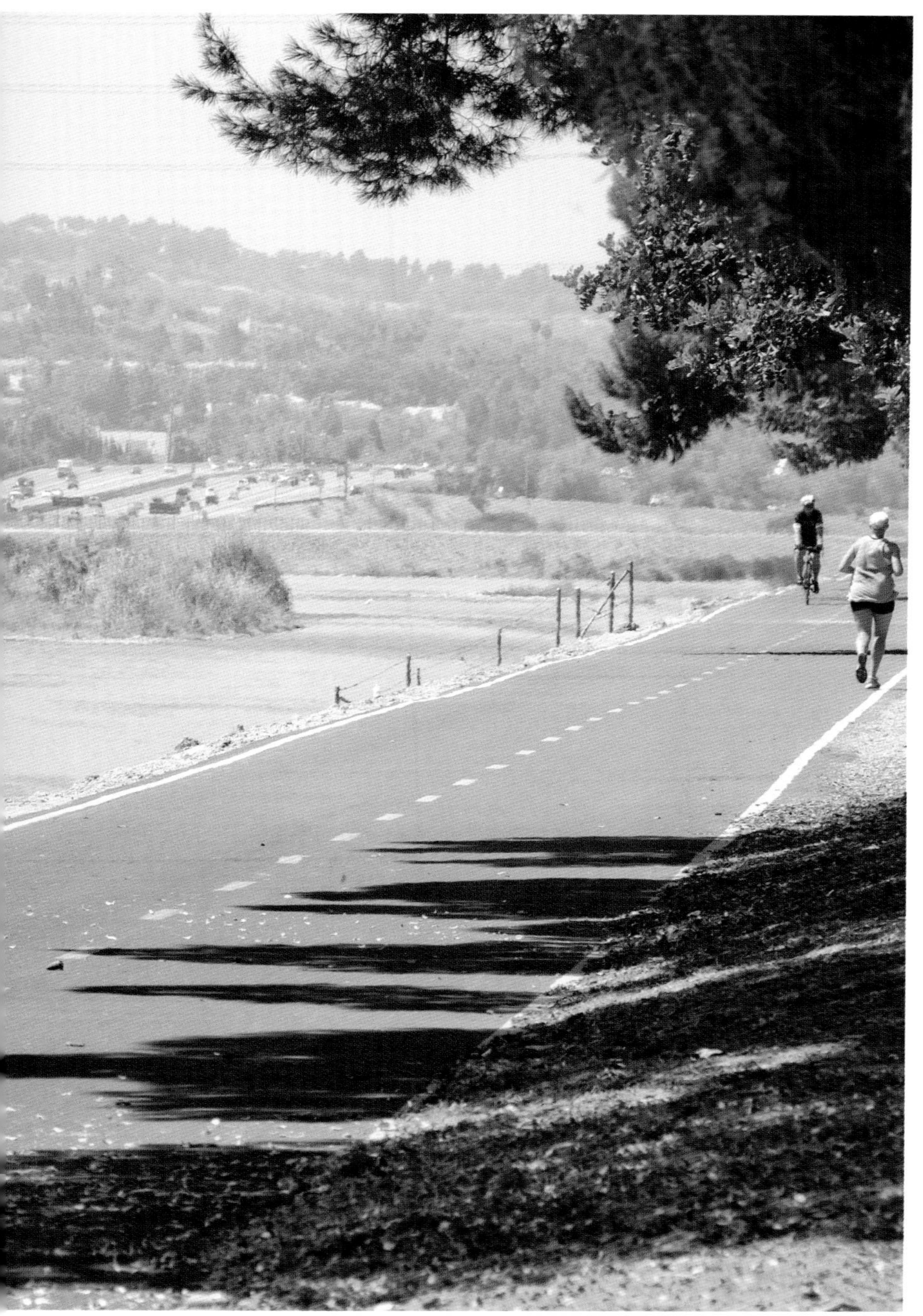

North Inland Overview

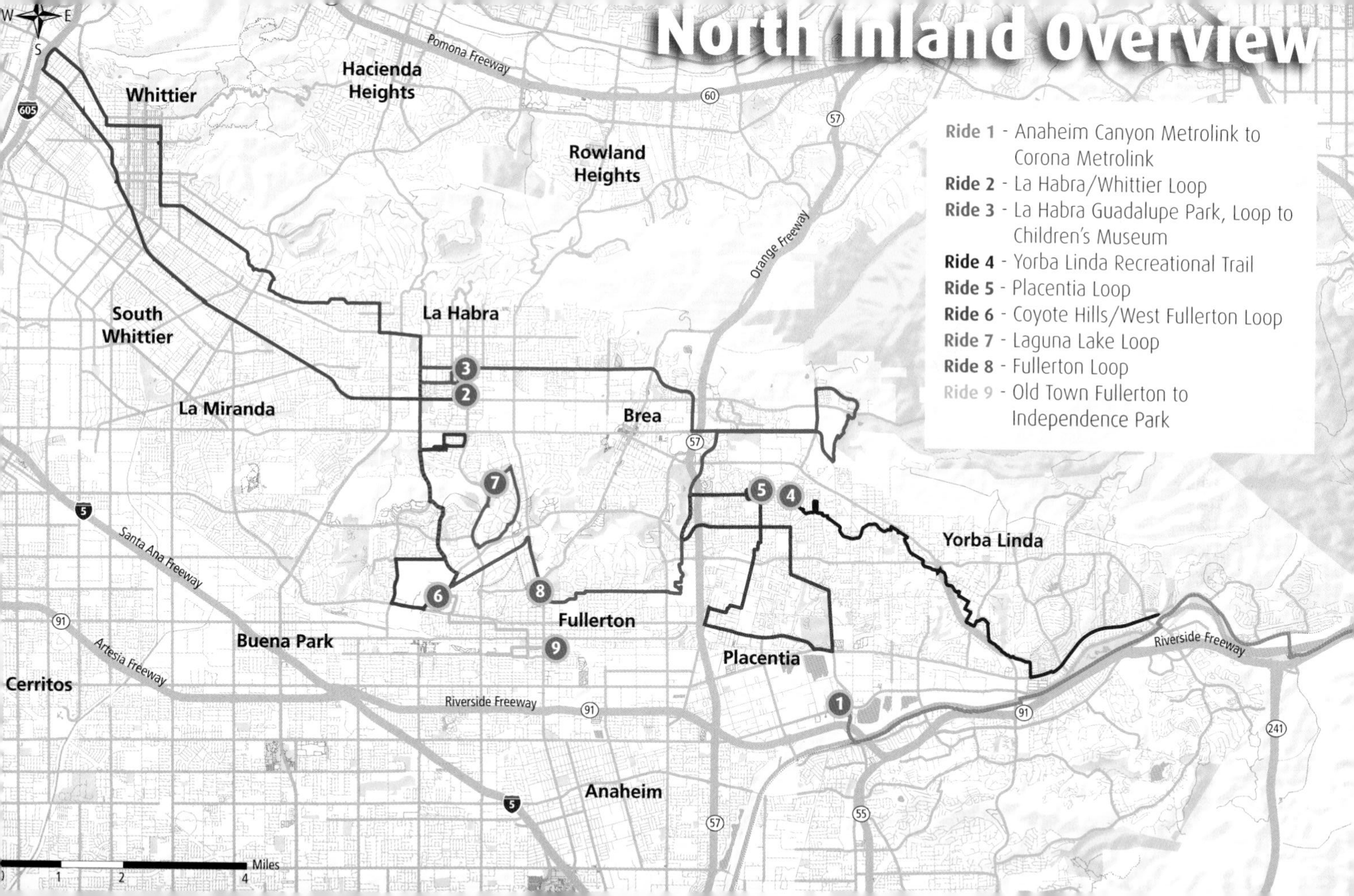

Ride 1 - Anaheim Canyon Metrolink to Corona Metrolink
Ride 2 - La Habra/Whittier Loop
Ride 3 - La Habra Guadalupe Park, Loop to Children's Museum
Ride 4 - Yorba Linda Recreational Trail
Ride 5 - Placentia Loop
Ride 6 - Coyote Hills/West Fullerton Loop
Ride 7 - Laguna Lake Loop
Ride 8 - Fullerton Loop
Ride 9 - Old Town Fullerton to Independence Park
Whittier
Hacienda Heights
Rowland Heights
South Whittier
La Habra
La Miranda
Brea
Yorba Linda
Fullerton
Buena Park
Placentia
Cerritos
Anaheim
Pomona Freeway
Orange Freeway
Santa Ana Freeway
Artesia Freeway
Riverside Freeway
Miles

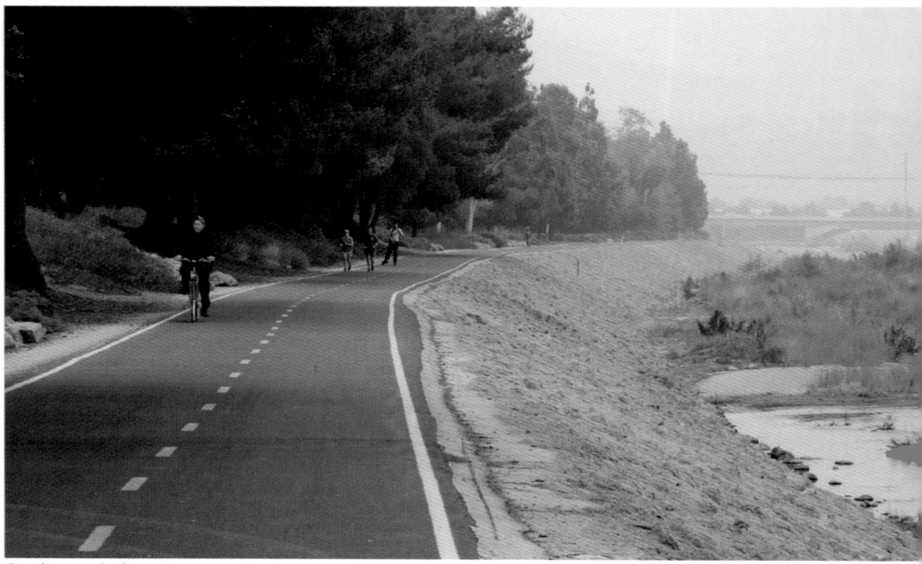

Be alert on the busy Santa Ana Trail.

At a Glance

partially

Distance 42.55 miles **Elevation Gain** 2982′

Terrain

About half this route travels bike paths that are smooth and flat. The other half of the ride has steep climbs along road bike lanes.

Traffic

On the Santa Ana River Trail expect heavy pedestrian traffic on the weekends. With the exception of the areas around the Metrolink stations, the roads traveled have light traffic.

How to Get There

By train, Metrolink's Inland Empire-Orange County line stops at both stations on the route.

By bus, OCTA buses 24, 28, 71, 167, 410, 411 all make stops at Anaheim Canyon Metrolink.

By car, take the 91 Freeway to exit 32, Tustin Avenue, heading north. After 0.2 miles turn left onto Pacific Center Drive and into Metrolink parking lot.

Food and Drink

Before you reach the Corona station at 80 West Gr you'll find Spice it Up Market and Grill which ser traditional Indian food. Also nearby the Metrolink tion at 300 Main Street is Lamppost Pizza Main St Brewery.

Side Trip

Along the way consider a ride through beautiful Yo Regional Park. Once in the Corona area explore city along one of the many bike paths that crissc this city.

Links to 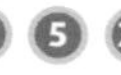    K7 K14

Where to Bike Rating 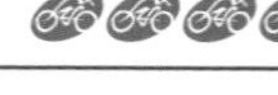

About...

This route travels through Santa Ana Canyon, connecting northern Orange County and the Inland Empire, going from Anaheim Canyon Metrolink to Corona Metrolink 21 miles away. Once in Corona board a train and return in style, or mount up and ride back to earn those bragging rights; 42 miles, 2900 feet of climbing. Whichever option you choose, you will ride through beautiful natural environments alongside Southern California's longest river before you reach a challenging climb, followed by a mellow downhill to Corona's train station.

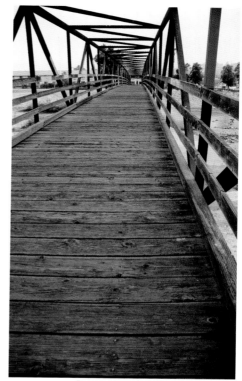

Pause midway along the pedestrian bridge and enjoy the view.

fter leaving the Anaheim Canyon station, you will ickly find yourself on the upper part of the Santa a River Trail. Through this stretch the river be- mes more natural and wild. As an important part of igratory patterns, keep an eye out for a wide variety birds as well as smaller animals, especially in the ornings. Traveling in late spring is a special treat as ture puts on a spectacular display of wild flowers and e blossoms.

At 5.99 miles the trail passes by Yorba Regional rk, 166 acres of greenery and lakes crisscrossed by les of bike paths. Kid's Ride 7 is located here and s park is a peaceful place to take a break and have icnic lunch.

Once you cross Gypsum Canyon Bridge, the ride rts climbing, first mild, rolling hills. At 14 miles that anges as a long challenging ascent over the next two les lies ahead. This climb along Green River Road is longest and most difficult in the North Inland sec- n. For those who would like to avoid this climb, at 21 miles turn left onto Palisade Drive, followed 1.7 es later by a left onto Serfas Club Drive. From there n right onto Sixth Street where it will rejoin this te where Sixth crosses Buena Vista Avenue. While this alternate route avoids the biggest climbs, it does land you on Sixth earlier and longer than the original route and this is a much busier street.

Corona, originally the self-proclaimed "lemon capital of the world", was as late as the 1990s primarily an agricultural city. High real estate prices lead to its transformation into a suburb of the Orange County suburbs. One of the great advantages of this later development is the inclusion of bike routes. Throughout this tidy city you will find painted bike lanes, signs and lots of bike sharrows.

If you are returning by train check the Metrolink schedule in advance. On the weekend, trains generally run only in the morning while during the week they run throughout the day. Prices fluctuate, but at the time of writing a one-way regular fare was $6.75 and the trip took about 20 minutes.

Ride Log

0.0 Begin ride at the Anaheim Canyon Metrolink parking lot.
0.05 Turn right on Pacific Center Dr.
0.10 Still on Pacific Center Dr, turn left at stop sign.
0.19 Turn right onto Tustin Ave.
0.45 Cross over 91 Freeway, watch for traffic.
0.67 Turn right onto Santa Ana River Trail.
0.71 Turn right, heading north, and pass under bridge.
1.93 Bear left and pass under Lakeview Ave.
3.49 Bear left and pass under Imperial Hwy.
3.63 Cross pedestrian bridge to other side of river.
3.73 Turn right onto trail.
4.93 Yorba Regional Park on your left.
6.28 Bear left, follow the painted path.
6.37 Bear right.
9.03 Bear left. Do not pass under Gypsum Canyon Bridge.
9.06 Turn right and cross bridge.
9.40 On other side of bridge, bear right.
9.48 Turn right back onto trail.
12.14 Trail ends. Continue straight on Green River Rd.
13.03 Bear right continuing on Green River Rd.
13.21 Cross bridge over 91 Freeway.
14.21 To take alternate route that avoids the climb ahead, turn left onto Palisades Dr.
16.71 Turn right onto Ontario Ave.
18.16 Cross Via Pacifica.
18.62 Cross Lincoln Ave.
18.94 Turn left on Buena Vista Ave.
20.28 Turn right on Sixth St.
20.47 Turn left on Grand Blvd.
20.88 Cross Main St.
21.30 Turn left in Corona Metrolink station. Turn around and return to Grand Blvd.
21.42 Cross Main St.
21.83 Cross Second St.
21.89 Turn right onto Third St.
22.02 Turn left onto Vicentia Ave.
22.23 Turn right on Sixth St.
22.36 Turn left onto Buena Vista Ave.
23.68 Turn right onto Ontario Ave.
23.99 Cross Lincoln Ave.
24.46 Cross Via Pacifica.
25.91 Turn left onto Paseo Grande which becom Green River Rd.
28.4 Cross Palisades Dr.
29.4 Cross over 91 Freeway.
30.50 Return to Santa Ana River Trail.
33.15 Turn left and follow path to cross Gypsum C yon Bridge.
33.57 Turn left back onto trail.
36.25 Bear left.
36.7 Yorba Regional Park on your right.
38.93 Turn left onto pedestrian bridge.
39.0 Turn right onto trail.
39.04 Bear right and pass under Imperial Hwy.
40.61 Bear right and pass under Lakeview Ave.
41.85 Bear left and exit trail.
41.86 Turn right onto Tustin Ave.
42.17 Cross 91 Freeway, watch for traffic.
42.35 Turn left onto Pacific Center Dr.
42.42 Still on Pacific Center Dr, turn right at stop si
42.49 Turn left into Anaheim Canyon Metrolink parking
42.55 End.

Anaheim Canyon Metrolink to Corona Metrolink

Please note: the profile for Ride 1 is depicted in 200ft vertical increments due to unusually high elevation.

Altitude ft: 1000, 800, 600, 400, 200
Distance miles: 0, 10, 20, 30, 40

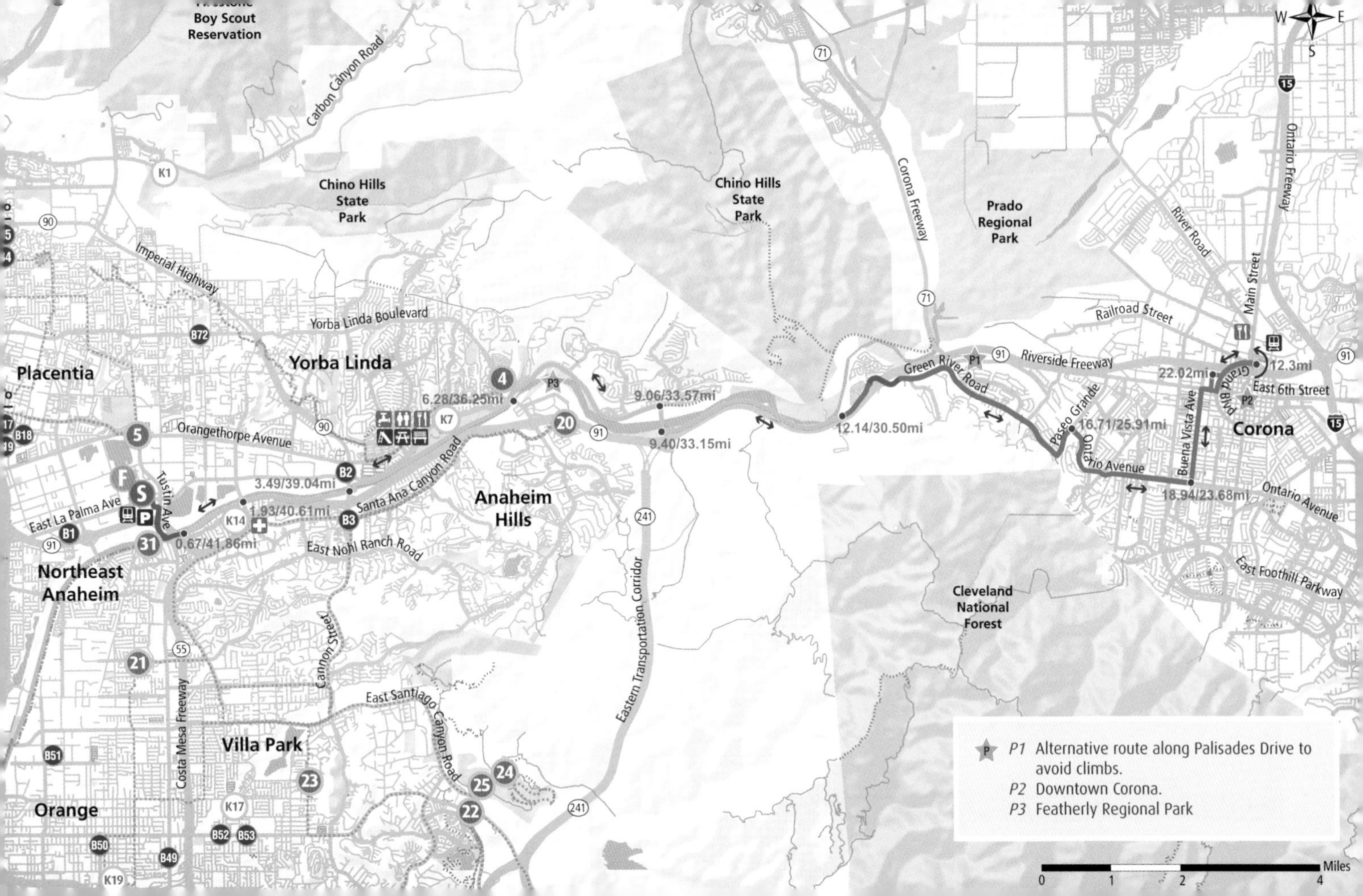
Boy Scout Reservation
Carbon Canyon Road
Chino Hills State Park
Chino Hills State Park
Corona Freeway
Prado Regional Park
River Road
Main Street
Ontario Freeway
Imperial Highway
Yorba Linda Boulevard
Railroad Street
Placentia
Yorba Linda
Riverside Freeway
Green River Road
P1
P2
P3
12.3mi
22.02mi
East 6th Street
Grand Blvd
Corona
6.28/36.25mi
9.06/33.57mi
9.40/33.15mi
12.14/30.50mi
16.71/25.91mi
18.94/23.68mi
Paseo Grande
Ontario Avenue
Buena Vista Ave
Ontario Avenue
East Foothill Parkway
Orangethorpe Avenue
3.49/39.04mi
1.93/40.61mi
0.67/41.86mi
Santa Ana Canyon Road
Tustin Ave
East La Palma Ave
East Nohl Ranch Road
Anaheim Hills
Northeast Anaheim
Eastern Transportation Corridor
Cleveland National Forest
Cannon Street
Costa Mesa Freeway
East Santiago Canyon Road
Villa Park
Orange
P1 Alternative route along Palisades Drive to avoid climbs.
P2 Downtown Corona.
P3 Featherly Regional Park
0
1
2
4
Miles

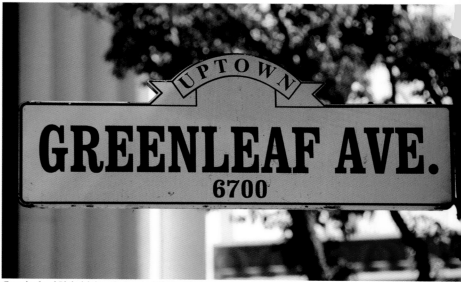

Greenleaf and Philadelphia, the heart of Uptown.

At a Glance

Distance 21.53 miles **Elevation Gain** 984′

Terrain

Mostly flat with a few gentle climbs. Bike paths account for four miles, the rest of this route travels city streets.

Traffic

For most of the ride traffic is moderate, although pedestrian traffic on Whittier Greenway Trail can be heavy, especially mornings and weekends.

How to Get There

By bus, take OCTA number 37 which stops at Portola Park.

By car, take the 91 Freeway to exit 23, Beach Boulevard, northbound. Drive 4.9 miles, turn right onto Imperial Highway. After 1.3 miles, turn left onto Euclid Street, Portola Park will be on the left after 0.8 miles.

Food and Drink

The best place to fuel up is at 13.12 miles, turning ri onto Philadelphia Street and stopping at Greenleaf A enue, the center of Whittier Uptown. Here you will f numerous coffee shops, restaurants and pubs.

Side Trip

In addition to wandering Uptown's eateries, there antique shops, a 1950s movie theater, and quirky b tiques. Also, there is a serious hill to be climbed those who think a perfect ride has to have at least o monster hill.

Links to 

Where to Bike Rating 

About...

With this section of Orange County pressed up against foothills, it is often difficult to find a ride of this length that does not include at least one serious climb. This ride accomplishes this mostly by running parallel to the old Union Pacific route, and for a good four miles, actually riding over those former tracks on the attractive Whittier Greenway Trail. The return trip meanders through historic Whittier before passing Whittier College and Uptown, also known as Whittier Village.

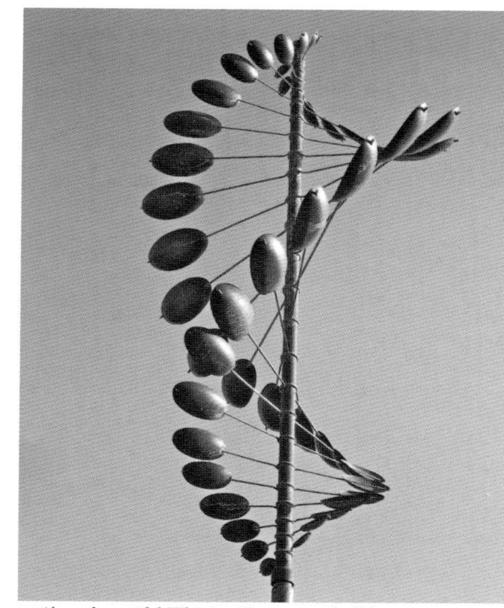

Along beautiful Whittier Greenway Trail keep an eye open for moving wind sculptures. Image Jon Riddle

he ride begins at La Habra's Portola Park. From here ɔu will find yourself traveling along Lambert Road hich runs parallel to the rail line. This road is mostly at and well maintained while traffic through here can brisk during rush hour. At 4.99 miles you will reach Iills Avenue and the entrance to Whittier Greenway ail.

The Whittier Greenway Trail is a right-of-way purased from Union Pacific in 2001, officially opened in)09, and has quickly become a favorite for commuts, strollers and joggers. On mornings and weekends ɔu will find pedestrian traffic at its heaviest as locals joy the beautifully landscaped, quiet path. Along the ute, stop at interpretive stations to learn the history the rail line, city founders and the region. Whittier pes to gain an easement along the active rail line ction so hopefully we will see this trail grow in the ture.

Once off the trail, the return leg travels through hittier's beautiful historic neighborhood. Here you ll find immaculately maintained California Craftsen homes side-by-side Spanish Colonial Revival mes as you ride under the shaded canopies of mature es. Painter Avenue is especially attractive and you may find yourself slowing down to imagine what it would be like to live along this road.

At 13.12 miles turn right on Philadelphia Street and travel two blocks to Greenleaf Avenue. You will find yourself at the center of picturesque Whittier Uptown, also known as Whittier Village. Park your bike and stroll through the "village".

Since there are a number of rides in this section that include serious climbs, I chose not to include one in this ride. However, for those who insist every good ride must have at least one heart-pounding climb, here is a side trip for you. At 16.23 miles the route turns right onto La Serna Drive. For a challenging climb turn left and follow La Serna to Youngwood Drive where you will turn left again. At Villaverde Drive turn right where the ascent begins in earnest. Turn right onto Mar Vista Street and climb until you reach Cerquita Drive before backtracking to resume ride. This detour will only add about 2.6 miles to the ride, but the 1.3 mile climb will probably burn more calories than the other 21.5 miles you will ride on this trip.

Ride Log

0.0 Begin on Euclid St at the entrance to Portola Park.
0.31 Turn right onto Lambert Rd.
1.04 Cross S Idaho St.
1.53 Cross Beach Blvd.
2.69 Cross First Ave.
3.0 Cross Leffingwell Rd.
4.4 Cross Colima Rd.
4.99 Turn right onto Mills Rd.
5.03 Turn left onto Whittier Greenway Trail.
5.35 Cross Gunn Ave.
5.70 Cross Calmada Ave.
6.13 Cross Laurel Ave.
6.40 Cross Painter Ave.
6.74 Cross Greenleaf Ave.
7.51 Bear left, cross Mar Vista St.
7.69 Cross Penn St.
7.96 Cross Philadelphia St.
8.09 Cross Bailey St diagonally back onto trail.
8.27 Cross Hadley St.
8.44 Cross Magnolia Ave.
8.59 Cross Broadway.
8.84 Cross Palm Ave.
9.2 Whittier Greenway Trail ends, turn right onto Pioneer Blvd.
10.22 Turn right on Beverly Blvd.
10.76 Cross Norwalk Blvd.
11.35 Cross Magnolia Ave.
11.60 Beverly bends left, turn right onto Hoover Ave. Railing prevents cars and other vehicles from turning right, you will need to lift bike over curb.

P1 Whittier Uptown
P2 Whittier College
P3 La Serna Rd, challenging uphill section
P4 Children Museum of La Habra

11.73 Left onto Broadway.
12.20 Broadway Park on your right, good place to r or use restrooms.
12.62 Turn right on Painter Ave.
13.12 Cross Philadelphia St. Whittier College on yo left and if you take Philadelphia to Greenleaf Ave y will reach Whittier's Uptown district.
13.49 Cross Mar Vista St.
13.85 Turn on La Quarta St.
14.17 Cross College Ave.
15.82 La Quarta ends, turn left onto Carretera Ave.
16.0 Cross Colima Rd.
16.23 Turn right on La Serna Dr. If you are interes in a climbing side trip, turn left here.
16.43 Turn left on Janine Dr.
16.91 Straight across Santa Gertrudes Ave.
18.31 Turn right on Macy St. Be aware, the only v ible sign reads Capulet Ave.
18.77 Turn left onto Whittier Blvd.
18.93 Cross Beach Blvd.
19.42 Turn on Idaho St.
19.94 Cross La Habra Blvd.
20.43 Turn left onto Lambert St.
21.2 Turn left onto Euclid St.
21.53 End

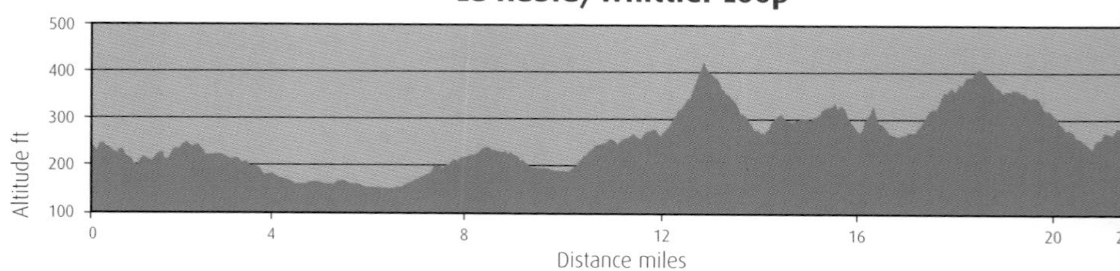

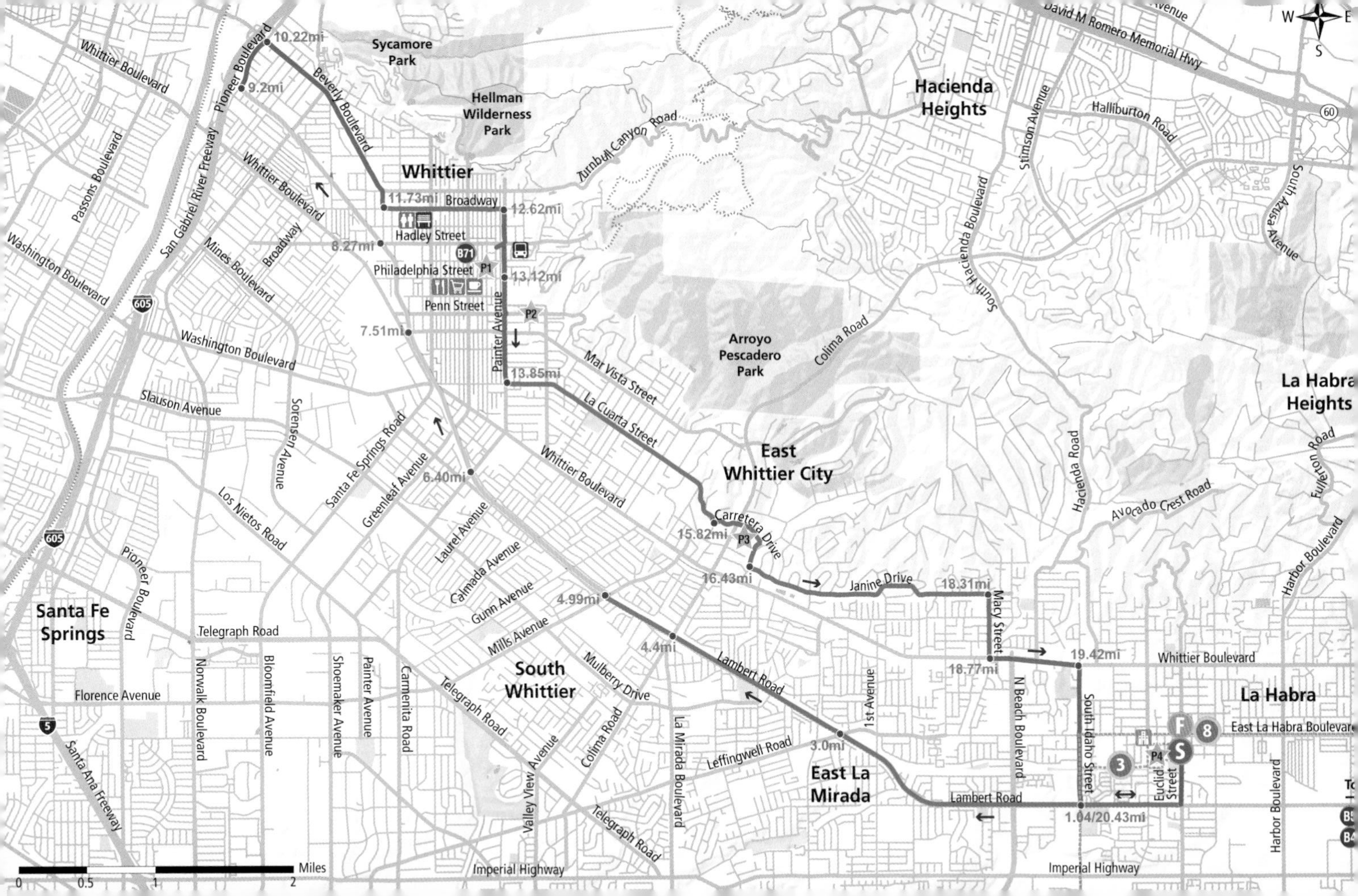
W
E
S
Whittier Boulevard
Pioneer Boulevard
10.22mi
9.2mi
Sycamore Park
Hellman Wilderness Park
Beverly Boulevard
Hacienda Heights
David M Romero Memorial Hwy
Halliburton Road
Stimson Avenue
60
Turnbull Canyon Road
Whittier
Passons Boulevard
San Gabriel River Freeway
Whittier Boulevard
11.73mi
Broadway
12.62mi
South Hacienda Boulevard
South Azusa Avenue
Hadley Street
8.27mi
Broadway
Mines Boulevard
B71
Philadelphia Street
P1
13.12mi
Washington Boulevard
605
Penn Street
P2
7.51mi
Painter Avenue
Washington Boulevard
Arroyo Pescadero Park
Colima Road
Mar Vista Street
13.85mi
La Habra Heights
Slauson Avenue
La Cuarta Street
Sorensen Avenue
Santa Fe Springs Road
East Whittier City
Hacienda Road
Fullerton Road
Greenleaf Avenue
6.40mi
Whittier Boulevard
Los Nietos Road
Avocado Crest Road
Carretera Drive
15.82mi
P3
Harbor Boulevard
605
Laurel Avenue
Calmada Avenue
16.43mi
Janine Drive
18.31mi
Pioneer Boulevard
Gunn Avenue
4.99mi
Macy Street
Santa Fe Springs
Telegraph Road
Mills Avenue
4.4mi
Whittier Boulevard
19.42mi
South Whittier
Mulberry Drive
Lambert Road
18.77mi
Florence Avenue
Norwalk Boulevard
Bloomfield Avenue
Shoemaker Avenue
Painter Avenue
Carmenita Road
Telegraph Road
1st Avenue
N Beach Boulevard
South Idaho Street
La Habra
5
F
8
East La Habra Boulevard
Colima Road
La Mirada Boulevard
3.0mi
P4
S
3
Euclid Street
Leffingwell Road
Santa Ana Freeway
Valley View Avenue
East La Mirada
Harbor Boulevard
Lambert Road
1.04/20.43mi
Telegraph Road
Miles
0
0.5
1
2
Imperial Highway
Imperial Highway
B5
B4

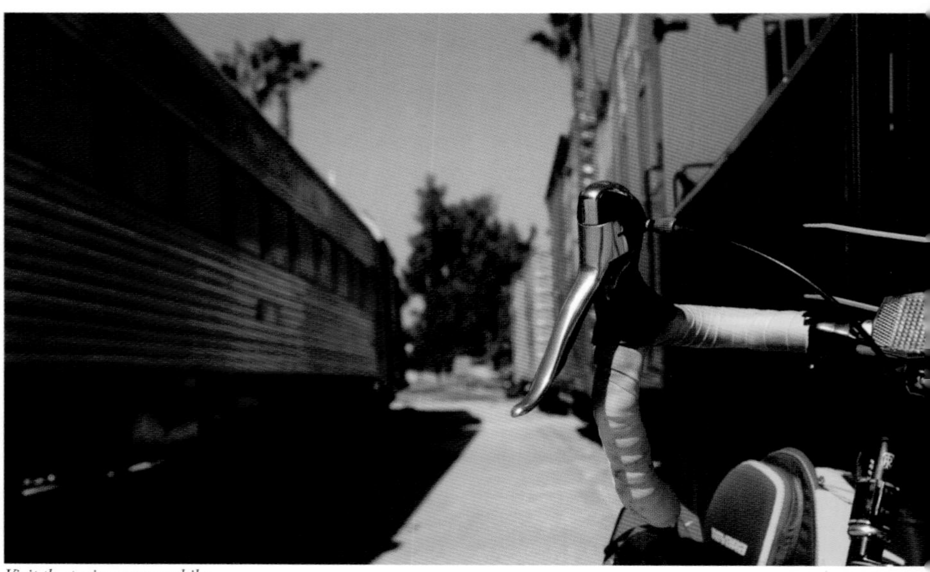

Visit the trains on your bike.

At a Glance

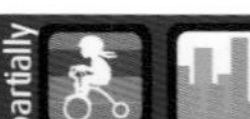

Distance 1.81 miles **Elevation Gain** 85′

Terrain

Flat, smooth trails and roads, with one small patch of gravel.

How to Get There

By bus, there are no buses to the ride's start, however OCTA bus 37, traveling along Euclid Street makes a stop at Portola Park.

By car, take the 91 Freeway to exit 23, Beach Boulevard, northbound. Drive 5.4 miles, before turning right onto Lambert Road. After a mile, turn left onto South Walnut Street, then drive 0.3 mile. Park entrance will be on your left.

Food and Drink

Bring a picnic and snacks and enjoy the park. Near Tacos y Mariscos La Fuente serves authentic Mexic food with large portions and reasonable prices.

Side Trip

The Children's Museum at La Habra as well as the D pot Theatre are located in Portola Park and are gr places to visit during this family ride.

Links to  

Where to Bike Rating 

About...

'Land of Gracious Living," the signs in Yorba .inda read. As you ride through this quiet, ɔrganized suburb with flowers planted along ɔike trails and crosswalk buttons placed high ɛnough that equestrians need not dismount or ean over, it is easy to see how the city came :o that description. As with most of this part of :he county, its history revolves primarily around ɔgriculture until a population boom in the 1970s and 80s led to the development of large 'esidential plots, bridle trails and bike paths.

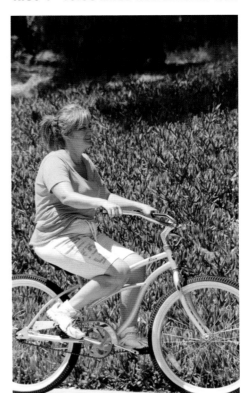

Cruising in the sun.

ɪis out-and-back ride is comprised of two distinctly fferent legs. The first is a mellow, meandering path ithout any climbs and is a perfect stretch for even the ɔst inexperienced cyclists. You will travel this sec- ɔn alongside joggers, horses and even a helicopter. At 63 miles, the trail ends and a challenging 4.5 miles ahead. Expect three steep climbs that will set your gs on fire and, naturally, three exhilarating descents.

Begin at Koch Park and from there travel along sidential streets in order to avoid a busy stretch of astanchury Road that is not family friendly. Once on e trail be aware that at every street intersection traf- : has the right of way. Make use of the pedestrian ossing lights.

As the trail approaches Yorba Linda Boulevard it ns alongside the Richard Nixon Presidential Library. ɪe library houses Nixon White House materials, the ixon Tapes as well as Nixon's birthplace. Here you ill also catch sight of the VH-3A Sea King, a heli- ɔpter that was part of the presidential fleet until its ɛcommission. Climb aboard and see how presidents ennedy, Johnson, Nixon and Ford traveled. Admis- on to library is $9.95 for adults, $3.75 for children -11, and free to kids aged six and under.

Once you reach Grandview Avenue the family friendly section ends and it is best to turn around if traveling with young or inexperienced riders. From here you can expect a more challenging ride. The next 0.89 miles travel along quiet residential streets, with the last few hundred yards culminating in a very steep section along Arroyo Canyon Drive. Near the peak of this climb, on your right, the bike path resumes. It is lacking a sign but easy to spot.

At 6.58 miles this section of the bike path ends and you head downhill to link up with the final stretch of bike trail at the bottom of the hill. Here, at Esperanza Road, you will have the choice of riding on a hard-packed, multi-use dirt trail, or along on-road bike lanes. Once you reach New River Road, turn around and head back to the start.

Ride Log

P1 Richard Nixon Library
P2 Carbon Canyon Regional Park
P3 Black Gold Golf Course

0.0 Begin ride at George Koch Park heading towards the entrance located at Royal Stewart Dr.

0.19 Turn right on Mathewson Ave.

0.42 Turn left on McCormack Ln.

0.59 Turn right on Williams Ave.

0.64 Turn right on Traynor Ave.

0.81 Traynor bends and becomes Spahn Dr.

0.93 Turn left onto Bastanchury Rd. This is a busy road, be careful.

1.03 Turn right onto bike path. Although there is no sign here, this is the beginning of the Yorba Linda Recreational Trail.

1.23 Cross Rose Dr.

1.59 Cross Prospect Ave.

1.85 Cross El Cajon Ave.

2.3 Cross Valley View Ave.

2.65 Cross Casa Loma Ave.

2.83 Turn right, head towards wooden pedestrian bridge.

3.17 Cross Eureka Ave.

3.41 Cross Yorba Linda Blvd. The Richard Nixon Library is located here.

3.68 Bear left and pass through bridge under Lakeview Ave. There is a narrow blind corner on the other side, be alert.

3.75 Turn right onto Lakeview Ave bike lane.

3.83 Turn right back onto Yorba Linda Trail.

4.63 This section of the Class 1 trail ends, turn right onto Grandview Ave.

4.76 Turn left, still on Grandview.

5.18 Turn left onto Kellog Dr. This can be a busy i tersection, be careful.

5.28 Turn right onto Arroyo Cajon Dr.

5.52 Turn right onto bike path.

6.58 Turn right onto Fairlynn Blvd.

6.83 Turn left onto Esperanza Rd. This road has bi lanes on the road or an off-the-road, multi-use path th is composed of hard-packed earth.

9.22 Turn around at New River Rd and follow cour back.

11.61 Turn right onto Fairlynn Blvd.

11.87 Cross over Fairlynn and return to bike path.

12.95 Bike path ends and turn right onto Arroyo Caj Dr.

12.97 Make U-turn and head down Arroyo Canyon I

13.22 Turn left onto Kellog Dr.

13.30 Turn right onto Grandview Ave.

13.72 Turn right, still on Grandview Ave.

13.75 Cross Grandview and return to Yorba Lin Trail.

14.68 Trail ends at Lakeview Ave, turn left onto sid walk and cross over bridge.

14.77 Hairpin turn onto trail and into tunnel. Wat for blind corner here.

17.53 Yorba Linda Recreational Trail ends, turn le onto Bastanchury Rd.

17.61 Cross Bastanchury onto Spahn Ln.

17.91 Turn left onto Williams Ave.

17.95 Turn left at McCormack Ln.

18.13 Right on Mathewson Ave.

18.35 Turn left onto Royal Stewart Dr.

18.55 End.

Yorba Linda Recreational Trail

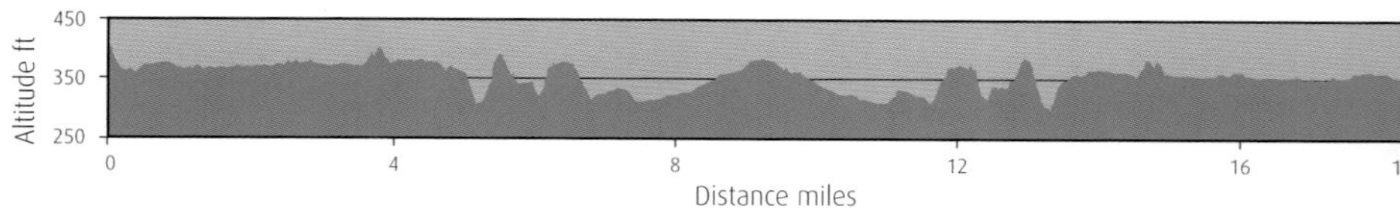

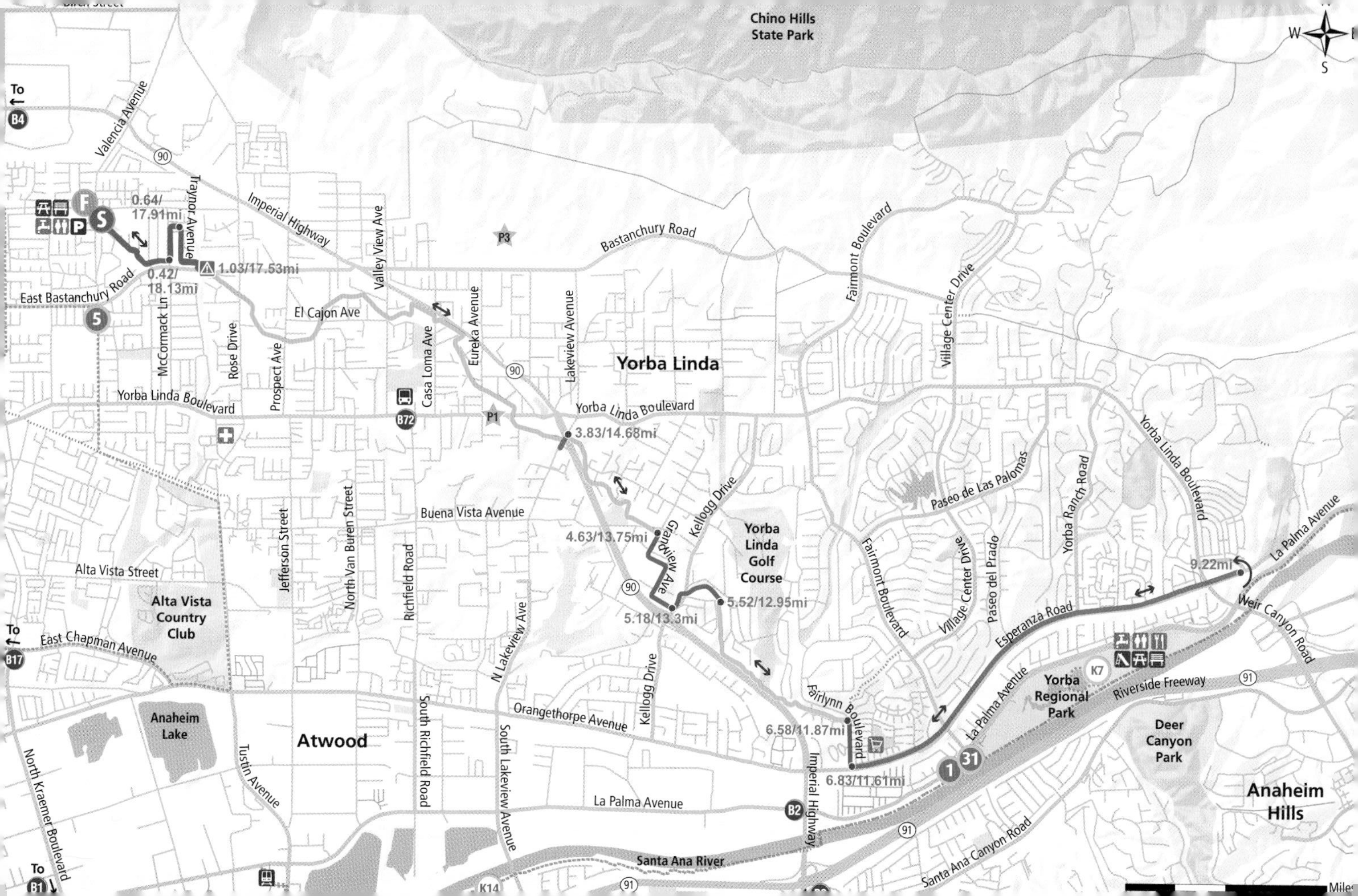

Chino Hills State Park
Yorba Linda
Atwood
Anaheim Hills
Yorba Linda Golf Course
Alta Vista Country Club
Anaheim Lake
Yorba Regional Park
Deer Canyon Park
Valencia Avenue
Imperial Highway
Traynor Avenue
Bastanchury Road
East Bastanchury Road
McCormack Ln
Rose Drive
Prospect Ave
El Cajon Ave
Valley View Ave
Casa Loma Ave
Eureka Avenue
Lakeview Avenue
Yorba Linda Boulevard
Fairmont Boulevard
Village Center Drive
Paseo de Las Palomas
Paseo del Prado
Yorba Ranch Road
Esperanza Road
La Palma Avenue
Weir Canyon Road
Riverside Freeway
Santa Ana Canyon Road
Santa Ana River
Fairlynn Boulevard
Kellogg Drive
Grandview Ave
Buena Vista Avenue
N Lakeview Ave
South Lakeview Avenue
Orangethorpe Avenue
Richfield Road
South Richfield Road
North Van Buren Street
Jefferson Street
Alta Vista Street
East Chapman Avenue
Tustin Avenue
North Kraemer Boulevard
0.64/17.91mi
0.42/18.13mi
1.03/17.53mi
3.83/14.68mi
4.63/13.75mi
5.18/13.3mi
5.52/12.95mi
6.58/11.87mi
6.83/11.61mi
9.22mi
To B4
To B17
To B1
B72
B2
K7
K14
P1
P3
W
S

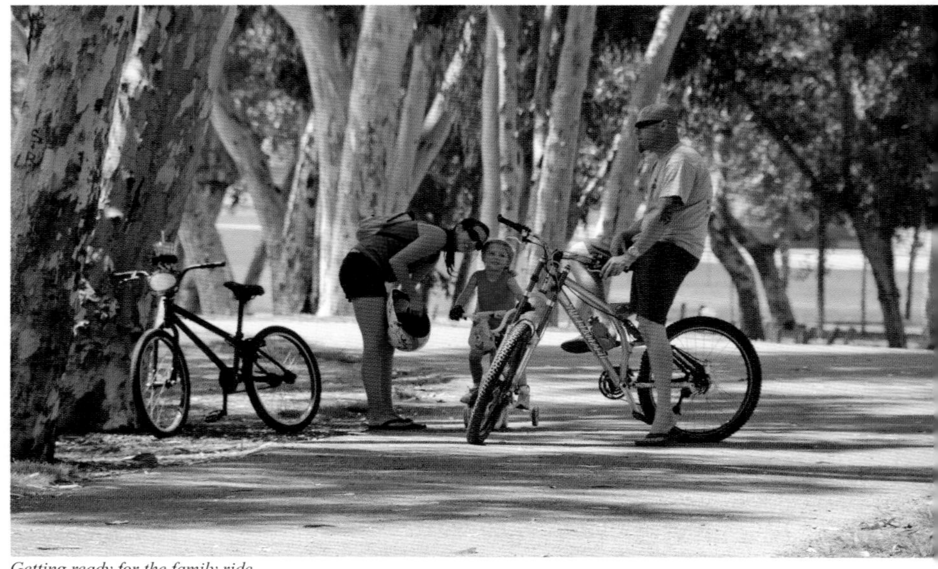

Getting ready for the family ride.

At a Glance

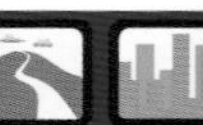

Distance 11.91 miles **Elevation Gain** 640′

Terrain

Mild, rolling hills along well maintained roads.

Traffic

This ride travels mostly along quite roads, although the western section of Chapman Avenue can be rather busy where it intersects with Placentia Avenue.

How to Get There

By bus, OCTA routes 24, 30, 71, 129 and 153 all intersect with this route.

By car, take the 57 Freeway to exit 9, Imperial Highway, eastbound. After one mile turn right on South Kraemer Boulevard, then turn right on Golden Avenue. Tri-City Park will be on your right after half a mile.

Food and Drink

There are a number of great Mexican food places at the Placita-Santa Fe District. El Farolito located at t corner of Bradford and Center streets is my favorite.

Side Trip

Along this ride are a number of wonderful parks, sta ing with Tri-City Park itself. Craig Regional Park, s of Kids' Ride 5, is a tree shaded valley with a numb of bike paths worthy of exploration. At 7.92 miles y will pass the Placita-Santa Fe District, Placentia's c town where you will find a number of restaurants a historic buildings.

Links to    KS

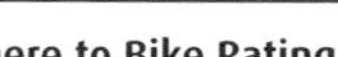 

Where to Bike Rating

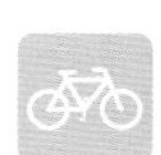    

About...

The city of Placentia, like so many in this part of Orange County, started out as agricultural land in the 1800s, first as land grants from Mexican governors, followed by American settlers arriving after the civil war. Citrus, walnuts and grapes were thriving by the time the Santa Fe Railroad company re-routed track through here and built a station in 1910. Placentia soon became an orange growing center and incorporated as a city in 1926. By 1960 the city had a population of 5000; by 1970, 25000. Today it stands at 45000 citizens.

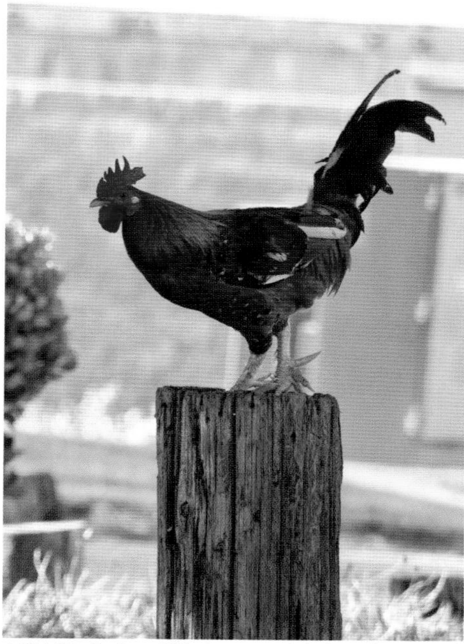

At Tri-City Park you'll find geese, and ducks and... roosters?

.s the city grew, agriculture made way for houses and arks. Today Placentia is primarily a bedroom commu-ity with wide streets, open spaces for recreation and lenty of bike routes. This ride starts at Tri-City Park, a eautiful green space that once was the main reservoir or what was to become the cities of Anaheim, Fuller-n and Placentia. A bike/walking path circles the park nd the ride finishes with a nice cool down lap along is path. Watch your speeds during the weekend as ere are lots of pedestrians here.

The route begins by cutting through the park to e Rolling Hills Drive entrance. At the bottom of is downhill stretch, along North Associated Road, Craig Regional Park which is the location of Kids' ide 5. This park also has a lake and a number of bike aths, making it a great place for a family outing. The asiest way to enter the park is to turn left as you would r this ride and on your right you will pass a bike path ading into the park. Ride 8 overlaps with this route re, traveling in the opposite direction.

At 6.5 miles the route travels along Chapman Av-ue which is an on-street bike lane. However, the retch beginning at 7.5 miles narrows and during rush ur this is a major artery for commuters heading towards the 57 Freeway. If traffic through this section is uncomfortably busy, consider a detour, turning right at Bradford Avenue which you will end up on at 9.32 miles anyway.

Located at 7.92 miles is the Placita-Santa Fe district, Placentia's old town. Although still a work in progress, the area is clean and attractive with a number of historical buildings including the Calvary Church, the Placentia Public Library and a water tower adorned with the Santa Fe Railroad emblem. It also features an on-street bike lane. What this area lacks in variety, it makes up for in a huge selection of Mexican restaurants. A local favorite is El Farolito serving authentic Mexican, generous portions and affordable prices.

Ride Log

0.0 Start at Tri-City Park entrance off of Golden Ave. Follow bike path the runs parallel to road.
0.36 Turn right off of path.
0.37 Turn left into parking lot.
0.39 Exit park and enter on-road bike lane on Rolling Hills Dr.
0.65 Continue straight across Placentia Ave.
1.25 Turn left onto N Associated Rd.
2.01 Turn left onto E Bastanchury Rd.
2.6 Straight across Hartford Ave.
2.88 Straight across Placentia Ave.
3.38 Straight across N Kraemer Blvd.
3.64 Straight across Brookhaven Ave.
3.88 Turn right on Valencia Ave.
4.37 Straight across Yorba Linda Blvd.
4.61 Left on E Palm Dr.
5.3 Right on N Rose Dr.
5.73 Straight across Alta Vista St.
6.27 Right on E Orangethorpe Ave.
6.56 Turn right on E Chapman Ave.
7.38 Passing Placentia City Hall and Civic Center.
7.92 Straight across Bradford Ave. The Placita, old town area, is located to your left and the Mexican restaurant Farolito is located here.
8.04 Kraemer Memorial Park on your right, this is an excellent place to take a break.
8.43 Turn right on N Placentia Ave.
8.71 Turn right onto Primrose Ave.

P1 Fullerton Arboretum
P2 Placentia-Santa Fe District
P3 El Farolito Restaurant
P4 Placentia Champions Sports Complex
P5 Fullerton Dam

8.99 Turn left on Orange Grove Ave. There is also sign here indicating this is the beginning of Diamon Rd.
9.07 Turn left onto Diamond Rd.
9.14 Right on Ruby Dr.
9.32 Left on Bradford Ave.
9.43 Straight across E Madison Ave.
10.04 Cross Yorba Linda Blvd.
10.22 Road ends but there is a pedestrian pass throug The street changes to La Salle Circle.
10.28 La Salle ends turn right onto Louise Dr.
10.34 Turn left onto Kingston Rd.
10.44 Turn right onto Livingston Ave.
10.47 Turn left onto N Kraemer Blvd.
10.72 Straight across E Bastanchury Rd.
11.24 Turn left into Tri-City Park.
11.28 Turn left at fork in the road and follow bike pa signs.
11.33 Turn left onto path that follows lake.
11.54 Bear left.
11.67 Bear left.
11.83 Cross road and turn right onto path.
11.91 End.

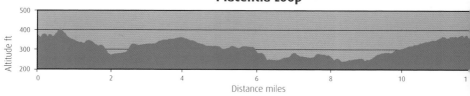

Placentia Loop

Altitude ft: 500, 400, 300, 200
Distance miles: 0, 2, 4, 6, 8, 10, 1

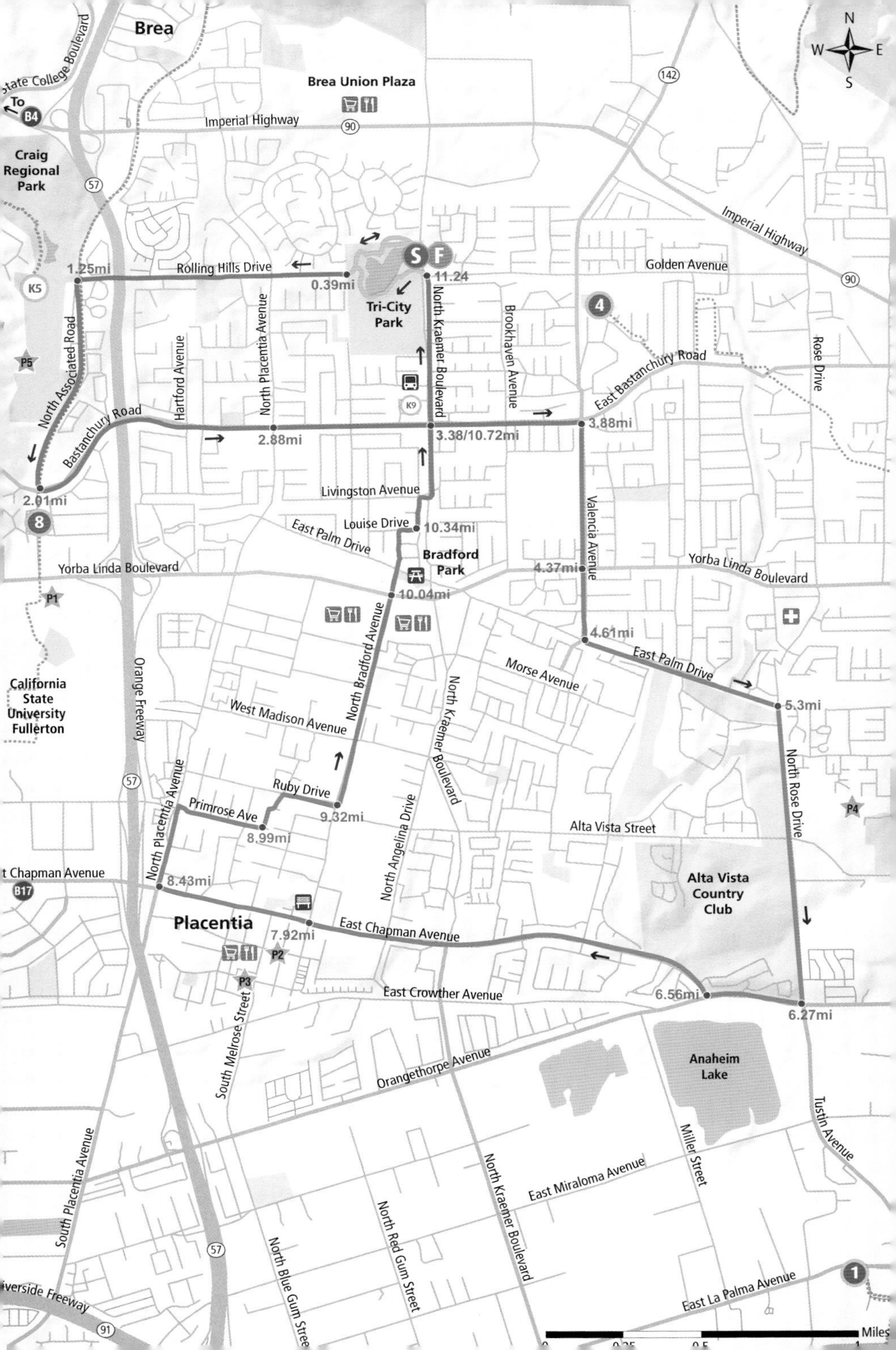
Brea
State College Boulevard
To B4
Brea Union Plaza
Imperial Highway
90
142
Craig Regional Park
57
K5
P5
1.25mi
Rolling Hills Drive
0.39mi
S F
11.24
Tri-City Park
Imperial Highway
Golden Avenue
90
4
North Associated Road
Hartford Avenue
North Placentia Avenue
North Kraemer Boulevard
Brookhaven Avenue
East Bastanchury Road
Rose Drive
K9
Bastanchury Road
2.88mi
3.38/10.72mi
3.88mi
2.01mi
8
Livingston Avenue
Louise Drive
10.34mi
East Palm Drive
Bradford Park
Valencia Avenue
Yorba Linda Boulevard
4.37mi
Yorba Linda Boulevard
P1
10.04mi
North Bradford Avenue
4.61mi
Morse Avenue
East Palm Drive
North Kraemer Boulevard
California State University Fullerton
Orange Freeway
West Madison Avenue
5.3mi
North Rose Drive
57
North Placentia Avenue
Ruby Drive
Primrose Ave
9.32mi
8.99mi
North Angelina Drive
Alta Vista Street
P4
t Chapman Avenue
8.43mi
B17
Placentia
7.92mi
East Chapman Avenue
Alta Vista Country Club
P2
P3
East Crowther Avenue
6.56mi
6.27mi
South Melrose Street
Orangethorpe Avenue
Anaheim Lake
Miller Street
Tustin Avenue
South Placentia Avenue
East Miraloma Avenue
North Red Gum Street
North Kraemer Boulevard
North Blue Gum Stree
57
iverside Freeway
91
East La Palma Avenue
1
N
W
E
S
Miles

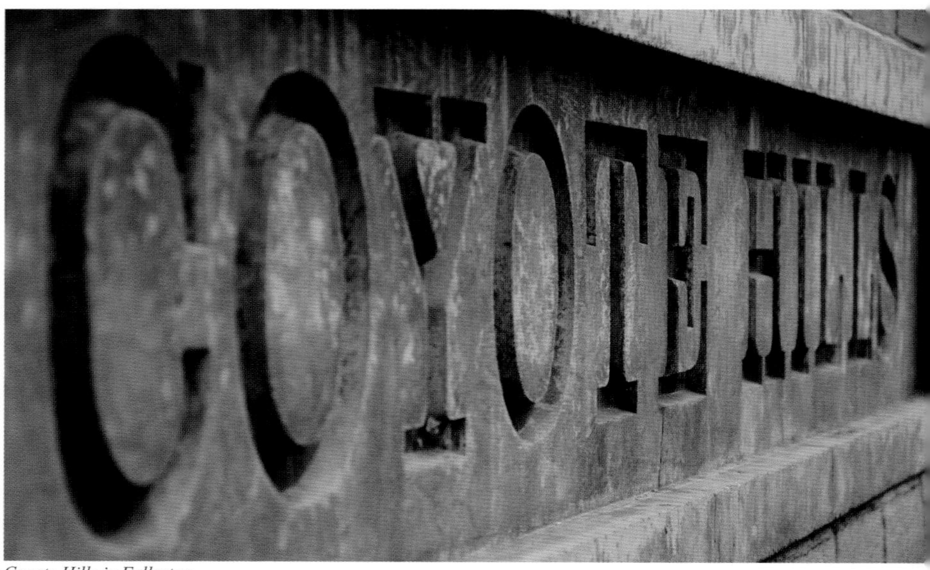

Coyote Hills in Fullerton.

At a Glance

Distance 8.94 miles **Elevation Gain** 1222′

Terrain

This ride is all about hills and for most of these miles you will either be climbing or descending a slope. Roads are well maintained, but there a couple of bumpy patches.

Traffic

This route travels along quiet streets with light traffic.

How to Get There

By bus, OCTA routes 24 and 37 intersect this ride.

By car, take Interstate Highway 5 to Beach Boulevard north. Travel two miles before turning right onto Malvern Avenue. Travel for another two and a half miles before turning left on Bastanchury Road. Turn left into Bastanchury Park.

Food and Drink

Near the ride's start is Amerige Heights town cen with a number of eating options. There are a cou of parks along the route to fill up on water as neede

Side Trip

For anyone owning a mountain bike, Robert E. Wa Nature Preserve offers an opportunity to explore a va ety of challenging trails that link up to a larger netwo throughout Fullerton. Bastanchury Park is an excelle place to picnic as well as the place that connects Ri 9 to this one.

Links to   

Where to Bike Rating 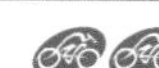

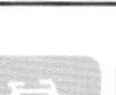  

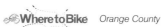

About...

or those looking to get off the beaten path nd explore a slice of nature, this ride fits the ill. Starting on the Bud Turner Trail at Laguna ake Park you will connect to the Juanita Cooke reenbelt Trail before looping back to the Bud urner Trail by residential streets. Along the way xpect to share your experience with nature overs, strollers, joggers and equestrians as you ass beautiful homes, cross old train bridges nd travel the land.

e trails that make up a large part of this route are ned after individuals who helped to develop Full-on's trail system. Both trails are relatively flat and y, they are, however, unpaved and a bit bumpy so rcise a bit more caution than usual. Also keep in nd that during wet periods this route will become ddy, with some sections becoming outright swamps, plan your ride accordingly.

This ride starts at Lake Laguna, a quiet, lush oasis that makes for a great little day trip get-a-way for the family. Built in 1952 and renovated in 2004 this park is nestled in a valley, surrounded by upscale homes. The lake is stocked throughout the year with rainbow trout, bluegill, bass and catfish. A fishing license is required at all times for those 16 and older. Nearby are restrooms and picnic tables.

Also nearby is the Equestrian Center complete with a riding ring, show ring and grandstands. The center is home to the Fullerton Recreation Riders, a club that organizes trail rides, campouts, and social events all geared towards families. Consider swapping your iron horse for the real McCoy.

These trails are part of a much larger system totaling 28 miles which pass through Fullerton, some of which are challenging and steep with lots of technical sections. If you are looking for something a little more demanding, consider following the Juanita Cooke Trail to its terminus near Harbor Boulevard near the start of Ride 8. To do this, instead of turning right onto West Laguna Road bear left onto North Morellia Avenue where the trail resumes after about a quarter mile. Keep in mind that it's all uphill coming back!

Some helpful reminders for sharing trails; cyclists yield to equestrians and pedestrians; pass on the left; stay on the marked trail. Most importantly, ride within your abilities.

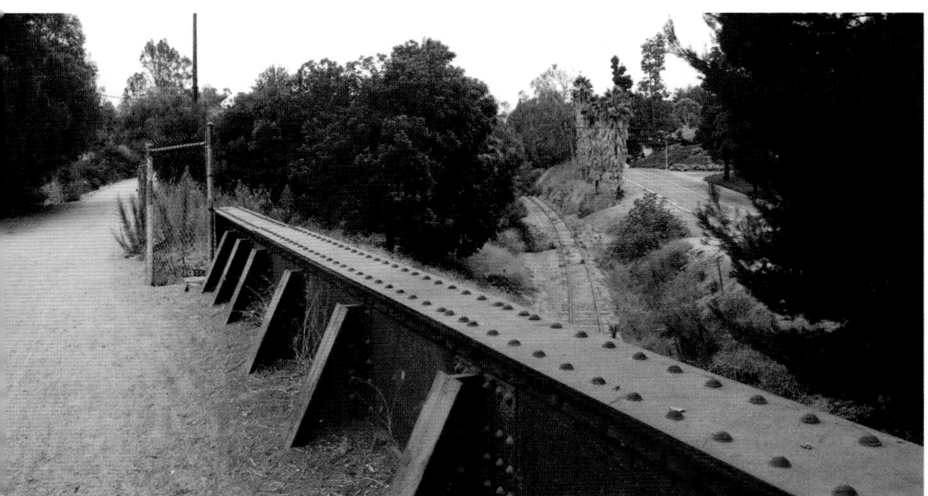

s bridge is an excellent place to pause along the Juanita Cooke Greenbelt Trail.

Ride Log

0.0 Start just outside the gate that leads into Laguna Lake.

0.33 Leaving Laguna Lake cross Lakeside Dr and turn right onto Juanita Cook Greenbelt Trail.

0.96 Old train bridge, path narrows.

1.24 Juanita Cook Trail ends, turn right onto W Laguna Rd.

1.32 Turn left onto N Domingo Rd.

2.04 Turn left onto Paseo Dorado.

2.05 Turn right onto N Euclid St.

2.49 Bud Turner Trail begins, move on to this.

2.74 Turn right at W Laguna Rd.

P1 Robert E. Ward Nature Preserve
P2 Nora Kuttner Recreational Trail
P3 Equestrian Center
P4 Brea Damn Trail
P5 Fullerton Municipal Golf Course

2.77 Turn left back onto Bud Turner Trail.

2.97 Bear left towards road.

3.09 Turn right onto Lakeview Dr.

3.20 Turn right onto W Clarion Dr.

3.26 Bear left onto trail, ride ends.

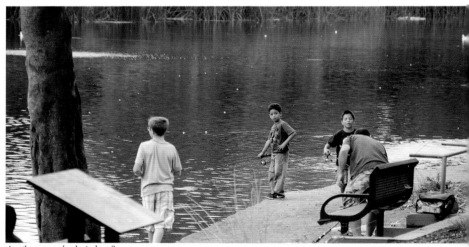

Are there any sharks in here?

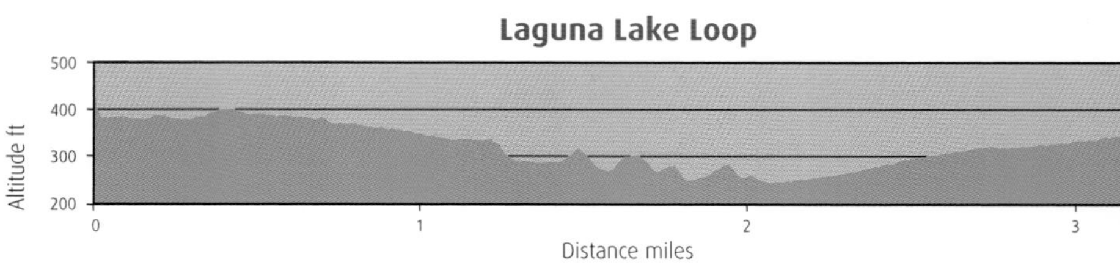

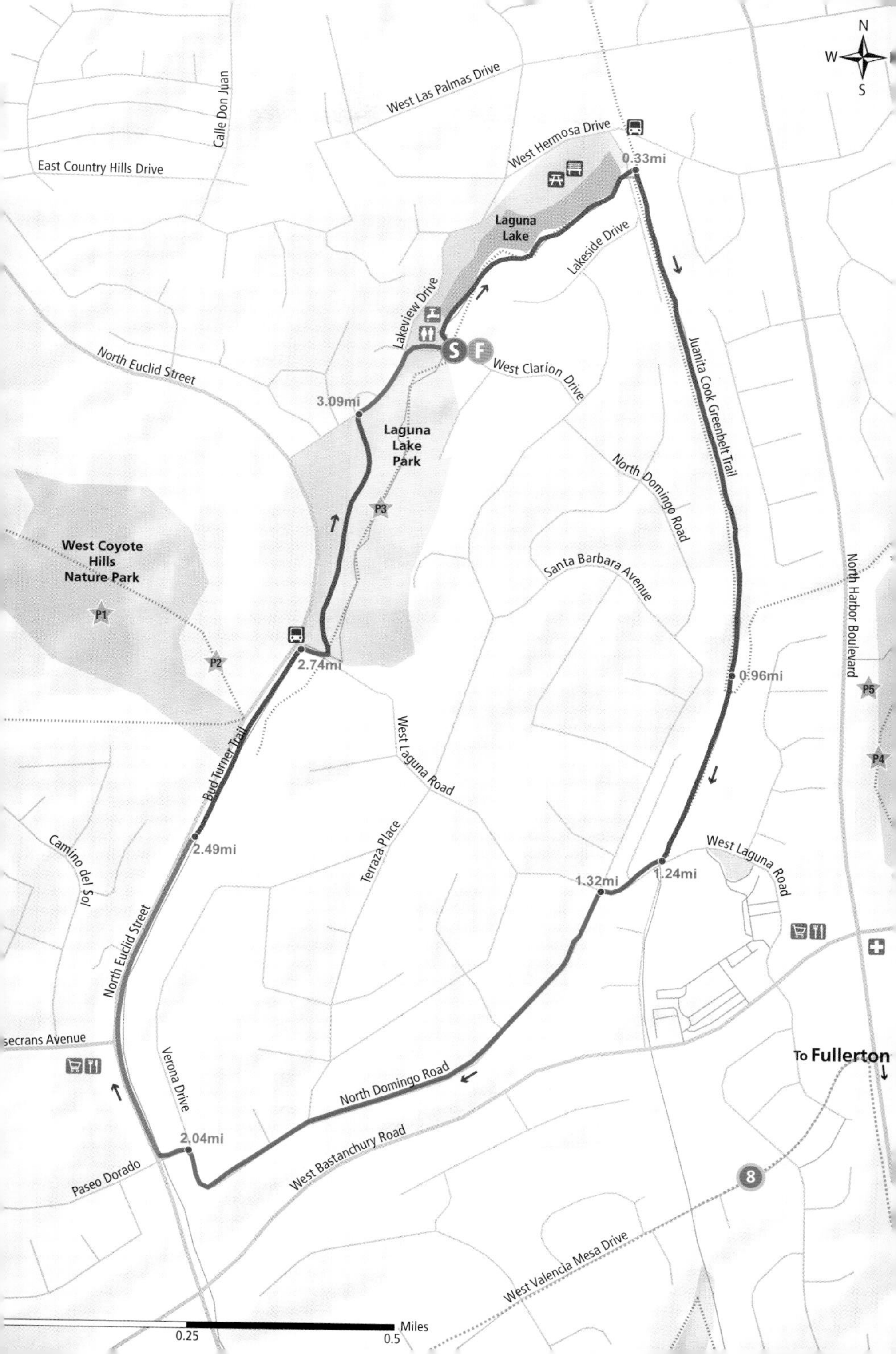

N
W
S
West Las Palmas Drive
Calle Don Juan
East Country Hills Drive
West Hermosa Drive
0.33mi
Laguna Lake
Lakeside Drive
Lakeview Drive
North Euclid Street
West Clarion Drive
3.09mi
Laguna Lake Park
Juanita Cook Greenbelt Trail
North Domingo Road
P3
West Coyote Hills Nature Park
P1
Santa Barbara Avenue
P2
2.74mi
0.96mi
North Harbor Boulevard
P5
West Laguna Road
Bud Turner Trail
P4
Camino del Sol
2.49mi
Terraza Place
West Laguna Road
1.32mi
1.24mi
North Euclid Street
secrans Avenue
Verona Drive
North Domingo Road
To Fullerton
2.04mi
West Bastanchury Road
Paseo Dorado
8
West Valencia Mesa Drive
0.25
0.5
Miles

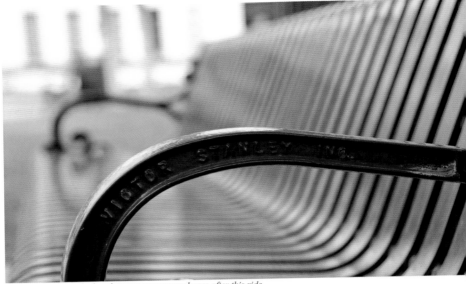

You're going to need a bench to rest your weary bones after this ride.

At a Glance

Distance 23.81 miles **Elevation Gain** 1715′

Terrain

Most of this ride is along on-road bike lanes with plenty of climbs and an especially steep section along South Idaho Street.

Traffic

Expect moderate to heavy traffic, especially if riding during morning or evening rush hour.

How to Get There

By bus, OCTA 43 makes a stop on Berkeley Avenue just north of the ride's start.

By car, take exit 28, Harbor Boulevard, off of the 91 Freeway and head north for 1.8 miles. Turn left onto North Berkeley Avenue and park in the lot on your left.

Food and Drink

Your best bet for food is near the ride's end. Heading down Harbor Boulevard, less than a quarter mile, you will find McClain's Coffeehouse with a relaxed v and great patio. On Chapman Avenue near the Har intersection is Chronic Tacos, a funky local food ch with tasty Mexican food.

Side Trip

Take a detour and visit the attractive campus of F erton College, or stop as you pass through Cal S Fullerton to explore Fullerton Arboretum. Near ride's finish, head to downtown Fullerton and en the vibrant atmosphere of this historic district.

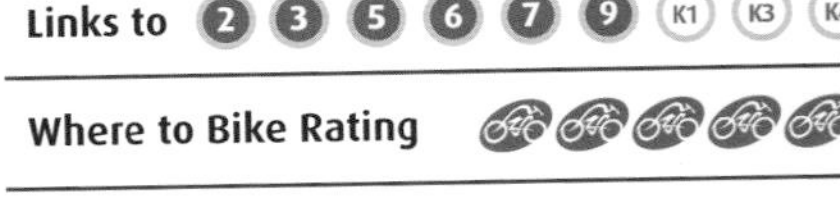

About...

This ride starts near the urban center of Fullerton and from there takes you out to the edge of suburban civilization as you traverse beautiful Carbon Canyon Regional Park. From there you will ride into the most northerly and western corner of Orange County before a challenging climb up Idaho Street returns you to Fullerton and eventually to the ride's finish. Between the mileage and climbs, this ride is sure to reward you with a real sense of achievement.

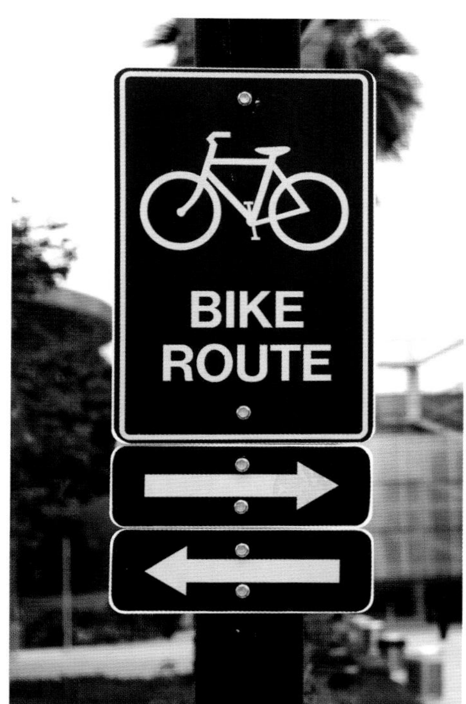

On Cal State Fullerton's campus, keep an eye out for the signs.

t mile 2.24 the route enters California State Uni-rsity of Fullerton campus. This school, once a vast ange grove, is now a campus of modern buildings d attractive landscaping. Be alert to pedestrian traf- and follow bike path signs as bicycling is allowed ly on specific paths. Located in the northeast corner the campus is the Fullerton Arboretum, 26 acres of tanical gardens with plants from around the world. e arboretum is open to the public and offers various sses throughout the year as well as offering unique d unusual plants for sale.

From here a few modest climbs lie ahead until you ch the Carbon Canyon bike path just off Rose Drive. is path sneaks up on your left so keep an eye out it or you will whizz right past it. The path is not ecially long but it is rather steep as it takes you up the top of Carbon Canyon Dam. Pause at the top g enough to enjoy the panoramic view before zip-g down into the park. If you are looking for a place picnic or even just rest for a bit, you won't find a ter venue than Carbon Canyon Regional Park, site Kid's Ride 1. Lush and green, with plenty of activi- to entice you, this is a wonderful park.

Once you leave the park you will find yourself nbing another steep hill as you pass through the Ol-inda Ranch neighborhood. This newer suburb is still in the process of being built, but already the backbone of a planned community can be seen. Enjoy the well-designed layout and attractive landscaping and look for many more bike paths in the future.

The most formidable part of this ride hits you at 18.56 miles as you ride Idaho Street and cross Imperial Highway. Depending on how you feel about climbing, this one mile is an exciting, thrilling, awesome challenge or a grisly, grueling, agonizing crawl. The first section up to Sandalwood Avenue is the steepest and the rest is comparatively easy. Remember, it is only one mile.

When the ride is done and you are looking for refreshments or are interested in shopping, head down Harbor Boulevard to historic downtown where you will find a huge selection of shops and eateries to choose from.

Ride Log

0.0 Begin near the parking lot on Berkeley Ave, near its intersection to Juanita Cooke Recreational Trail.

0.13 Cross Harbor Blvd.

0.39 Cross Lemon St, Fullerton College will be on your right.

0.66 Turn left onto Homet Way.

0.76 Turn right onto Dorothy Ln.

0.94 Turn right, still on Dorothy Ln.

2.24 Cross State College Blvd and enter the campus of California State University Fullerton.

2.29 Bear right, follow bike path signs throughout campus.

2.5 Bear left.

2.74 Bear right.

2.8 Turn right.

2.89 Cross road and pick up path through athletic fields.

3.21 Turn right.

3.26 Turn left towards campus exit.

3.33 Cross Yorba Linda Blvd onto N Associated Rd.

3.64 Cross Bastanchury Rd.

4.92 Cross Imperial Hwy.

5.50 Turn right onto E Birch St.

7.12 Cross Valencia Ave. Here Birch turns into N Rose Dr and bears right.

7.72 Cross over to your left and enter the Carbon Canyon Regional Park Trail. If you cross Vesuvius Dr you have gone too far on Rose.

7.77 Pass through gate into park.

8.16 Sharp right turn downhill.

8.60 Path ends, turn right into parking lot.

8.69 Turn left and head towards park exit.

8.79 Exit park and cross Carbon Canyon Rd ont Santa Fe Rd.

9.06 Olinda Museum on your right.

9.72 Turn left onto Valencia Ave.

9.99 Cross Lambert Rd.

10.39 Turn right onto Birch St.

11.3 Cross Kraemer Blvd.

12.0 Cross N Associated Rd.

12.39 Turn right onto State College Blvd.

12.89 Cross Lambert Rd.

13.77 Cross Brea Blvd, State College turns into Central Ave.

14.5 Cross Berry St.

15.03 Cross N Puente St.

15.52 Cross S Palm St.

16.02 Cross Harbor Blvd. Central turns into E L Habra Blvd.

16.78 Cross Euclid St.

17.75 Turn left onto S Idaho St.

18.05 Cross Lambert Rd.

18.56 Cross Imperial Hwy.

19.69 Turn left onto Castlewood Dr.

19.96 Turn right onto N Parks Rd.

20.45 Cross Rosecrans Ave.

21.11 Turn right onto Bastanchury Rd.

21.33 Turn left onto Valencia Mesa Dr.

21.91 Cross Euclid St.

22.00 Turn right onto Harbor Blvd.

23.57 Turn right onto Valley View Dr.

23.63 Turn left onto N Berkeley Ave.

23.81 End.

Fullerton Loop

Please note: the profile for Ride 8 is depicted in 200ft vertical increments due to unusually high elevation.

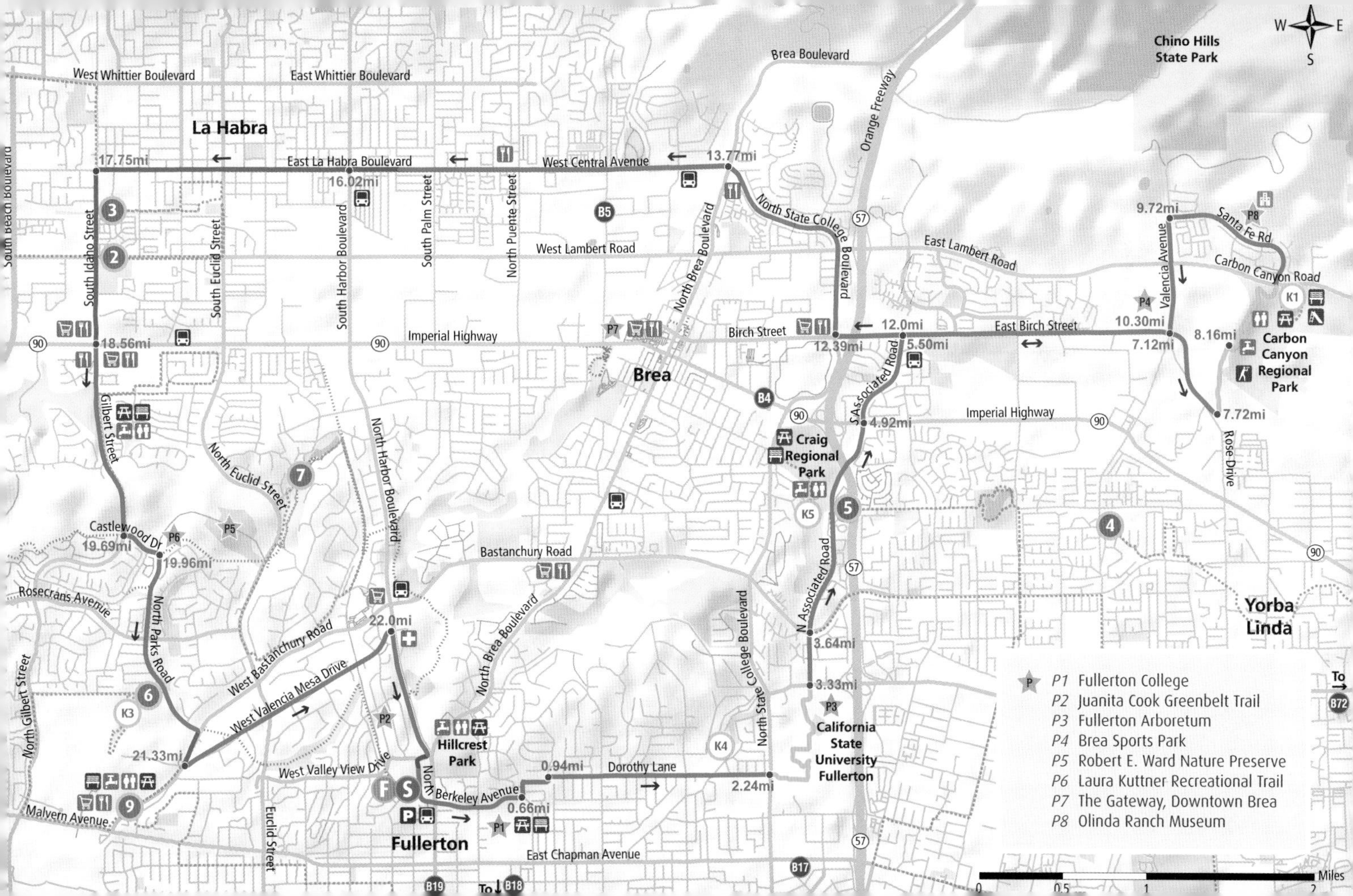
Chino Hills State Park
La Habra
Brea
Fullerton
Yorba Linda
Carbon Canyon Regional Park
Craig Regional Park
Hillcrest Park
California State University Fullerton
West Whittier Boulevard
East Whittier Boulevard
Brea Boulevard
Orange Freeway
East La Habra Boulevard
West Central Avenue
North State College Boulevard
South Beach Boulevard
South Idaho Street
South Euclid Street
South Harbor Boulevard
South Palm Street
North Puente Street
West Lambert Road
East Lambert Road
North Brea Boulevard
Santa Fe Rd
Carbon Canyon Road
Valencia Avenue
Imperial Highway
Birch Street
East Birch Street
S Associated Road
N Associated Road
Rose Drive
Gilbert Street
North Euclid Street
North Harbor Boulevard
Castlewood Dr
Bastanchury Road
Rosecrans Avenue
North Parks Road
West Bastanchury Road
West Valencia Mesa Drive
West Valley View Drive
North Gilbert Street
Malvern Avenue
Euclid Street
North Berkeley Avenue
Dorothy Lane
East Chapman Avenue
17.75mi
13.77mi
16.02mi
9.72mi
10.30mi
12.0mi
12.39mi
18.56mi
8.16mi
7.12mi
5.50mi
4.92mi
7.72mi
19.69mi
19.96mi
22.0mi
21.33mi
3.64mi
3.33mi
0.94mi
2.24mi
0.66mi
P1 Fullerton College
P2 Juanita Cook Greenbelt Trail
P3 Fullerton Arboretum
P4 Brea Sports Park
P5 Robert E. Ward Nature Preserve
P6 Laura Kuttner Recreational Trail
P7 The Gateway, Downtown Brea
P8 Olinda Ranch Museum
To B72
To B18
Miles
0
0.5
1
2

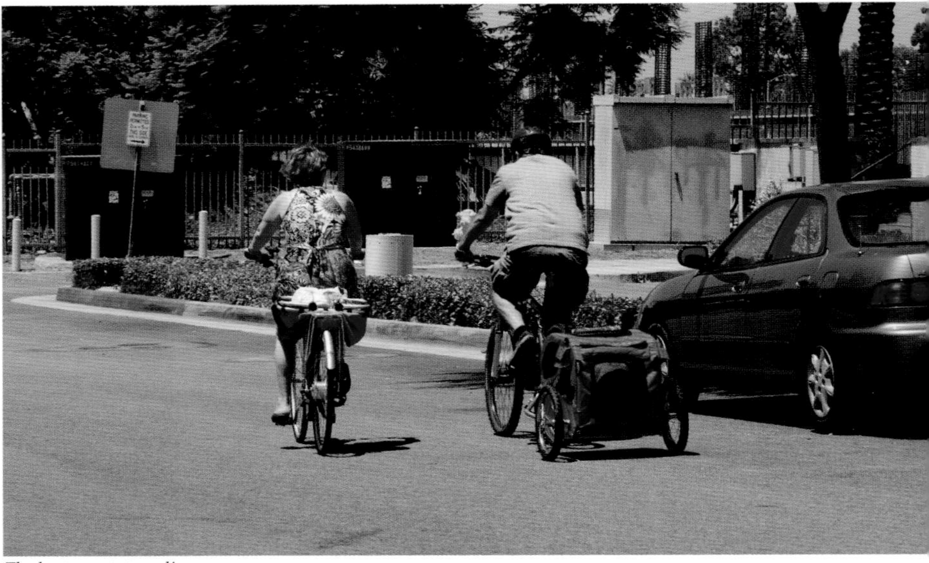

The best way to travel!

At a Glance

Distance 7.86 miles **Elevation Gain** 209′

Terrain

Mostly flat with a couple of modest climbs and a few bumpy sections.

Traffic

This route travels along quiet streets but does cross a few busy thoroughfares.

How to Get There

By train, both Metrolink and Amtrak's Surfliner make regular stops at Fullerton station.

By bus, OCTA routes 26, 43, 47, 143 and 213 all make stops at Fullerton Transportation Center.

By car, take the 91 Freeway to the Harbor Boulevard exit north bound for one mile, turn left onto West Valencia Avenue, then right on South Highland Avenue. Make a quick right onto East Walnut Avenue and park adjacent to Fullerton station.

Food and Drink

Downtown Fullerton is chock full of opportunities dine and drink. Two of my favorites are the Pint Hou and nearby Tranquil Tea House. For those looking a casual, family friendly atmosphere, try the Old Sp ghetti Factory.

Side Trip

Along the route are two excellent parks, Independen Park and Bastanchury Park at either end of the ri There is also revitalized downtown Fullerton with colorfully painted storefronts, wonderful selection eateries and quirky shops.

Links to 6 8

Where to Bike Rating 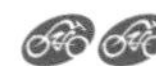

  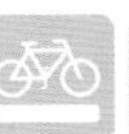  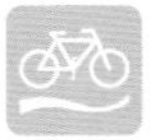

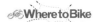

About...

This is a tour of Fullerton that starts in the urban area around downtown and the train station and then meanders through quiet neighborhoods until it reaches more suburban parts of the city before returning to the station. There is something for everyone on this ride whether it be shopping and dining, gelato and playgrounds for the kids, museums, or trainspotting. For those whom Fullerton is the birthplace of the Fender Stratocaster, a vibrant music scene still exists and in recent years a number of theater companies have had great success.

This is where your ride begins.

ullerton was founded in 1887 and as you begin this de near Track 3 at Fullerton station, it is easy to imgine what things might have looked like back then. he station's Spanish architecture, rolling freight, train histles and boarding passengers will transport you ack to another era. Nearby downtown, located along arbor Boulevard on the other side of the station, only inforces this sensation with its restored, early 20th ntury buildings and narrow, "main street Americana" ok.

In keeping with its transportation hub reputation, bicle paths abound throughout Fullerton. At the ride's art you will find yourself traveling parallel to train acks on your right and buildings that were once wareuses and factories but are now converted offices and p urban living spaces. This first leg takes you to Inpendence Park with an excellent playground, swiming pool and community center.

Downtown Fullerton is split by Harbor Boulevard ich is not a safe road for cyclists. However, Wilshire enue, which is part of this route, intersects downvn and is a safe way to enter the area. Once here, nsider walking through this compact space. One of favorite restaurants is the Pint House, located at 136 Wilshire Avenue which has an excellent selection of micro-brews as well some of the standard names. Check out the well-appointed patio for the best dining experience. Located close by is Tranquil Tea Lounge with a healthy approach to food, a vast selection of teas and tea drinks and an atmosphere that is...well, tranquil.

The Fullerton Museum Center, located at 301North Pomona Avenue, is a small but proud museum surrounded by a beautiful courtyard area complete with a playground, a unique water fountain kids can play in, and a wonderful place to enjoy a picnic lunch. Located around the corner to the north is the Fox Theater, a local landmark designed by the same firm that designed Grauman's Chinese Theatre in Hollywood. Currently under renovation, this unique building once renovated is expected to resume its place as an entertainment center for Fullerton and the surrounding area.

Ride Log

0.0 Ride begins on E Walnut Ave near pedestrian bridge that crosses over train tracks.
0.35 Cross Highland Ave and continue straight.
0.61 Highland ends, turn left onto S Richman Ave.
0.72 Turn right onto W Valencia Ave.
0.99 Turn right into Independence Park parking lot.
1.11 Turn left onto W Valencia, heading back the way you came.
1.48 Cross Richman and continue straight.
1.75 Turn left onto Highland.
1.89 Cross E Walnut, continue straight.
2.03 Continue straight across W Commonwealth Ave. City hall is on your left.
2.17 Turn left onto W Wilshire Ave.
2.68 Turn right onto N Woods Ave.
2.78 Turn left onto W Chapman Ave.
3.03 Continue straight across N Euclid St.
3.54 Turn right onto N Basque Ave.
3.66 Cross W Malvern Ave. This intersection is busy with some odd angles so stay alert. Once across the road, Basque turns into Carhart Ave.
3.99 Turn left onto W Fern Dr.
4.48 Turn right onto N Adlena Dr.
4.55 Turn left onto Adlena Pl.
4.58 Turn left onto W Bastanchury Rd.
4.63 Turn right into Bastanchury Park. Water and clean restrooms are here.
4.69 Turn around.
4.75 Left onto Bastanchury Rd.
4.8 Turn right onto Adlena Pl.

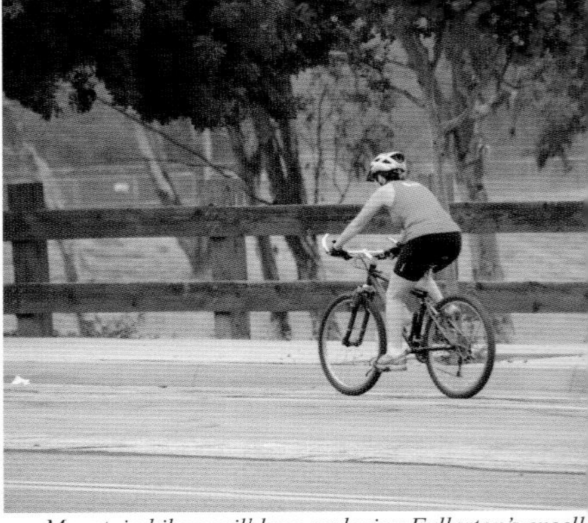

Mountain bikers will love exploring Fullerton's excell[...] trail syste[...]

4.83 Turn right onto Adlena Dr.
4.91 Left onto Fern Dr.
5.39 Turn right onto Carhart.
5.71 Cross Malvern where Carhart turns into Basque Ave.
5.84 Turn left onto Chapman.
6.35 Straight across Euclid St.
6.6 Turn right on Woods Ave.
6.71 Turn left onto Wilshire Ave.
7.22 Turn right on Highland Ave. Continuing straig[...] here will take you to downtown Fullerton full of sh[...] and an excellent place to grab a bite.
7.35 Straight across Commonwealth Ave.
7.48 Turn left onto Walnut Ave.
7.86 End.

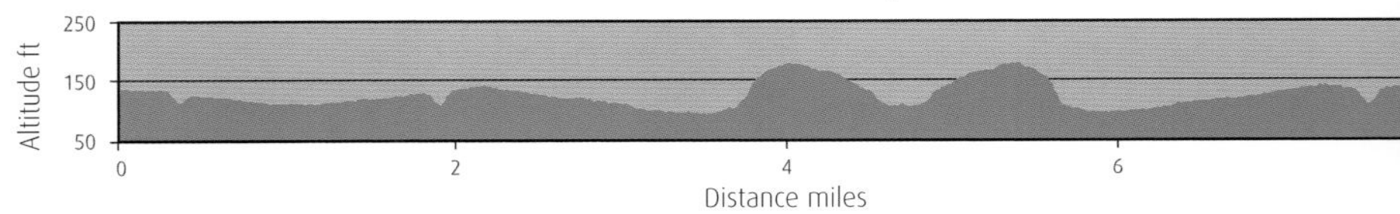

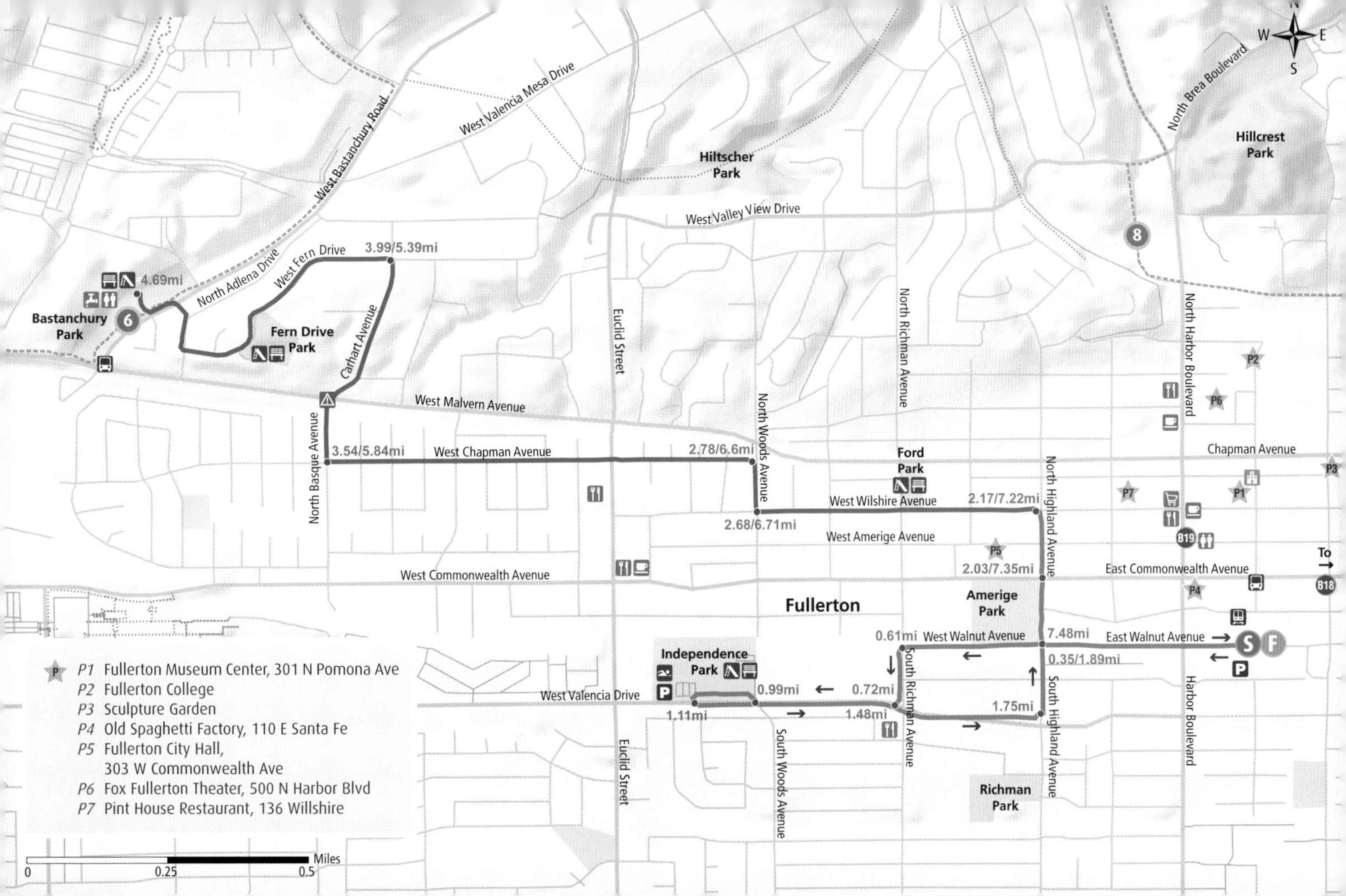

Hillcrest Park
North Brea Boulevard
Hiltscher Park
West Valencia Mesa Drive
West Bastanchury Road
West Valley View Drive
Bastanchury Park
North Adlena Drive
West Fern Drive
4.69mi
3.99/5.39mi
Fern Drive Park
Carhart Avenue
West Malvern Avenue
North Basque Avenue
3.54/5.84mi
West Chapman Avenue
2.78/6.6mi
North Woods Avenue
Euclid Street
North Richman Avenue
Ford Park
West Wilshire Avenue
2.17/7.22mi
2.68/6.71mi
West Amerige Avenue
North Highland Avenue
2.03/7.35mi
North Harbor Boulevard
Chapman Avenue
West Commonwealth Avenue
East Commonwealth Avenue
To
B18
B19
Fullerton
Amerige Park
0.61mi
West Walnut Avenue
7.48mi
East Walnut Avenue
0.35/1.89mi
Independence Park
West Valencia Drive
0.99mi
0.72mi
1.11mi
1.48mi
1.75mi
South Woods Avenue
South Richman Avenue
South Highland Avenue
Harbor Boulevard
Richman Park
P1 Fullerton Museum Center, 301 N Pomona Ave
P2 Fullerton College
P3 Sculpture Garden
P4 Old Spaghetti Factory, 110 E Santa Fe
P5 Fullerton City Hall, 303 W Commonwealth Ave
P6 Fox Fullerton Theater, 500 N Harbor Blvd
P7 Pint House Restaurant, 136 Willshire
Miles
0
0.25
0.5

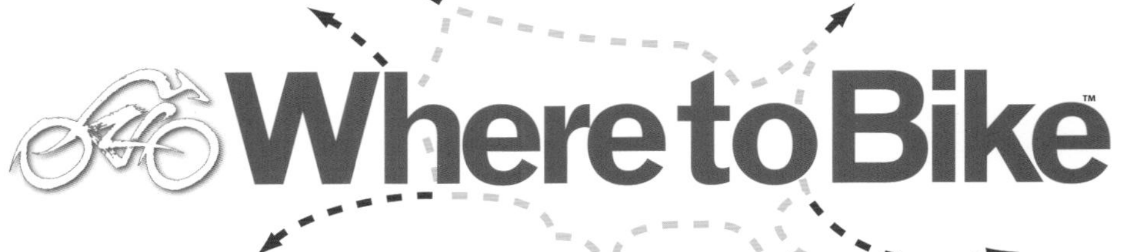

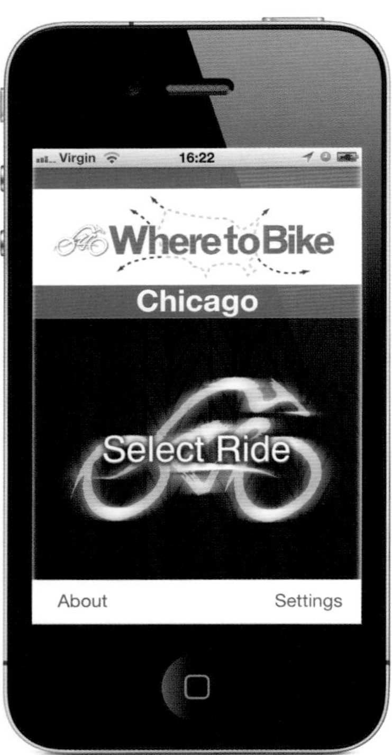

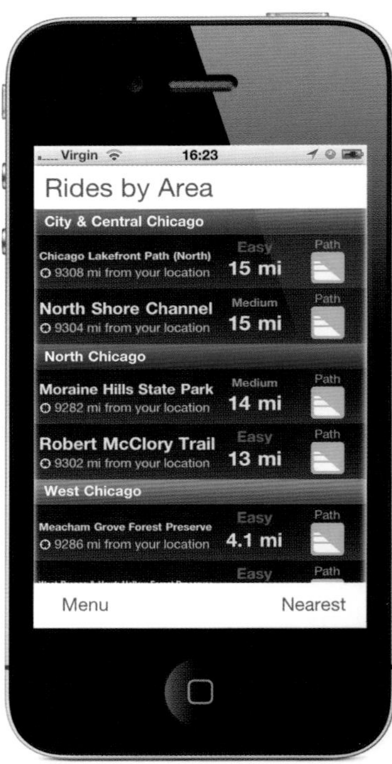

Getting Started

Step 1. Download the *Where to Bike* app for your city on the iTunes App Store. Once you load the app, you'll see this main page where you can select your ride, learn more about us, or configure settings. In the settings menu you can choose between miles and km, whether you want to display your speed, and whether you'd like a fixed or rotating map.

Select Your Ride

Step 2. Tap 'select ride' from the main screen and you will arrive at this page, where you will see a list of great rides organized into sections. These are the same as you will find in your *Where to Bike* book guide. In the bottom right-hand corner you will also see an option to arrange the rides based on their proximity to your current location.

Our *Where to Bike* apps are the perfect companion for your next ride. Don't leave home without it!

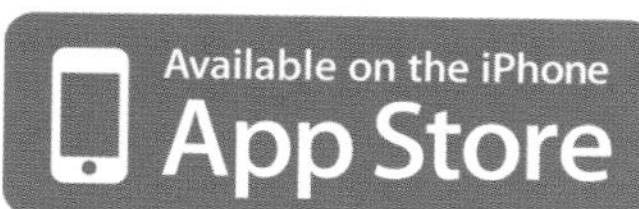

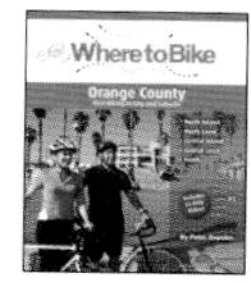

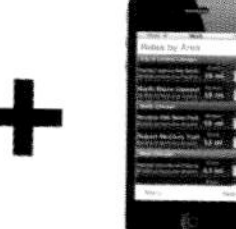

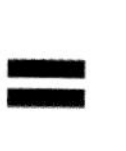

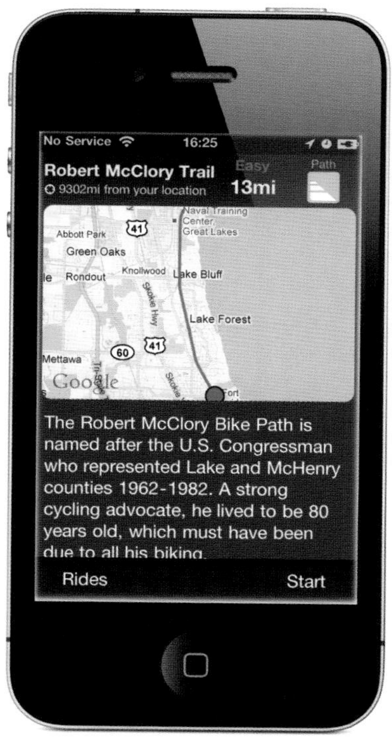

Ride Overview

Step 3. Once you select a ride, you'll be taken to this ride overview screen. Here you'll see a thumbnail map of the route, and a short description of the ride. You will also see important information such as ride difficulty, total distance, as well as how far you currently are from start of the ride. When you are ready, tap the 'Start' button to commence the ride.

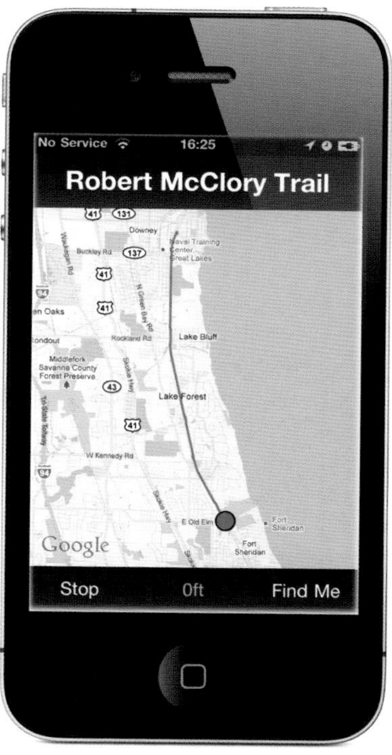

Ready to Ride

Step 4. Now you are ready to ride, it really is that simple! Your current position will be displayed by the red dot icon. You can slide your finger to scroll anywhere on the map, and if you lose your place, simply tap 'Find Me' to return to the ride route. If you feel like taking a break, simply tap the 'stop' button and you can continue again whenever you like. Have fun!

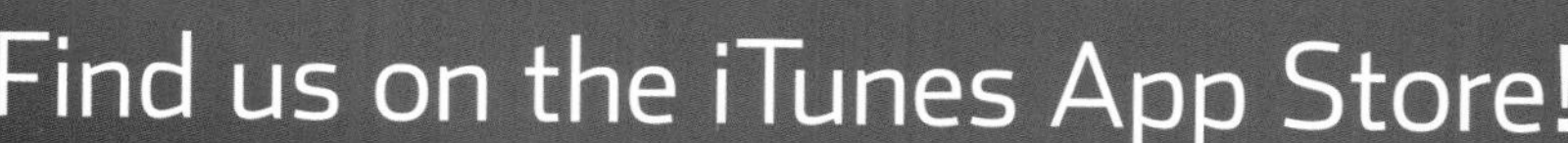

North Coast

The North Coast section is bounded by the Los Angeles County along the San Gabriel River, Interstate 5 along its inner edge and the Santa Ana River to the south. This landscape is comprised primarily of coastal flood plains and as a result all the rides in this section are flat and mostly coastal.

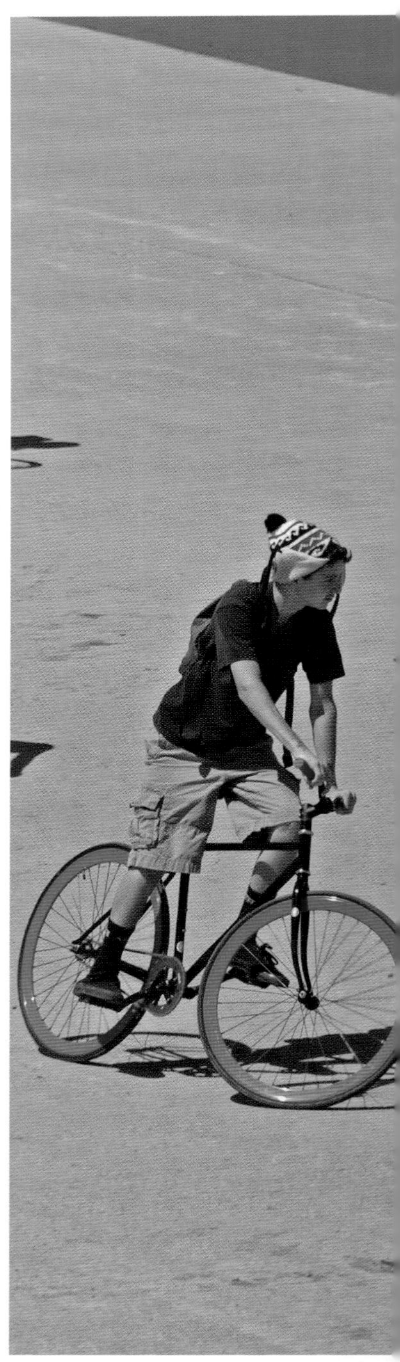

Pacific Coast Highway is the primary road through this section and not surprisingly is popular with cyclists. Rides 14, 18 and 19 spin alongside or parallel this road connecting the beach-side communities of Seal Beach, Sunset Beach and Huntington Beach. More experienced cyclists will prefer the fast energetic rides that travel along on-road lanes through these cities, while families and those looking for a leisurely ride will enjoy the Bolsa Chica Bike Path.

The San Gabriel River Trail also figures prominently into a number of rides in this section. Not as well-known as its larger, southerly cousin, the Santa Ana River, it is the backbone of numerous trails that meander between the two counties and as a result you will often find yourself weaving in and out of Los Angeles and Orange County. Car-free and well-maintained, the river trail is a safe place to ride for bicyclists of all levels. Explore Rides 10, 12 and 13 to get to know this area better.

The two premier family-friendly rides in this section are a great way for novice riders to get more comfortable on the bike. Ride 12 travels through El Dorado Park and is a beautiful, safe ride that is ideal for the most inexperienced of riders. Electric Avenue, Ride 15, travels through Seal Beach and is a short ride that offers all-day fun. After the ride, swim and surf, or stroll the pier and Main Street to take advantage of a plethora of shopping and dining opportunities.

While the coastal cities in this section have embraced the bike as part of their transportation plans and included hundreds of miles of bike lanes, the interior cities here have moved a bit slower to provide bike routes and lanes. Two exceptions are the cities of Cypress and La Palma, both of which have painted bike lanes on nearly all of their primary thoroughfares. Ride 11 is a very pleasant looping ride connected to the San Gabriel River that allow commuters and explorers to navigate the inner part of the North Coast section.

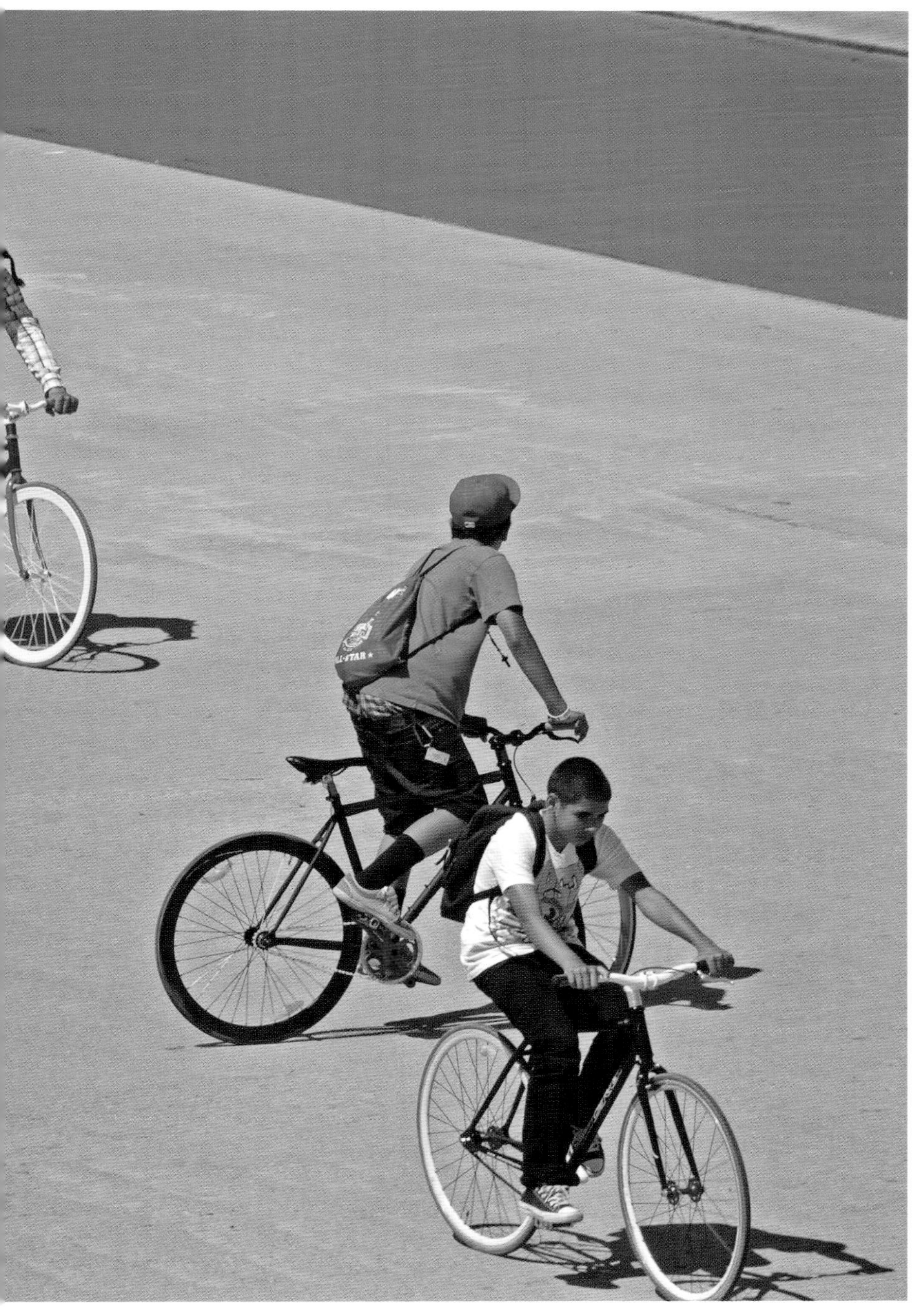
ALL-STAR ★

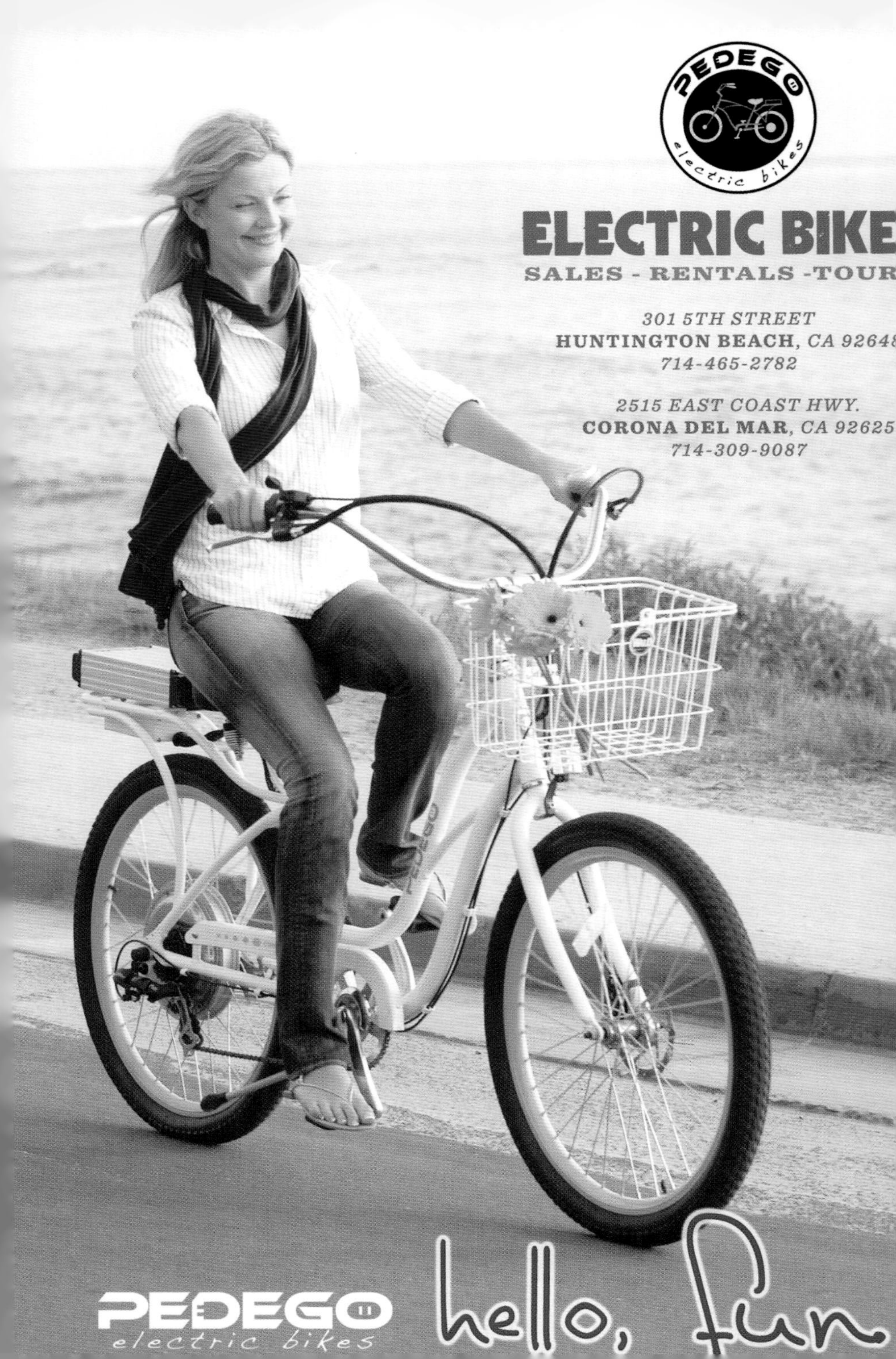
PEDEGO
electric bikes
ELECTRIC BIKE
SALES - RENTALS -TOUR
301 5TH STREET
HUNTINGTON BEACH, CA 9264
714-465-2782
2515 EAST COAST HWY.
CORONA DEL MAR, CA 92625
714-309-9087
PEDEGO
electric bikes
hello, fun

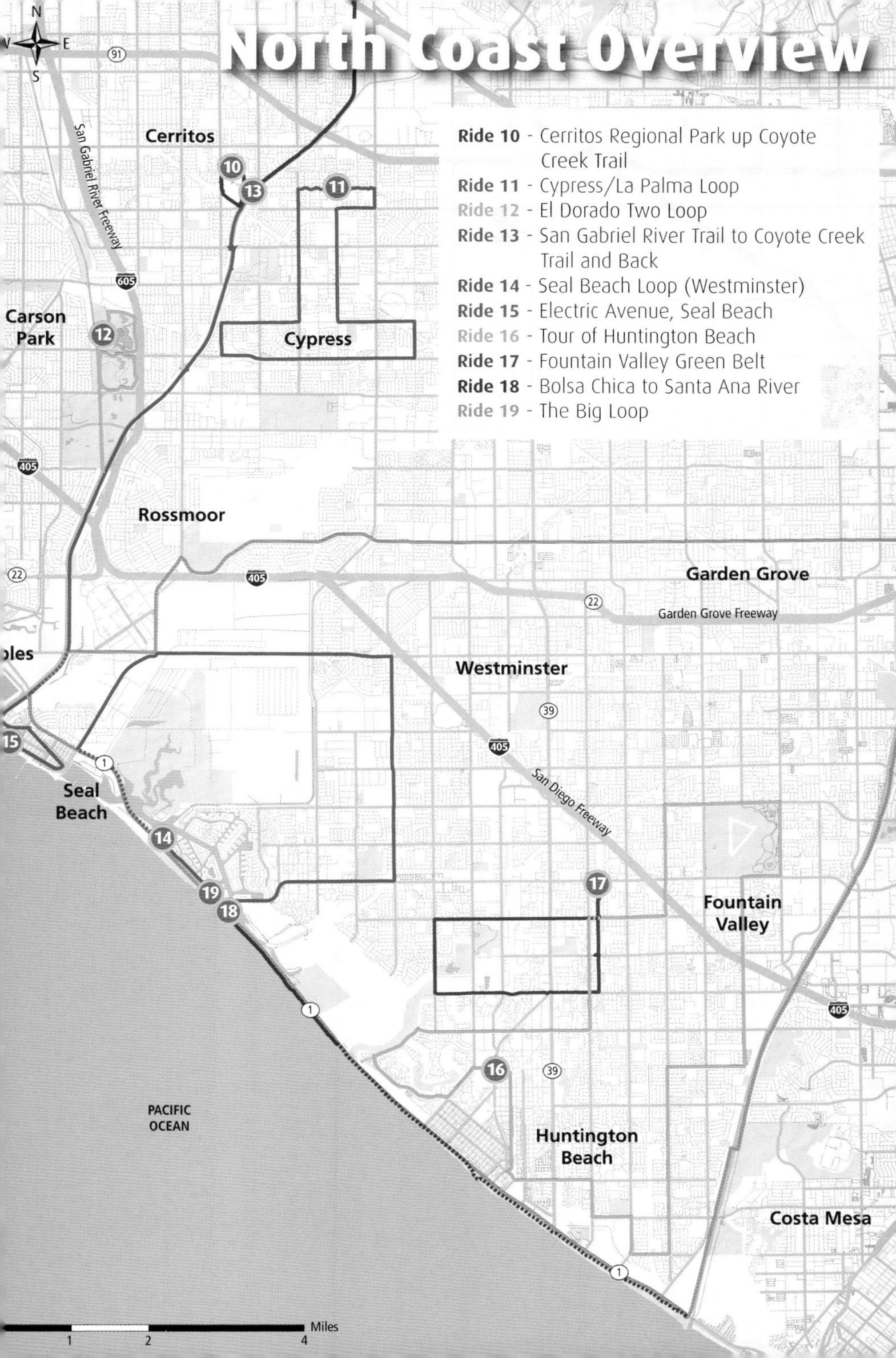
North Coast Overview
Ride 10 - Cerritos Regional Park up Coyote Creek Trail
Ride 11 - Cypress/La Palma Loop
Ride 12 - El Dorado Two Loop
Ride 13 - San Gabriel River Trail to Coyote Creek Trail and Back
Ride 14 - Seal Beach Loop (Westminster)
Ride 15 - Electric Avenue, Seal Beach
Ride 16 - Tour of Huntington Beach
Ride 17 - Fountain Valley Green Belt
Ride 18 - Bolsa Chica to Santa Ana River
Ride 19 - The Big Loop
Cerritos
San Gabriel River Freeway
Carson Park
Cypress
Rossmoor
Garden Grove
Garden Grove Freeway
Westminster
San Diego Freeway
Seal Beach
Fountain Valley
PACIFIC OCEAN
Huntington Beach
Costa Mesa
Miles
1
2
4

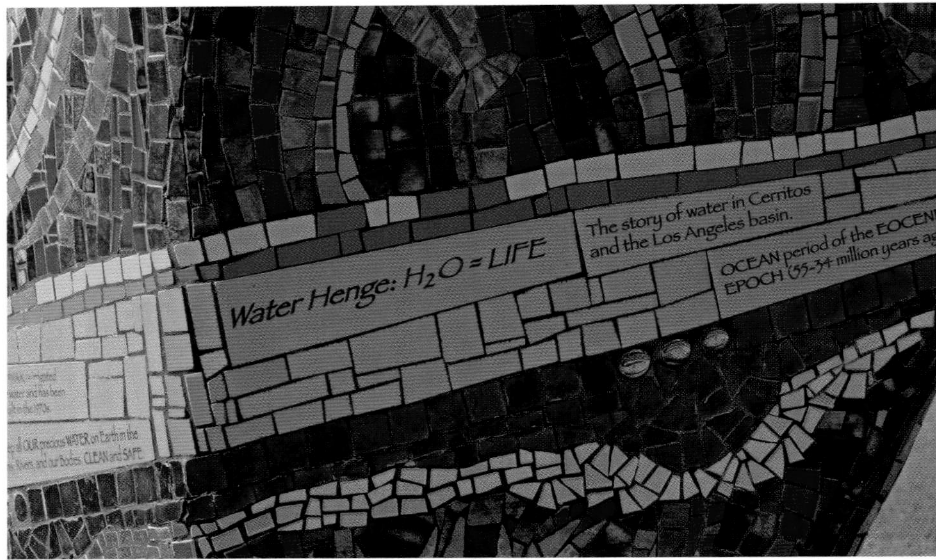

Water Henge. A public art sculpture that can teach you something as well.

At a Glance

Distance 11.29 miles **Elevation Gain** 240′

Terrain

Flat, smooth bike path for almost the entire route.

Traffic

Except for the beginning and end in the park, there are no cars at all and very little cyclist traffic as well.

How to Get There

By bus, OCTA route 30 or 38, to Cerritos on Wheels (COW) route 1 or 2. Get off at Cerritos Regional Park.

By car, take the 91 Freeway west, exit south onto Bloomfield Avenue. Travel one mile and turn left on 195th Street. Park in the first lot on your right.

Food and Drink

Along this route there is no food or drink available.

Side Trip

Cerritos Regional Park, the start and finish for this rid is an excellent place to spend a good part of the da Along the ride, if you are into bargain shopping ar haggling, the Santa Fe Springs Swap Meet is locate right off the bike path at Alondra Avenue.

Links to  

11 13

Where to Bike Rating 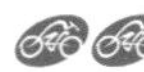

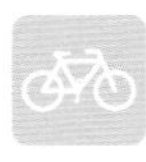    

About...

This ride starts at Cerritos Regional Park which connects to Coyote Creek Trail. One of the many Southern California waterways turned into a flood control channel, traveling along the trail allows completely uninterrupted riding and no car traffic to contend with. Although connected to Ride 13, this route does not suffer quite the same blistering winds as along the lower San Gabriel River. The ride finishes with a cool down loop around the park.

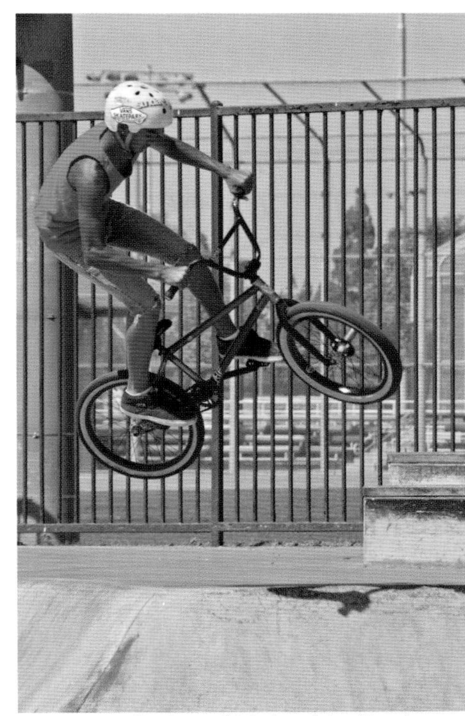

Don't even think about doing this unless your insurance is all paid up.

errritos Regional Park is a much used and beloved .rk and if you arrive in the morning on any given day ›u will find hundreds of walkers and joggers on the .rk's paths. Cerritos Regional Park is the anchor for is ride as well as Ride 13. Packed into 54 acres, it has all; an incredibly beautiful setting, tennis courts, bas-·tball courts, soccer fields, and baseball fields. Play-ounds, a skate park, a swimming pool and an outdoor ness center. There are three man-made lakes stocked ith fish and plenty of picnic tables and barbecues for army of people. And of course bike paths run all ·ross the park.

Also in the park is Water Henge, an interesting civic t project designed to tell the story of water in Cerritos ıd the Los Angeles Basin. Installed in an open green ›ace of the park, five pieces with stone-like shapes e arranged in a circular pattern, reminiscent of Stone-enge. On each "rock" are colorful blue mosaics with ords and information about how water once flowed ere and the role it now plays. The largest piece, 13 et high, also marks the spring and fall equinox.

While the park can be quite busy, Coyote Creek rail is underutilized, especially the northern section at comprises this ride. With spectacularly smooth surfaces and an uninterrupted riding experience, it's always a surprise to see so few people traveling this route. Enjoy it while you can; it's not likely to remain a secret for much longer.

For you bargain hunters, the Santa Fe Springs swap meet runs year round Tuesday through Sunday. Located at the Alondra exit, 3.62 miles from the start, this former drive-in theater is now permanently a swap meet. The cost to enter is $2 on the weekends when they have live performances with free admission the rest of the week. Beer and food are served and if you think "county fair" you'll have an idea of the menu. Popcorn, cotton candy, burgers and hot dogs. I always have a soft spot in my heart for a good churro. As far as shopping goes, kitschy is the order of the day: electronics, bags, shoes, drink coasters, parasols, tools and similar such products at truly bargain prices. Someone needs to get in there and sell some fun bike products!

Ride Log

0.0 Start on 195th St bike path beside first parking lot.

0.59 Turn right and head up slight incline to enter Coyote Creek Trail.

0.60 Watch for bicycle traffic in both directions. Turn left.

1.17 Continue straight under Carmenita Rd.

1.39 Continue straight under South St.

1.87 Continue straight under Marquardt Ave.

2.60 Continue straight under Artesia Blvd.

3.5 Continue straight under Firestone Blvd.

3.62 Continue straight under Alondra Blvd. Exit here to visit the Santa Fe Springs swap meet.

4.8 Continue under Rosecrans Ave.

5.36 End of path, turn around.

5.79 Straight under Rosecrans Ave.

7.09 Straight under Alondra Blvd.

7.20 Straight under Firestone Blvd.

7.99 Straight under Artesia Blvd.

8.73 Straight under Marquardt Ave.

9.21 Straight under South St.

9.41 Straight under Carmenita Rd.

10.1 Exit path, bear left onto path that runs parallel to Coyote Creek.

10.3 Cross road connecting parking lots and ride into Cerritos Regional Park, next to tennis courts.

10.4 At skateboard park turn left.

10.6 Bear right.

10.9 Bear right onto serpentine path.

11.1 Park entrance, watch for traffic as you cross.

11.2 Bear right.

11.29 End.

- P1 Santa Fe Springs swap meet
- P2 Skate Park in Cerritos Regional Park
- P3 Cerritos Center for the Performing Arts, 12700 Center Court Dr
- P4 Heritage Park, 18600 Bloomfield Ave
- P5 Cerritos City Hall, 18125 Bloomfield Ave
- P6 La Palma City Hall
- P7 San Gabriel River Trail
- P8 Norwalk Golf Course

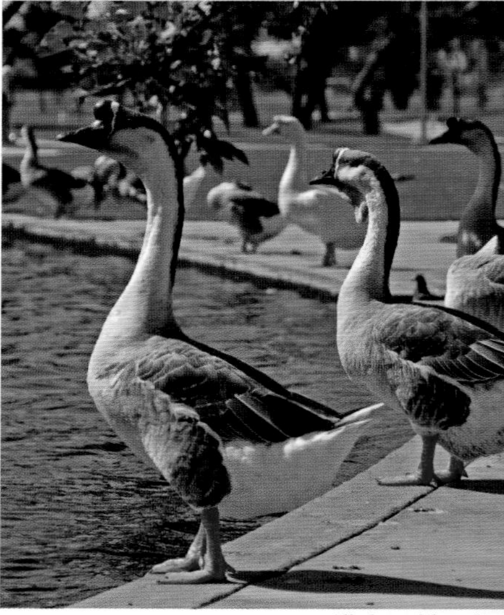

All cleared for takeo

Cerritos Regional Park up Coyote Creek Trail

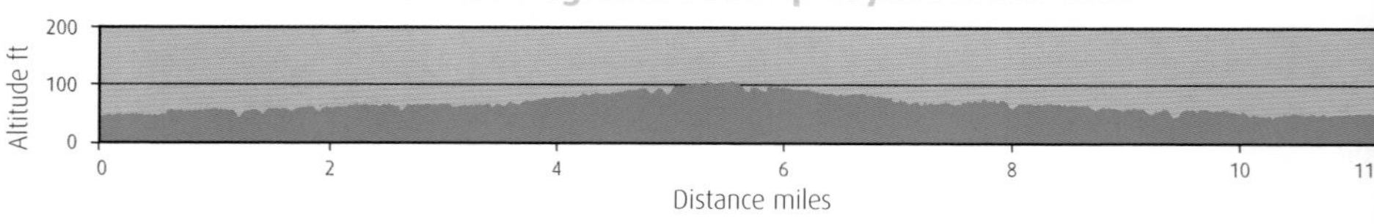

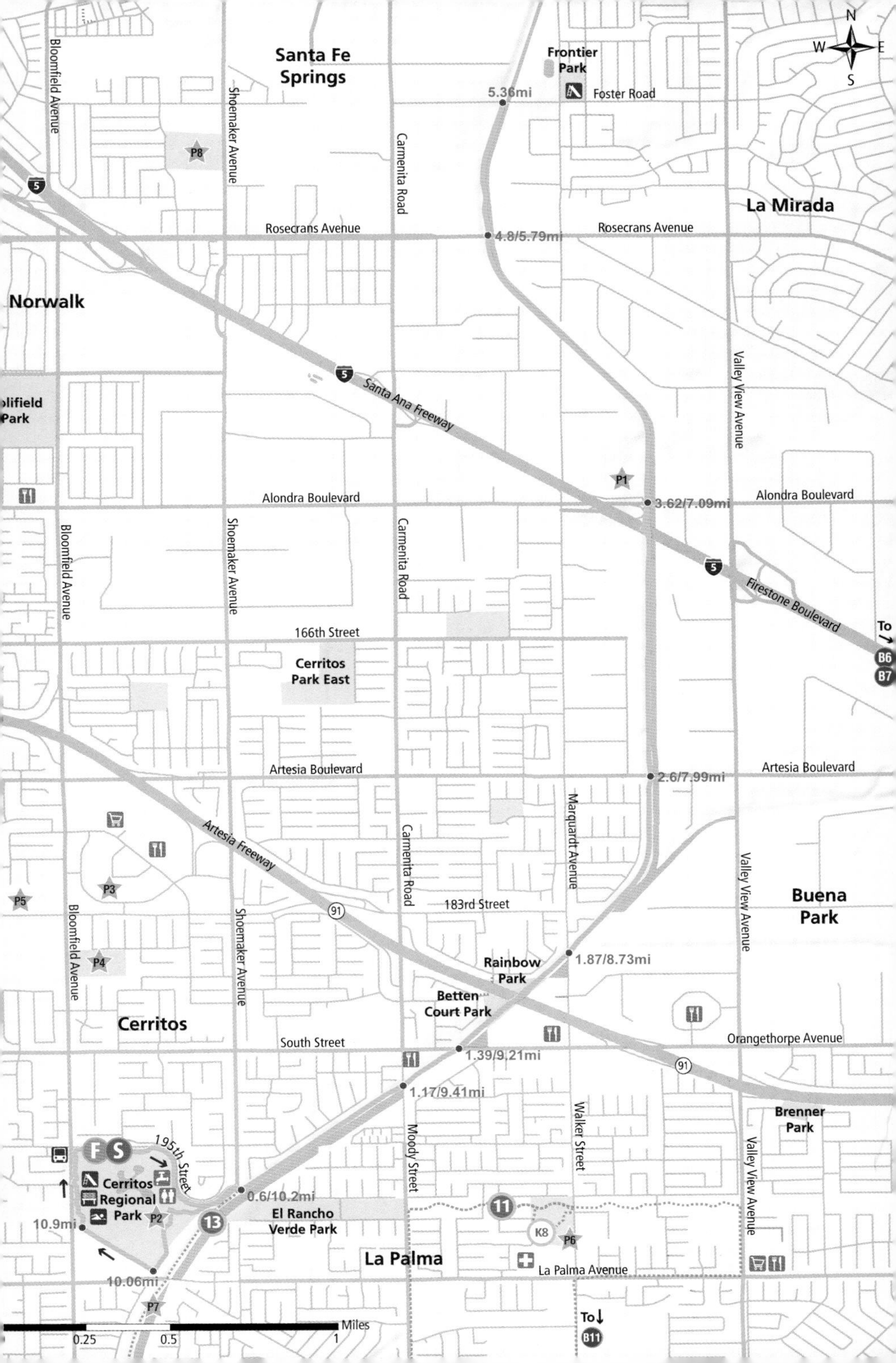

Santa Fe Springs
Frontier Park
Foster Road
5.36mi
La Mirada
Norwalk
Bloomfield Avenue
Shoemaker Avenue
Carmenita Road
P8
Rosecrans Avenue
4.8/5.79mi
Rosecrans Avenue
Santa Ana Freeway
Valley View Avenue
P1
Alondra Boulevard
3.62/7.09mi
Alondra Boulevard
Firestone Boulevard
To
B6
B7
166th Street
Cerritos Park East
Artesia Boulevard
2.6/7.99mi
Artesia Boulevard
Artesia Freeway
Marquardt Avenue
183rd Street
Buena Park
P3
P5
P4
Rainbow Park
1.87/8.73mi
Betten Court Park
Cerritos
South Street
1.39/9.21mi
Orangethorpe Avenue
1.17/9.41mi
Brenner Park
Moody Street
Walker Street
195th Street
Cerritos Regional Park
P2
10.9mi
0.6/10.2mi
El Rancho Verde Park
K8
P6
La Palma
La Palma Avenue
10.06mi
P7
Miles
0.25
0.5
1
To
B11

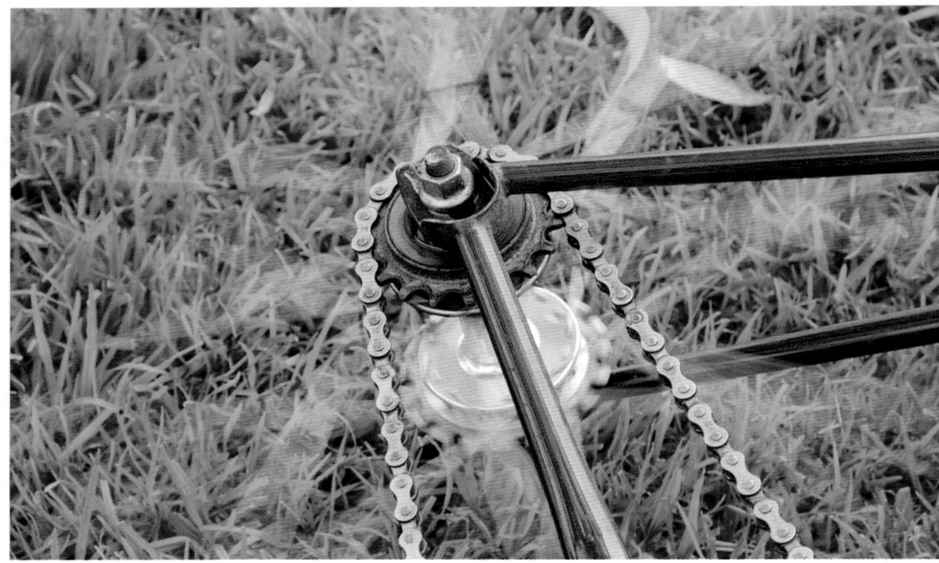
The greatest invention ever?

At a Glance

Distance 10.6 miles **Elevation Gain** 59′

Terrain

Although this ride begins and ends on a smooth, cement bike path, most of the ride travels across city streets.

Traffic

Moderate car traffic.

How to Get There

By bus, OCTA routes 21, 38, 42, 46 intersect with this route, however there is no bus that connects to the ride's beginning.

By car, take the 91 Freeway to the Orangethorpe exit, westbound. Turn left on Walker Street and drive half a mile before turning left in Central Park parking lot.

Food and Drink

In La Palma you will find plenty of Asian restaurant especially Korean and Mongolian barbecue. In Cy press, the fare is more mainstream American with lo of larger chain restaurants.

Side Trip

Cypress College Swap Meet takes place on weekend year round and is a fun place to shop for collectible plants and entertain the kids with bounce houses. Ve erans Park is a great place for a picnic and has a ska park for the kids.

Links to   

Where to Bike Rating 

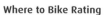

About...

Originally dairy land, both the cities of La Palma and Cypress grew into quiet suburbs in the shadow of the larger metropolitan centers of Los Angeles and Long Beach. Neither city has a hill or any significant incline unless you count a couple of bridges and both have been proactive in maintaining and developing bicycle paths as part of their overall transit plans. These two facts make this area a real pleasure to ride through. Paths are plentiful and well-marked and I found motorists to be courteous and polite at crossings and in general.

his ride begins on El Rancho Verde bike path near a Palma's Central Park, site of Kid's Ride 8. Almost very thoroughfare in these two cities has a bike lane nd they are used most often as commuter routes. This eans that bike lanes, and roads, will be busiest during eekday rush hours. If you ride through on the week-nd you are likely to have a very peaceful ride, full of olitude.

As you travel along Orange Avenue, Cypress Col-ge rolls into view. From here you are looking at the ack side of the campus with lots of green space and running track, all open to the public. The campus uildings have a futuristic look with lots of concrete nd glass as well as a campanile that sits at the cam-us center. Near the main entrance off of Valley View treet, the swap meet takes place on Saturdays and undays year round. You'll find collectibles, food and n activities for the kids here.

At 6.31 miles is Veteran's Park, an excellent loca-on to make a detour and enjoy a snack in the park. here is also a skate park located here. Nearby is the ypress Nature Park which is home to hummingbirds, estrels, a fox, opossums and a variety of trees and in-ects. Originally a flood control basin, the park is open

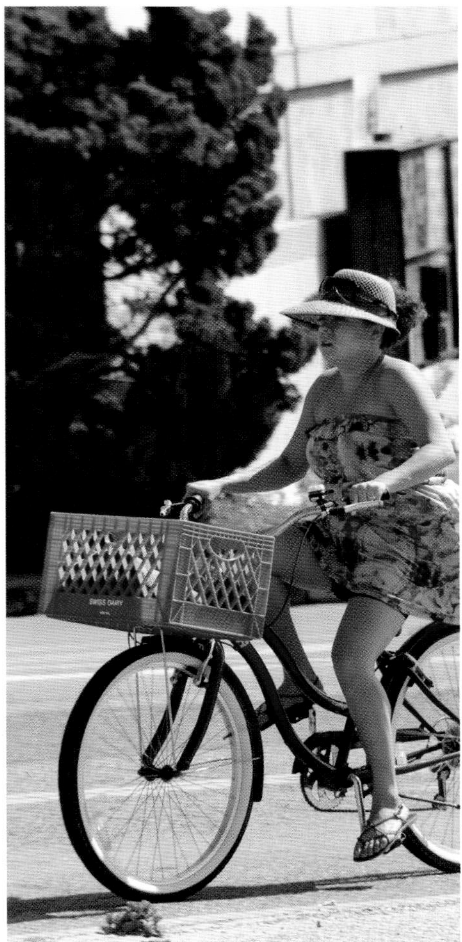

Hat, dress and bike all match. Now that's accessorizing!

primarily during summer months.

On La Palma Avenue, near the intersection with Moody Street, is Jangmo Jip a Korean restaurant that serves a sullungtang (soup of oxtail broth, noodles and chives) that has achieved legendary status. It is just around the corner from the ride's finish and is a perfect meal after a long spin, especially on a cold day. On the other hand, if you are looking to undo all that good work you did for your body by pedaling your bike all those miles, Johnnie's Jr. Burger is just the place to do it. Try the breakfast burrito, you can't go wrong.

Ride Log

P1 La Palma City Hall, 7822 Walker St
P2 San Gabriel River Trail
P3 Coyote Creek Bikeway
P4 Los Alamitos Army Airbase
P5 Cypress Swap Meet (Saturdays and Sundays)

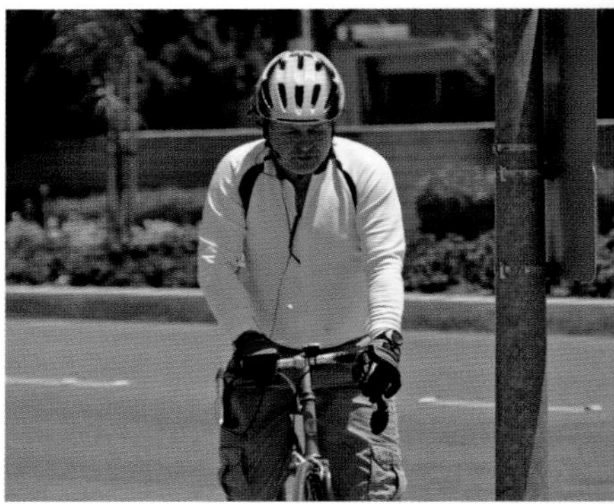

The mobile office. It's the wave of the futu

0.0 Cross Walker St to other side of El Rancho Verde bike path.

0.26 Cross residential street, Furman Rd.

0.53 Path ends at Valley View St, turn right.

0.79 Turn right onto La Palma Ave.

1.29 Turn left on Walker St.

1.81 Cross Crescent Ave.

2.3 Cross Lincoln Ave.

2.82 Turn left onto Orange Ave.

2.95 Cypress community center and park on your right.

3.3 Cross Valley View St.

3.5 Cypress College on your left.

3.8 Turn right onto Holder St.

4.34 Turn right on Ball Rd.

4.79 Cross Valley View St.

5.29 Cross Walker St.

5.8 Cross Moody St.

6.31 Cross Denni St. Veteran's Park is located here and is a pretty spot to take a break.

6.48 Cypress Nature Park located on your right.

6.80 Turn right on Bloomfield Ave.

7.24 Turn right onto Orange Ave.

8.25 Turn left onto Moody St.

8.77 Cross Lincoln Ave.

9.26 Cross Crescent St.

9.77 Cross La Palma Ave.

10.0 Turn right onto bike path through El Rancho Verde.

10.3 Cross residential road Laurelwood Ln.

10.6 End before crossing Walker St.

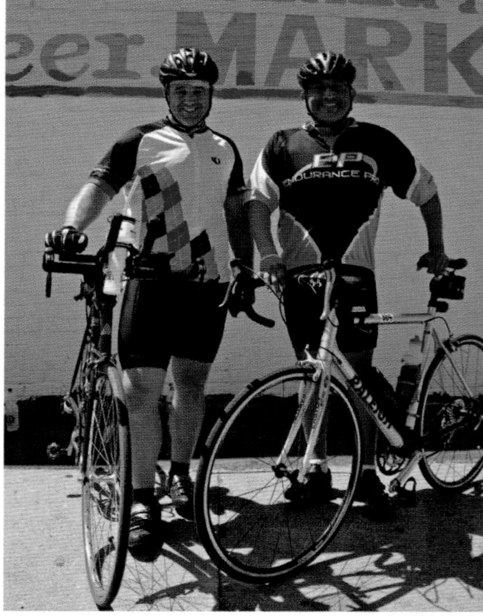

Riding buddies taking a break at the halfway mar

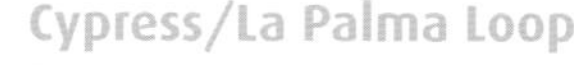

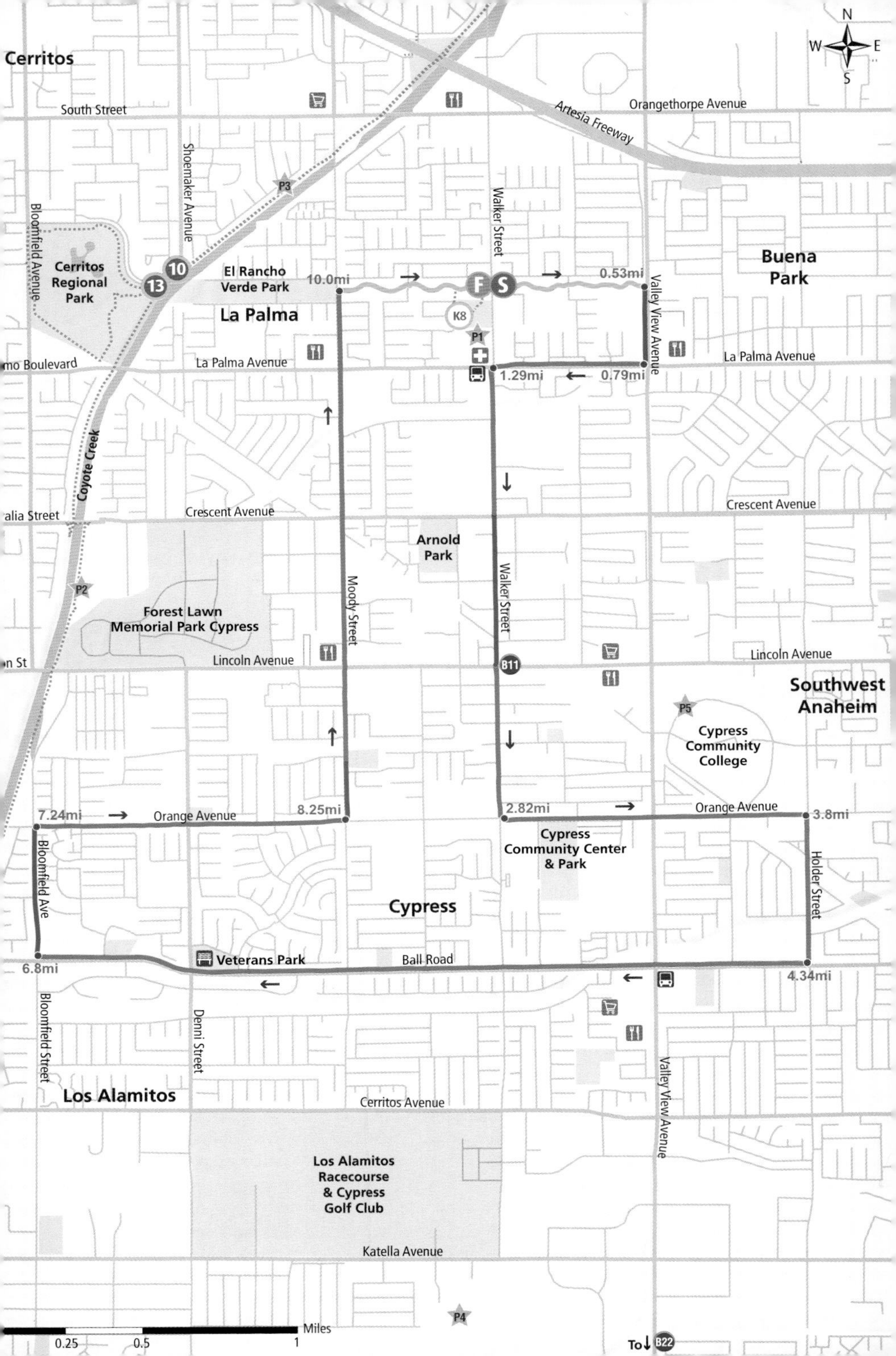

N
W
E
S
Cerritos
South Street
Orangethorpe Avenue
Artesia Freeway
Shoemaker Avenue
Bloomfield Avenue
Cerritos Regional Park
13
10
P3
El Rancho Verde Park
10.0mi
F
S
0.53mi
Walker Street
Valley View Avenue
Buena Park
La Palma
K8
P1
mo Boulevard
La Palma Avenue
La Palma Avenue
1.29mi
0.79mi
Coyote Creek
alia Street
Crescent Avenue
Crescent Avenue
Arnold Park
P2
Forest Lawn Memorial Park Cypress
Moody Street
Walker Street
n St
Lincoln Avenue
Lincoln Avenue
B11
Southwest Anaheim
P5
Cypress Community College
7.24mi
Orange Avenue
8.25mi
2.82mi
Orange Avenue
3.8mi
Cypress Community Center & Park
Bloomfield Ave
Holder Street
Cypress
6.8mi
Veterans Park
Ball Road
4.34mi
Bloomfield Street
Denni Street
Valley View Avenue
Los Alamitos
Cerritos Avenue
Los Alamitos Racecourse & Cypress Golf Club
Katella Avenue
P4
Miles
0.25
0.5
1
To
B22

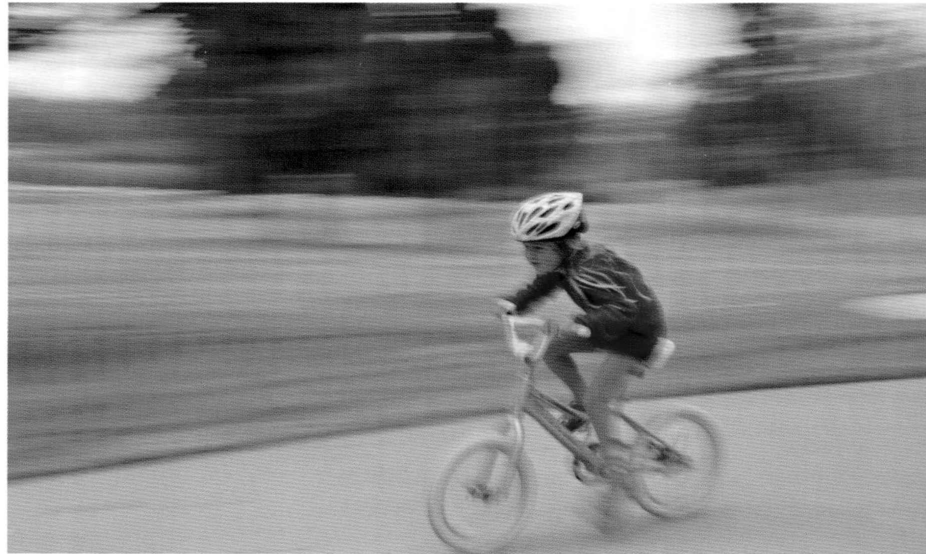

She's blazing fast!

At a Glance

Distance 7.66 miles **Elevation Gain** 91′

Terrain

Flat. Mainly bike paths through green grass park.

Traffic

Very little traffic.

How to Get There

By bus, the Long Beach Transit Bus #173 stops on Studebaker Street near Spring Street at the park's edge. From there ride east on Spring to the park entrance.

By car, take Interstate 605, exit west on Spring Street, the park entrance is on the right. When you enter the park you will be in Area 2. Follow signs to Area 3, where you will find the Golden Groves parking lot, adjacent to the ride start, on your immediate left after passing under the bridge.

Food and Drink

Although there are plenty of drinking fountains throughout the park, food is virtually nonexistent. Yo best bet is to pack a lunch or take advantage of many barbeques found throughout the park.

Side Trips

This is a giant park with many fun activities. In Are and 3 there are lakes stocked with fish and paddle bo for rent. In Area 3, keep an eye out for the El Dora Express, a miniature steam train. In Area 1 there is excellent Nature Center with nature trails and a lea ing center. There is also the Proportional Planet Tr right on the bikepath in Area 2.

Links to  

Where to Bike Rating 

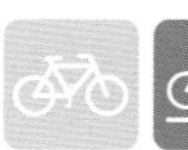  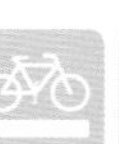  

About...

El Dorado Regional Park is a huge green space on the edge of Orange County, 815 acres in total. Two stocked lakes, a nature center, archery range, steam engine train, playgrounds, picnic shelters and lots of paved bike paths make this an ideal place to load up the bikes and spend a day picnicking in the park.

must confess to a soft spot in my heart for this park s I grew up close enough to ride here often as a child nd it is now a favorite destination for my kids. There re over four miles of bike routes within the park and is connected to the nearby San Gabriel River Trail, llowing for miles and miles of riding car-free. Bird atchers will be pleased to find an amazing array of pecies, including Blue Herons, Snowy White Egrets, wallows, Golden Eagles a number of different hum-ingbirds, and Red Tail Hawks.

The park is divided into three areas which are sepa-ated by city streets. If you have gone under a bridge, ou have traveled into a new area. Area 2 is the largest and includes the main entrance, an archery range (used by the 1984 Olympics), two stocked lakes, playgrounds and plenty of parking. Along the bike path at mile 3.73, the section that runs parallel to the San Gabriel River, you will find the Proportional Planet Trail complete with information markers that explain the planets' orbits, distance from the sun and each other. On the ground near each marker look for painted planets to indicate when you have reached the next planet.

Area 3 is probably the quietest, least used area and is the location of Kids' Ride 9. Tucked in the south-east corner of Area 3 is Caboose Corner where the El Dorado Express operates Saturdays and Sundays year round. Kids ride for $2, adults and infants are free. For $8 per half hour you can travel across the lake on pad-dle boats. The playground in Golden Grove (the one nearest the tunnel to Area 2) is the newest and 'funnest' in the park. Nearby is a large area with picnic tables and barbeque pits.

Area 1 is the smallest of the three but boasts the Nature Center, complete with naturally wooded areas, meadows and a running brook that feeds the small lake. The learning center, located at the front, is full of information on local flora and fauna as well as hands-on exhibits. There are two main hikes through the park. On the longer hike there is a pine/redwood grove that is a stopover for Monarch Butterflies on their long migra-tion. This is a great park to visit throughout the year as plants and animals that are present change seasonally.

North Coast

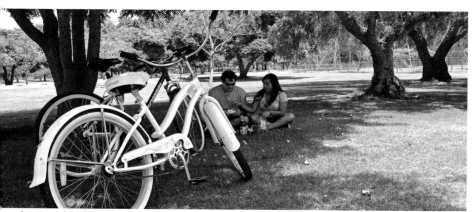

couple enjoys a bike date and lunch in the park.

Ride Log

0.0 Begin ride on bike path next to parking lot in Golden Grove, Area 3.

0.26 Continue straight past joining path from left.

0.38 Fork in the road, bear right.

0.61 Class 1 bikeway ends. Turn left onto roadway which is a one way loop.

0.9 On your right is the miniature train ride, great for the kids.

1.72 Fork in the road, bear left. The Long Beach Police Academy is in front of you and the roadway becomes a two lane road with traffic in both directions.

1.96 Follow bike route signs and cross road back on to bike path.

2.13 Completion of the first loop, you should be back where you started. Here you are going to take the path to the right.

2.15 Intersection with the road, traffic both directions. Ride straight across to where the path continues.

2.25 Intersection with another bike path. Continue straight, but watch to your right where sometimes cyclists coming down the San Gabriel River Trail are moving quite fast. Head under bridge.

2.36 On the other side of the bridge there is an intersection with another path and the road. Cars have a stop sign. Take a hard left here. Watch again for speeding cyclists coming at you from the San Gabriel.

2.57 Stop sign. Cross road to continue on path.

2.71 Bumpy bridge, careful.

3.45 Crossing road that leads to the park entrance/exit. This is definitely the busiest intersection in the park, be careful.

3.71 Intersection with road. Cross to continue.

3.73 Proportional Planet Walk begins here. Sign on left with an explanation.

4.21 Completion of second loop. If you wish to stay inside the park, continue straight on path heading under bridge. Official ride continues by making a hairpin left turn and heading up slight incline onto San Gabriel. Beware of high speed cycling traffic.

4.69 Bear left heading slightly downhill. Path does continue straight but dead ends.

4.83 Bear right. Turning left here would take you to the Nature Center for a side trip.

5.84 End of the San Gabriel section of ride. Turn around and head back up river. Cross bridge to join Ride 13.

6.82 Heading towards bridge, slightly downhill. Beware blind corner as you bear left.

6.96 Stay left, on River Trail.

7.41 Heading downhill, another blind corner. Stay on path under bridge.

7.54 Bear right off of River Trail and onto bike path.

7.64 Intersection with road. Travel straight across.

7.66 End.

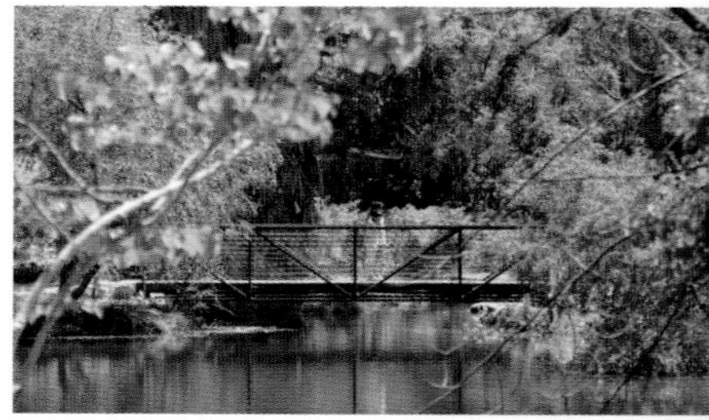

Lots of lakes at El Dorado Park

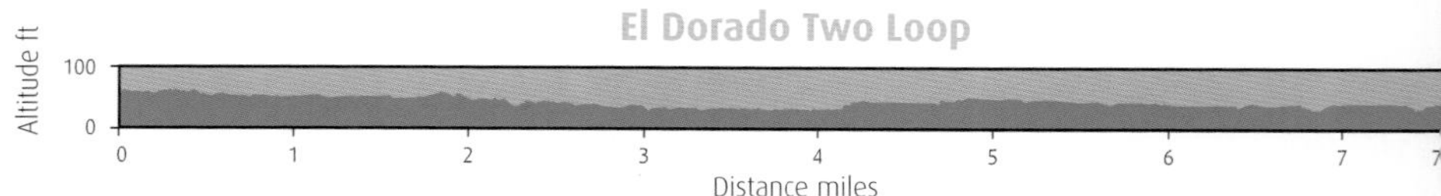

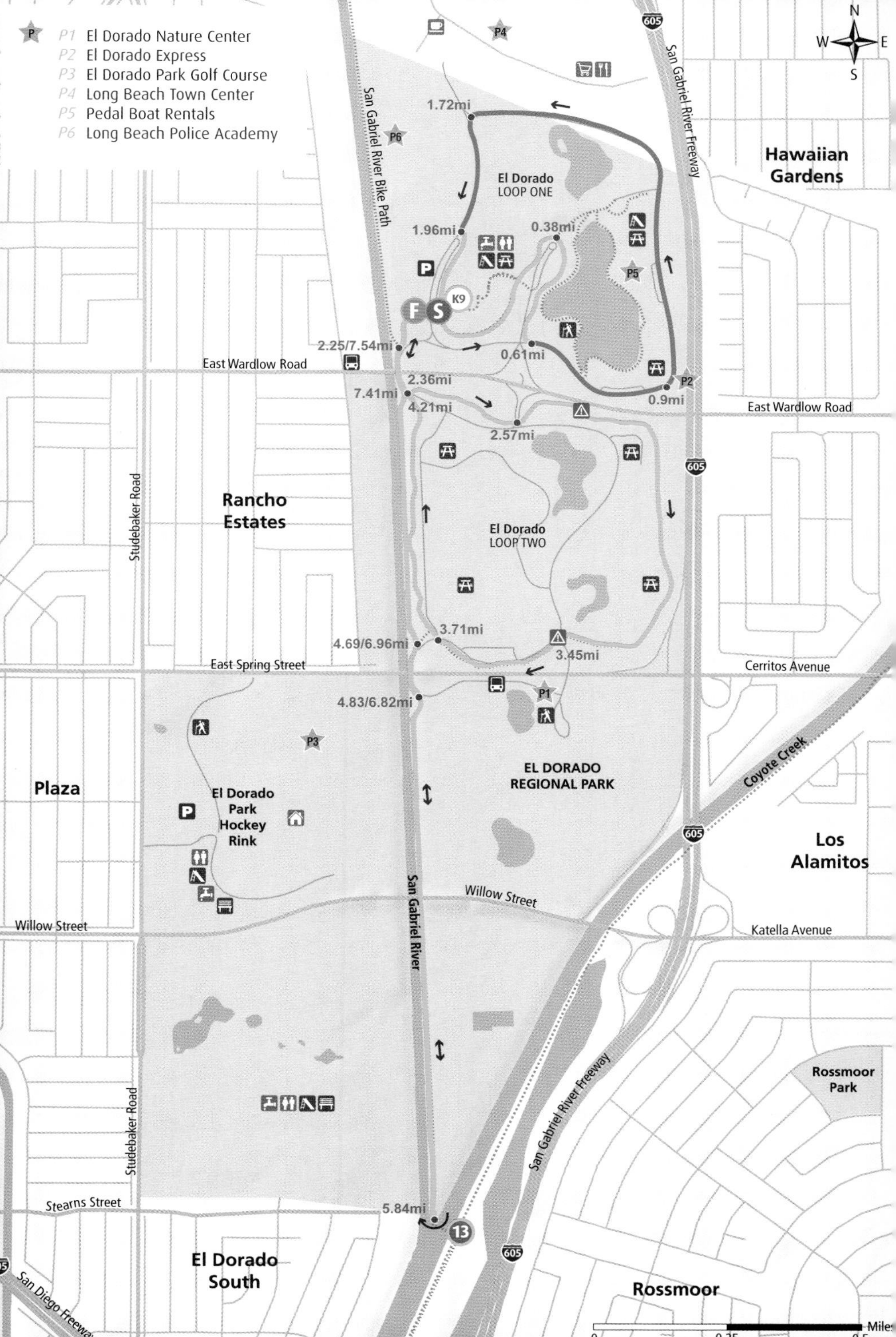

P1 El Dorado Nature Center
P2 El Dorado Express
P3 El Dorado Park Golf Course
P4 Long Beach Town Center
P5 Pedal Boat Rentals
P6 Long Beach Police Academy
N
W
E
S
San Gabriel River Bike Path
San Gabriel River Freeway
Hawaiian Gardens
El Dorado LOOP ONE
1.72mi
1.96mi
0.38mi
0.61mi
0.9mi
2.25/7.54mi
K9
East Wardlow Road
2.36mi
7.41mi
4.21mi
2.57mi
East Wardlow Road
Rancho Estates
Studebaker Road
El Dorado LOOP TWO
3.71mi
4.69/6.96mi
3.45mi
East Spring Street
Cerritos Avenue
4.83/6.82mi
Coyote Creek
EL DORADO REGIONAL PARK
Plaza
El Dorado Park Hockey Rink
Los Alamitos
San Gabriel River
Willow Street
Willow Street
Katella Avenue
Rossmoor Park
Studebaker Road
San Gabriel River Freeway
Stearns Street
5.84mi
13
El Dorado South
Rossmoor
San Diego Freeway
605
0
0.25
0.5

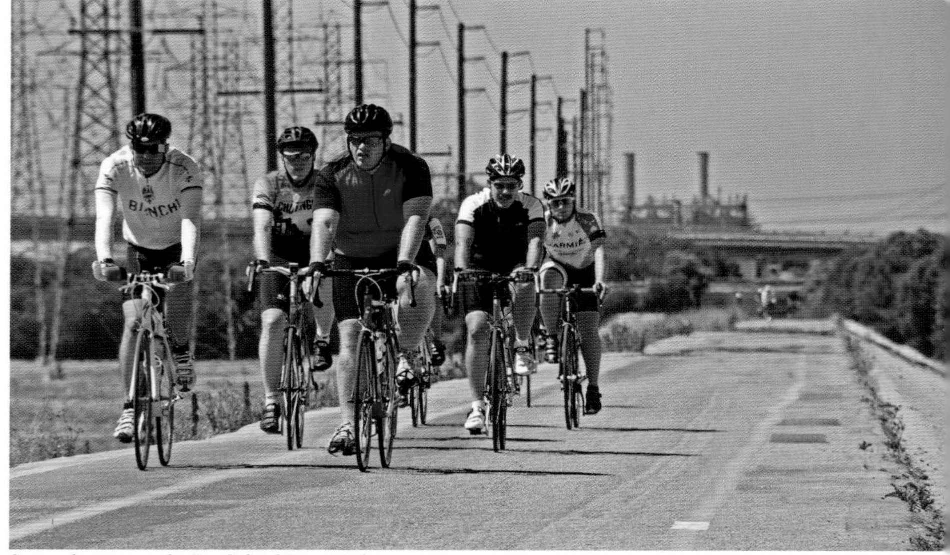

Serious business on the San Gabriel River Trail.

At a Glance

Distance 17.3 miles **Elevation Gain** 244′

Terrain

Mostly well maintained bike path with one potholed, cracked stretch.

Traffic

This is a nearly car-free route, with only a single street to cross. However, it is heavily traveled by cyclists on weekends.

How to Get There

By bus, OCTA route 30 or 38, to Cerritos on Wheels (COW) route 1 or 2. Get off at Cerritos Regional Park.

By car, take the 91 Freeway west, exit south onto Bloomfield Avenue. Travel one mile and turn left on 195th Street. Follow along Cerritos Regional Park to the last set of parking lots beside the tennis courts, turn right into lot and park.

Food and Drink

The River's End Café at the turnaround point is an excellent place to stop and rest your wind-seared body. Enjoy Mexican influenced breakfast and lunch dishe with a view of the beach and the river's end.

Side Trip

At the ride's start is Cerritos Regional Park, 83 acre of athletic fields, basketball courts, a fishing lake an numerous playgrounds. At the other end is quaint Sea Beach with a sleepy main street waiting to be explored

Links to 10 11 12 14 15 19

Where to Bike Rating 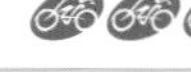

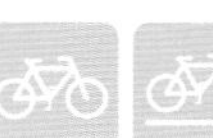 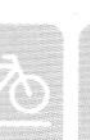 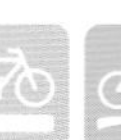 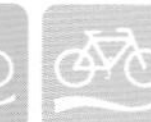

About...

long this route you'll see countless cyclists, power plant, seabirds, water, the beach and naybe even a sea turtle, but the most notable eature of this ride is the wind. Through some nexplicable set of odd circumstances, the wind oming off the ocean gets funneled through this ide with an unbelievable fierceness. Even on ays with no wind anywhere else, there will e wind on this ride. For this reason, I start the ide inland, battle against the wind and earn a pectacular push on the return.

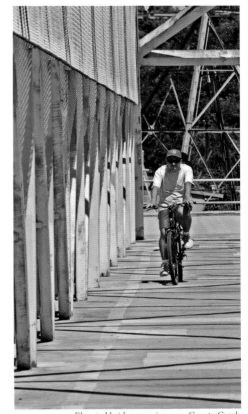

Elevated bridge crossing over Coyote Creek.

is excellent ride travels along two flood control annels, otherwise known as rivers. The ride starts Cerritos Regional Park and heads downriver along yote Creek Bikeway, a well maintained and lightly veled path. At 4.7 miles Coyote Creek joins the ger San Gabriel River and the two channels are con-cted by a pedestrian bridge. Be alert here as there n be quite a bit of traffic crossing over, or into, your e. Once you have joined the San Gabriel River Trail pect an increase in cycling traffic, as well as the oc-sional jogger, especially on weekends.

Just south of the bridge the concrete channel ends d is replaced with a soft bottom, lending the river a ore natural look. The bike path along this stretch is t at its best and you are sure to encounter potholes d cracks. Be alert. Even more challengingly, for the xt few miles your battle with the wind will be at its ost fierce. Searing, unrelenting, unforgiving. Here where you imagine the sand between your toes, the nch you're going to have or the dessert you are earn-g. But best of all, remember how much fun, and fast, e ride back is going to be.

Through this section you may also expect to see os-eys, herons and egrets hunting and fishing. As you approach the massive electric power plants, keep an eye out for Green Sea Turtles swimming upriver, attracted by the warm water discharged from the plant. Some of these creatures can weigh up to 500 pounds.

When you reach the sea take a much deserved rest. The River's End Café is located here and serves up Mexican inspired dishes. The best seats are on the patio and if you can get seated in the raised section you will be treated to a view of the ocean and Seal Beach Pier in one direction and in the other, Alamitos Bay and the Long Beach skyline.

A note about the wind. It is always present, but when Santa Ana wind conditions prevail, consider starting at Seal Beach to Cerritos and back as the wind blows just as hard, if not harder, out to sea.

North Coast

Ride Log

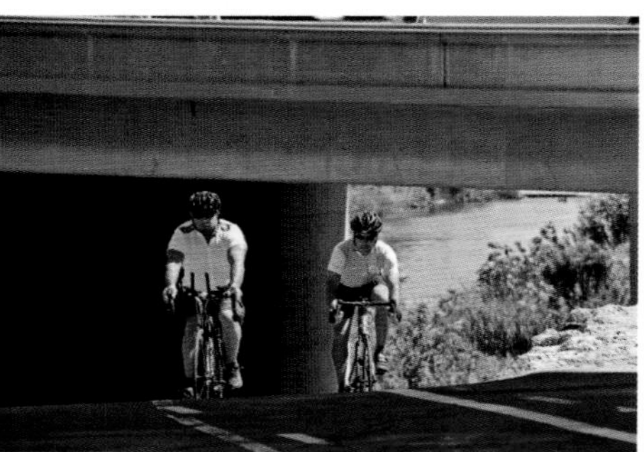
Putting in the miles.

P1 Alamitos Bay Landing
P2 Los Alamitos Race Track
P3 Heartwell Park
P4 Anaheim Bay
P5 Leisure World
P6 Seal Beach Pier

0.0 Begin ride on bike path near tennis courts, under the power line tower.

0.12 Up small rise, through gates onto Coyote Creek Bikeway, turn right. Watch for bicycle traffic in both directions.

0.52 Stay on path under Del Amo Blvd.

1.01 Stay on path, under Centralia St. On opposite side of bridge you will double back to cross to other side of the river.

1.18 Turn right, cross bridge.

1.26 Turn right, rejoin path.

1.56 Cross pedestrian bridge, bear right.

1.71 Stay on path under Lincoln St.

2.79 Stay on path under Ball Rd.

3.05 Pedestrian bridge, cross over then bear right.

3.08 Stay on path under Los Alamitos Blvd.

4.01 Stay on path under Katella Ave.

4.7 This is where Coyote Creek joins the San Gabr River.

6.05 Stay on path under Seventh St.

7.0 Stay on path under Westminster Blvd.

7.8 Stay on path under Pacific Coast Hwy.

8.01 Cross Marina St, watch for cars.

8.34 End of San Gabriel River Trail, turn around.

8.61 Cross Marina St, watch for cars.

9.11 Stay on path under Pacific Coast Hwy.

9.82 Stay on path under Westminster Blvd.

10.9 Stay on path under Seventh St.

12.5 You are now back on the Coyote Creek Bikew

13.1 Stay on path under Katella Ave.

14.1 Stay on path under Los Alamitos Blvd.

14.2 Pedestrian bridge, cross and bear right.

14.4 Stay on path under Ball Rd.

15.4 Stay on path under Lincoln St.

15.7 Pedestrian bridge, cross and bear right.

16.0 Stay on path under Centralia St and on other si of bridge double back.

16.1 Turn right, cross bridge to other side of river.

16.2 Turn right back onto bikeway.

16.7 Stay on path under Del Amo Blvd.

17.2 Exit Coyote Creek Bikeway through the gate a turn left.

17.3 End.

San Gabriel River Trail to Coyote Creek Trail and Back

Altitude ft: 0, 100
Distance miles: 0, 3, 6, 9, 12, 15, 1

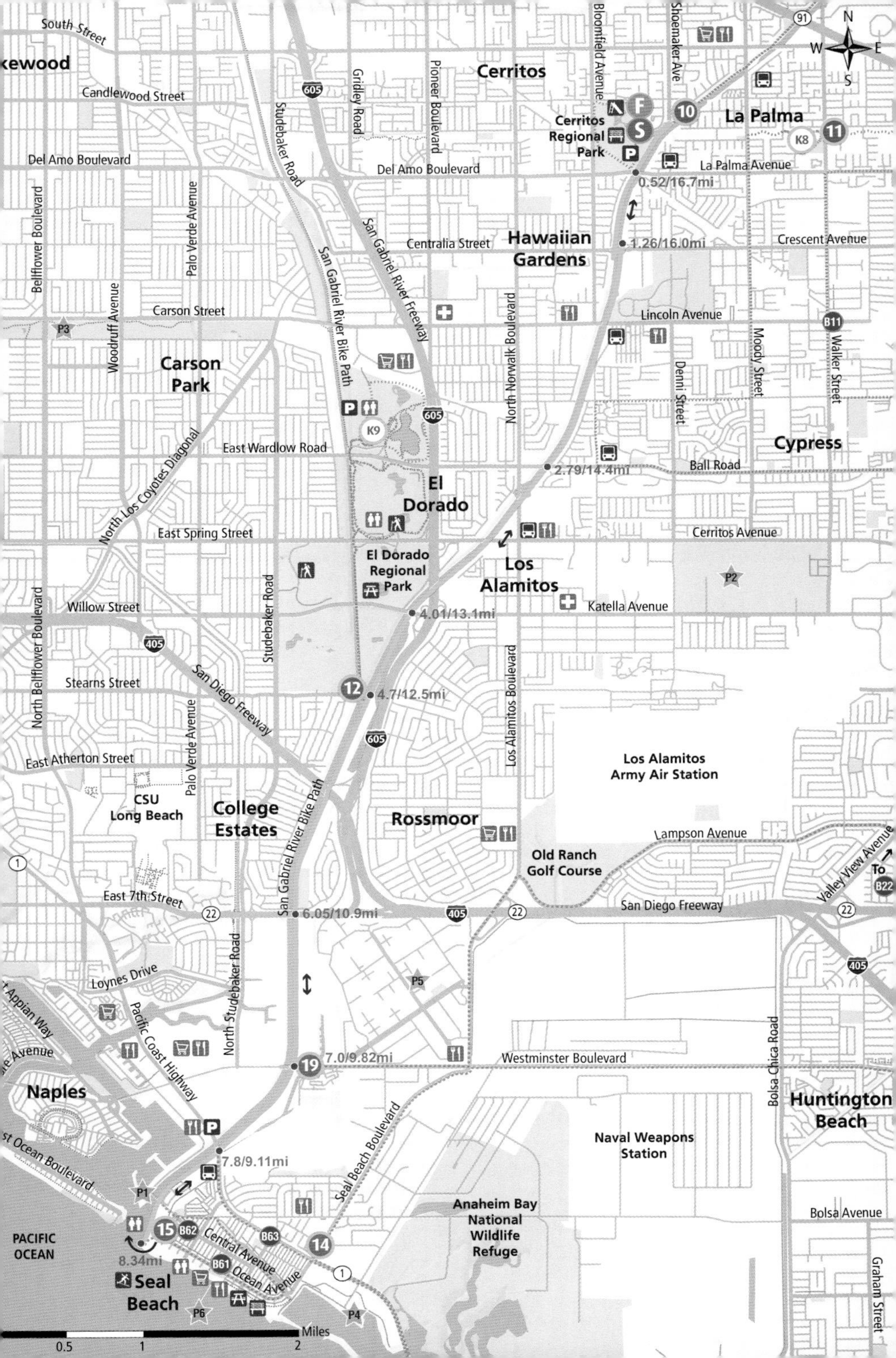

South Street
kewood
Candlewood Street
Cerritos
Cerritos Regional Park
La Palma
Del Amo Boulevard
La Palma Avenue
0.52/16.7mi
Studebaker Road
Gridley Road
Pioneer Boulevard
Bloomfield Avenue
Shoemaker Ave
Bellflower Boulevard
Palo Verde Avenue
San Gabriel River Freeway
San Gabriel River Bike Path
Centralia Street
Hawaiian Gardens
1.26/16.0mi
Crescent Avenue
Carson Street
Lincoln Avenue
Woodruff Avenue
Carson Park
North Norwalk Boulevard
Denni Street
Moody Street
Walker Street
Cypress
East Wardlow Road
Ball Road
2.79/14.4mi
North Los Coyotes Diagonal
El Dorado
East Spring Street
Cerritos Avenue
El Dorado Regional Park
Los Alamitos
Willow Street
Katella Avenue
4.01/13.1mi
North Bellflower Boulevard
Stearns Street
San Diego Freeway
4.7/12.5mi
Los Alamitos Boulevard
East Atherton Street
Los Alamitos Army Air Station
CSU Long Beach
College Estates
Rossmoor
Lampson Avenue
Old Ranch Golf Course
Valley View Avenue
To
East 7th Street
6.05/10.9mi
San Diego Freeway
Loynes Drive
North Studebaker Road
Appian Way
Pacific Coast Highway
Westminster Boulevard
7.0/9.82mi
Naples
Seal Beach Boulevard
Bolsa Chica Road
Huntington Beach
Naval Weapons Station
Ocean Boulevard
7.8/9.11mi
Anaheim Bay National Wildlife Refuge
Bolsa Avenue
PACIFIC OCEAN
8.34mi
Central Avenue
Ocean Avenue
Seal Beach
Graham Street
0.5
1
2
Miles

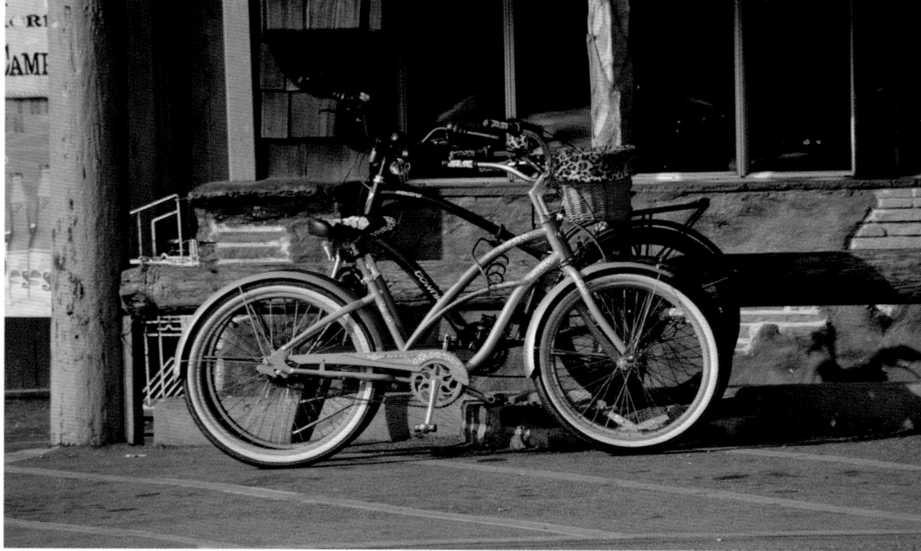

50 points for style. Don't you just love the faux leopard lining in the basket?

At a Glance

Distance 13.0 miles **Elevation Gain** 132′

Terrain

Mostly flat, well maintained city streets. Almost the entire route travels along on-road bike paths.

Traffic

Although the route does travel along streets, most of the roads are wide and easily accommodate cyclists and motorists. Pacific Coast Highway is a busy stretch with plenty of traffic so remain especially alert through here.

How to Get There

By bus, OCTA routes 1, 21, 25, 42, 60 and 72 all intersect with this route. Route 1 is the closest to the ride's start/finish.

By car, take Pacific Coast Highway towards Sunset Beach. Find parking along Pacific Coast Highway between Warner Avenue and 25th Street, or consider parking in nearby Bolsa Chica State Beach.

Food and Drink

There are a ton of wonderful places to explore in Sur Beach. Two of my favorites are Harbor House Café a Woody's Diner, both located just across from the ride's st Another good option, especially for breakfast, is Good D Café, located at 10.4 miles on Warner, which seems to c lect bicyclists on their way to or from the beach.

Side Trip

Consider renting a kayak or stand up paddle board a exploring the waterways and mansions of Hunting Harbor. Also nearby, at 11.8 miles, is the Bolsa Ch Wetlands Interpretive Center.

Links to 13 15 18 19

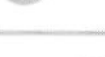

Where to Bike Rating

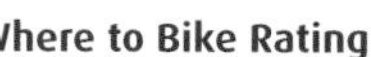

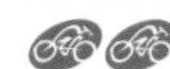

  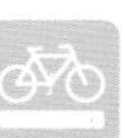  

About...

This ride begins and ends in picturesque Sunset Beach, famous for its giant beachfront homes and eclectic, independent streak. A popular bicycling route, don't be surprised if you get caught up in a peloton of Lycra and flashy bikes as the local cycle club zooms by. At times challenging, often panoramic, this ride is blissful.

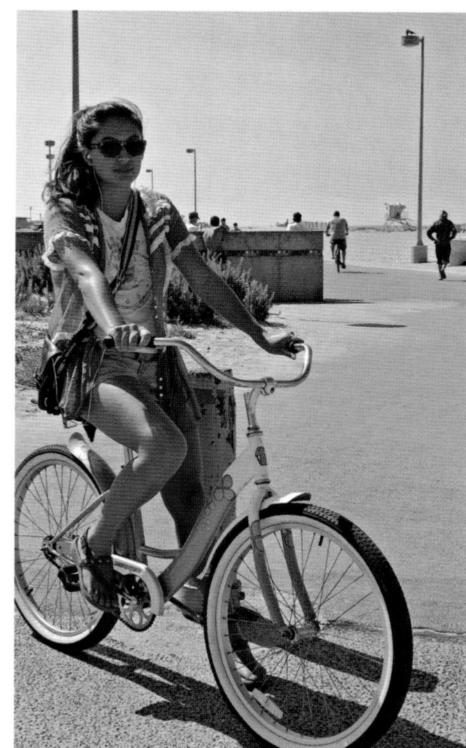

She's ready to cruise!

e ride starts in front of Out-Spoken bike shop, which rents bikes, and across the street from Woody's Diner along Pacific Coast Highway. This stretch along the highway is without a doubt the busiest section of the ride. You will leave Sunset Beach and enter Seal Beach by passing over a bridge that is just high enough to offer a spectacular, panoramic view that might make you interrupt your ride to appreciate the moment. To your left, across the bridge, the Pacific Ocean stretches out from the Huntington Harbor's opening. To your right is the Seal Beach Naval Weapons Station and the Anaheim Bay National Wildlife Refuge, a vast space of some 5000 acres of wetlands and roads bounded on the right by Huntington Harbor.

When the route turns onto Seal Beach Boulevard traffic decreases significantly and is very quiet except during morning rush hour as beach residents make their way to the 405 Freeway. A left turn onto Seal Beach Boulevard will take you to Electric Avenue and Ride 15. Along this section, at 2.43 miles, you will pass the Naval Weapons Station entrance and beside it the World War II Submarine Memorial.

Westminster Boulevard is oddly a perfectly straight two mile stretch that bisects the Weapons Station. To your left and right, open space seems to extend forever, an unusual experience for this part of Orange County. Expect blustery gusts of wind through this section as you travel through emptiness.

Near the route's end along Warner Avenue is the Bolsa Chica Wetlands Interpretive Center. Newly refurbished, the building houses aquariums, touch tanks and exhibits. Behind the building are trails to the wetlands. Nearby is also Bolsa Chica State Beach and routes 18 and 19.

At 12.3 miles along Pacific Coast Highway are locations where you can rent kayaks and stand up paddle boards. Behind the wall of one story buildings lining this stretch of highway are countless channels and waterways that make up Huntington Harbor. Spend a whole morning or afternoon exploring the harbor and its beautiful homes, boats and wildlife. Rentals start at $15/hour and include boats, paddles, lifejackets and basic instruction.

Ride Log

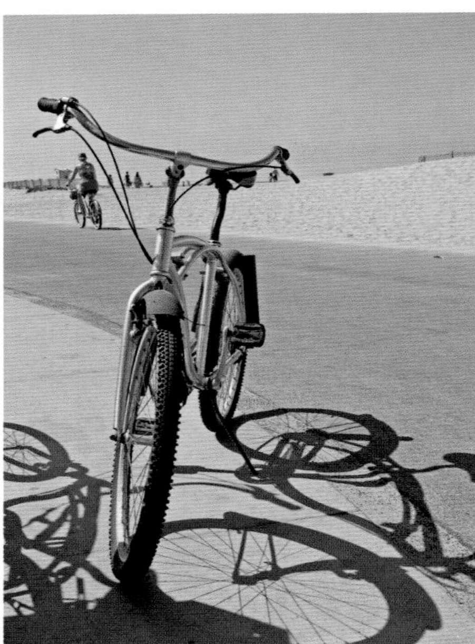

The perfect beach ride.

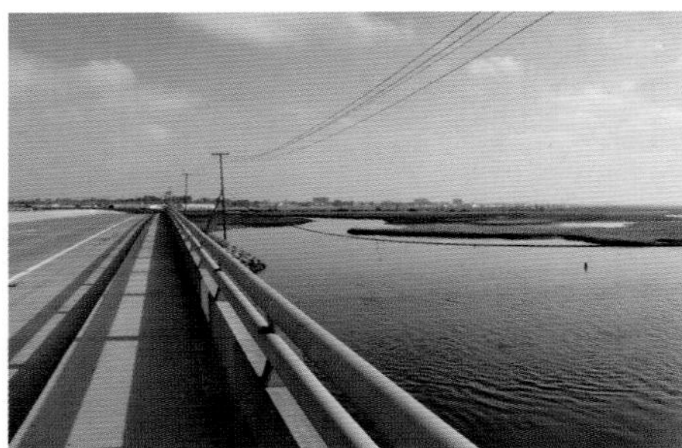

With such an amazing view, don't get distracted.

P1 Huntington Harbor Mall
P2 Bolsa Chica Conservancy
P3 Leisure World
P4 Seal Beach Pier
P5 Red Car Museum
P6 Paddle Board and Kayak Rentals

0.0 Start ride on Pacific Coast Hwy, in front of O Spoken bike shop.

0.5 Begin ascent over bridge.

1.7 Turn right on Seal Beach Blvd.

2.43 Pass entrance to Naval Weapons Station.

3.41 Turn right on Westminster Blvd.

5.42 Cross Bolsa Chica St. Avoid this street as it is safe for cyclists.

6.46 Turn right onto Springdale St.

7.45 Cross Bolsa Ave.

7.95 Cross McFadden Ave.

8.46 Cross Edinger Ave.

8.96 Cross Heil Ave. Carr Park located across street makes for a pleasant rest stop if needed.

9.45 Turn right onto Warner Ave.

9.94 Cross Graham St.

10.4 Cross Bolsa Chica St. Good Day Café loca here.

10.9 Cross Algonquin St.

11.8 On your left is the Bolsa Chica Wetlands Int pretive Center.

11.82 Turn right onto Pacific Coast Hwy. This i very busy intersection, exercise extreme caution.

12.1 Cross Fifth St.

12.3 Kayak rental location on your right.

12.4 Cross Broadway Ave.

12.7 Cross 19th St.

13.0 End.

Seal Beach Loop (Westminster)

Altitude ft: 0, 100
Distance miles: 0, 2, 4, 6, 8, 10, 12

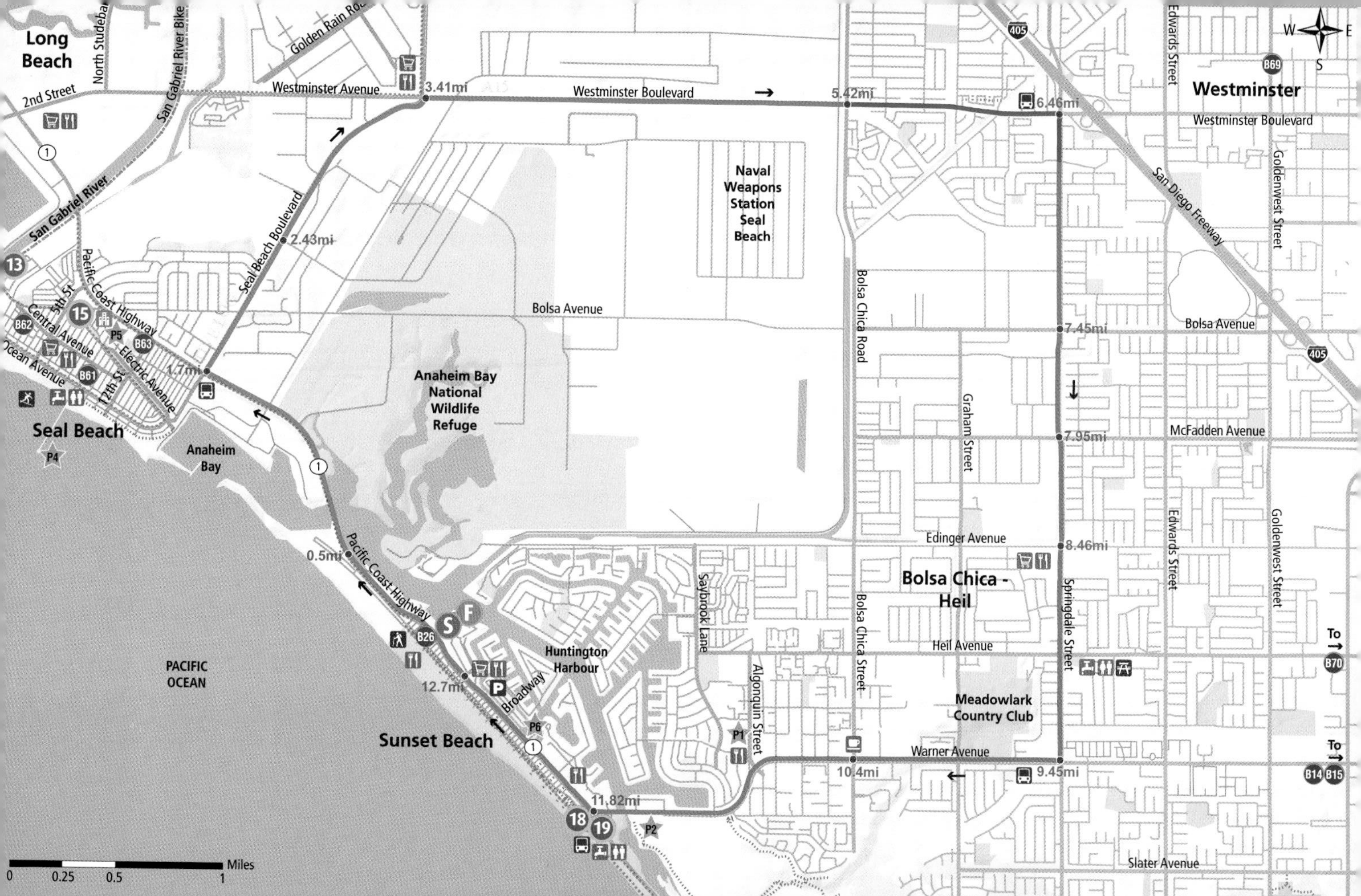

Long Beach
Westminster
Naval Weapons Station Seal Beach
Anaheim Bay National Wildlife Refuge
Bolsa Chica - Heil
Huntington Harbour
Meadowlark Country Club
Seal Beach
Sunset Beach
Anaheim Bay
PACIFIC OCEAN
2nd Street
North Studeba
San Gabriel River Bike
San Gabriel River
Golden Rain Ro
Westminster Avenue
Westminster Boulevard
San Diego Freeway
Goldenwest Street
Edwards Street
Seal Beach Boulevard
Bolsa Avenue
Bolsa Chica Road
Bolsa Chica Street
Graham Street
Springdale Street
McFadden Avenue
Edinger Avenue
Heil Avenue
Warner Avenue
Slater Avenue
Saybrook Lane
Algonquin Street
Pacific Coast Highway
Broadway
5th St
12th St
Central Avenue
Electric Avenue
Ocean Avenue
3.41mi
5.42mi
6.46mi
7.45mi
7.95mi
8.46mi
9.45mi
10.4mi
11.82mi
12.7mi
0.5mi
1.7mi
2.43mi
405
1
B69
B70
B14
B15
B26
B61
B62
B63
P1
P2
P4
P5
P6
13
15
18
19
S
F
P
To
W
E
S
Miles
0
0.25
0.5
1

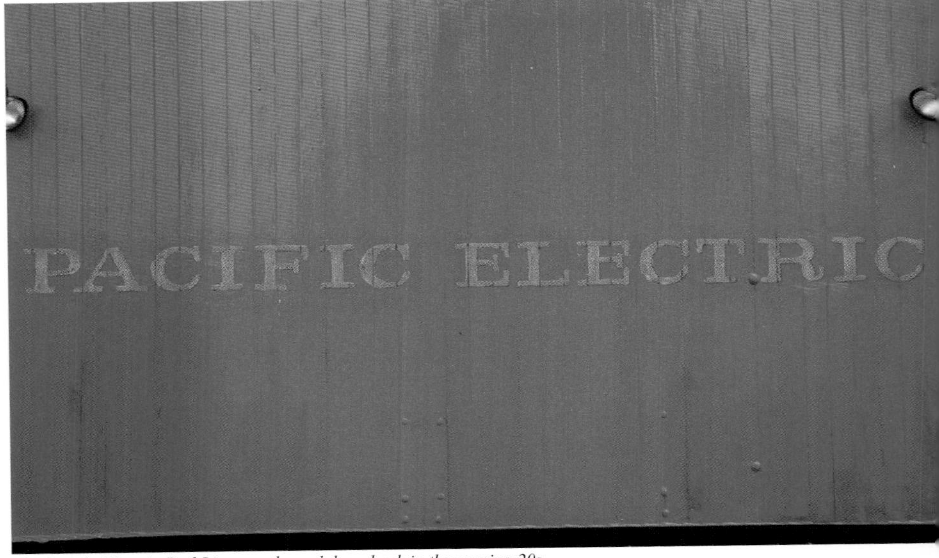

The Pacific Electric Rail Line ran through here back in the roaring 20s.

At a Glance

partially

Distance 2.49 miles **Elevation Gain** 43′

Terrain

Flat, well maintained paths and roads.

Traffic

Light residential traffic. The route has a number of stop signs and a single traffic light to navigate. During summer months do be aware of increased traffic from tourists and beachgoers.

How to Get There

By bus, OCTA Bus 42 and Long Beach Transit Bus 131 both stop on Electric Avenue, just past Main Street.

By car, take Pacific Coast Highway (Route 1) to First Street and follow First until it ends at the public parking lot.

Food and Drink

The River's End Café is at the start/finish of the lo It's Mexican inspired breakfast and lunch fare. Ma Street offers everything from coffee shops, to Th food, to pubs to barbeque. There is even a burger jo at the end of the pier.

Side Trips

There are no shortage of side trips, including the R Car Museum, a visit to the many shops on Main Stre the beach and a stroll on the Seal Beach Pier. Near pier, Bogart's Coffee House on Ocean is a bike frien meet up spot.

Links to 13 14 19

Where to Bike Rating 

  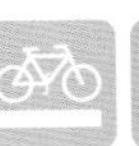 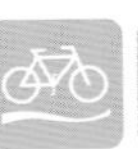 

About...

This ride begins at Westmont Park and travels through a series of connected parks that make up a giant greenbelt. This straight, mostly flat stretch is a favorite of joggers and dog walkers. From there you will ride on bike paths along city streets. There are a couple of modest climbs on this ride and one especially fun descent on Edwards Street. The ride finishes at Westmont Park, so bring a soccer ball or Frisbee and enjoy a restful, play day at the park.

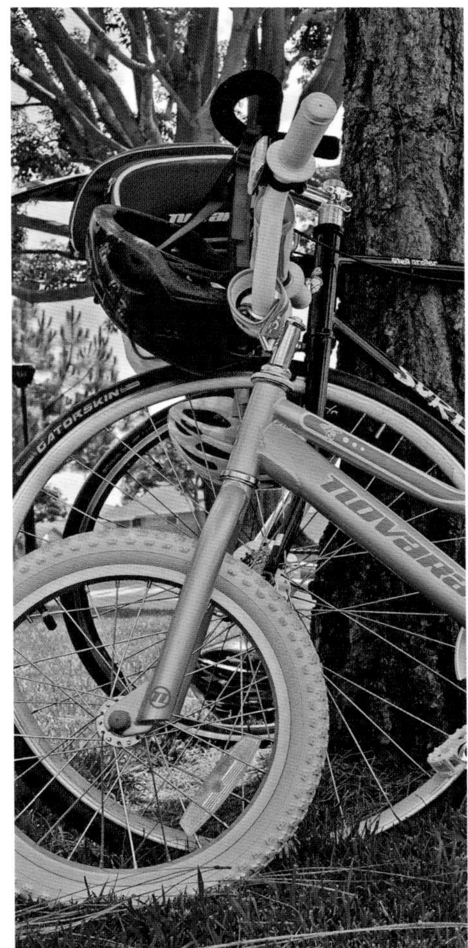

Bikes, like their owners, come in many sizes.

his stretch of land was originally part of a large arsh until the Santa Ana River was tamed and the ea drained. It then became farmland and by the early 00s the Courreges family, Basque farmers, had herds sheep grazing on this land. A park and street still ar the family's name and Courreges Ranch is listed an Orange County Historical Site. By the 1960s the operty around the ranch was changing as neighbor-od homes popped up creating a suburb of active milies. Only this long stretch remains as a reminder the green pastureland that used to exist here.

This route passes two entrances into Huntington each's Central Park. With 350 acres to explore, two kes, a disc golf course, an equestrian center, a sports mplex and the Central Library, this park could keep ou entertained all day. In the park, along Goldenwest reet, is the Park Bench Café, a quaint restaurant with utdoor tables arranged near the lake. The library sits op a hill overlooking the park and while libraries and ke rides don't usually go together, the view from in-de is worth a quick stop.

Near the start at Westmont Park is Casa Inka, a Pe-vian restaurant, great for lunch or dinner. Their sig-ature dish is lomosaltado, beef sautéed with onions, tomatoes and served with French fries and rice. Make sure you order some garlic bread, not at all like the Italian version. Their empanadas, small stuffed meat pies, are also good and they offer a number of fish dishes as well.

Although most of the ride is a well maintained path there are a few areas that are hard packed dirt. The section just after Talbert is also rather steep. For experienced riders this should pose no problem but for small children or the inexperienced it is recommended that you walk your bike.

Ride Log

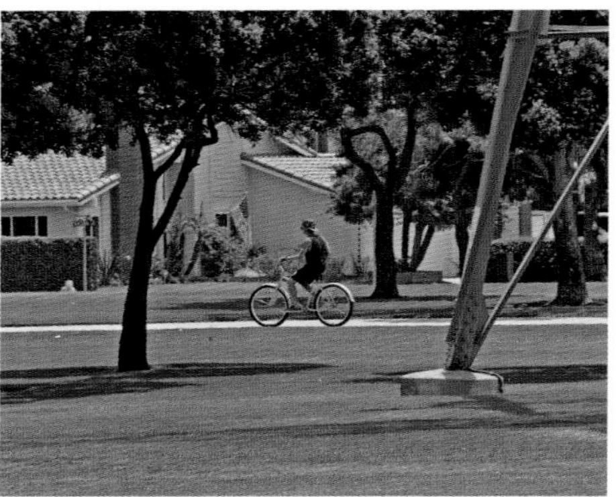

Sun, grass, bike, path. Ingredients for a perfect day in the park.

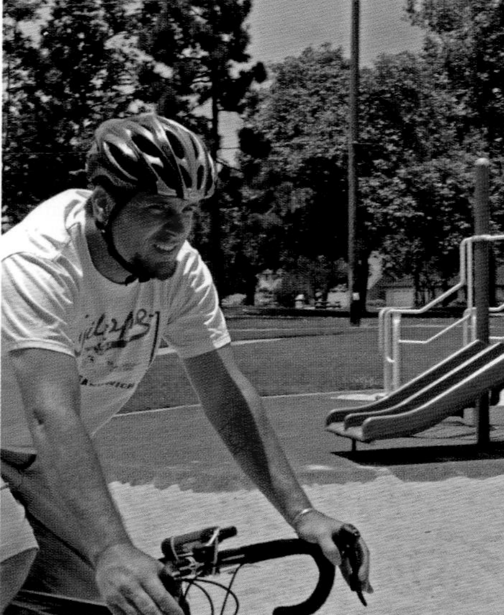

Is it time for the slides yet?

0.0 Start at the northern portion of the greenbelt Westmont Park near El Rancho Ave.

0.24 Cross residential street La Fiesta Ave.

0.43 Cross Slater Ave.

0.62 Cross El Lago Ave.

0.82 Path becomes a hard packed dirt road.

0.94 Path hits Talbert Ave, turn right.

0.98 Cross Talbert Ave and turn back towards pat Courreges historical ranch is here.

1.03 Turn right back onto bike path. This section is har packed dirt and there is a small downhill right here.

1.24 Cross Rogue River Ave.

1.53 Turn right onto Ellis Ave.

1.65 Cross Newland St.

2.14 Cross Beach Blvd. Do not travel along this roa as it is not safe for cyclists.

2.2 Ellis Ave bends across Main St here, then turn right.

2.79 Cross Gothard St.

3.16 Cross Goldenwest St.

3.66 Ellis ends, turn right on Edwards St.

3.75 Entrance to western edge of Central Park an wonderfully shady spot to take a break.

4.65 Turn right onto Slater Ave.

5.13 Cross Goldenwest St.

5.23 Another entrance into Central Park.

5.51 Cross Gothard St.

6.13 Cross Beach Blvd

6.65 Cross Newland Ave.

6.79 Turn left back onto the greenbelt trail.

6.99 Cross La Fiesta Ave.

7.24 End at El Rancho Ave.

Fountain Valley Green Belt

Altitude ft: 100, 0

0 1 2 3 4 5 6 7 7.

Distance miles

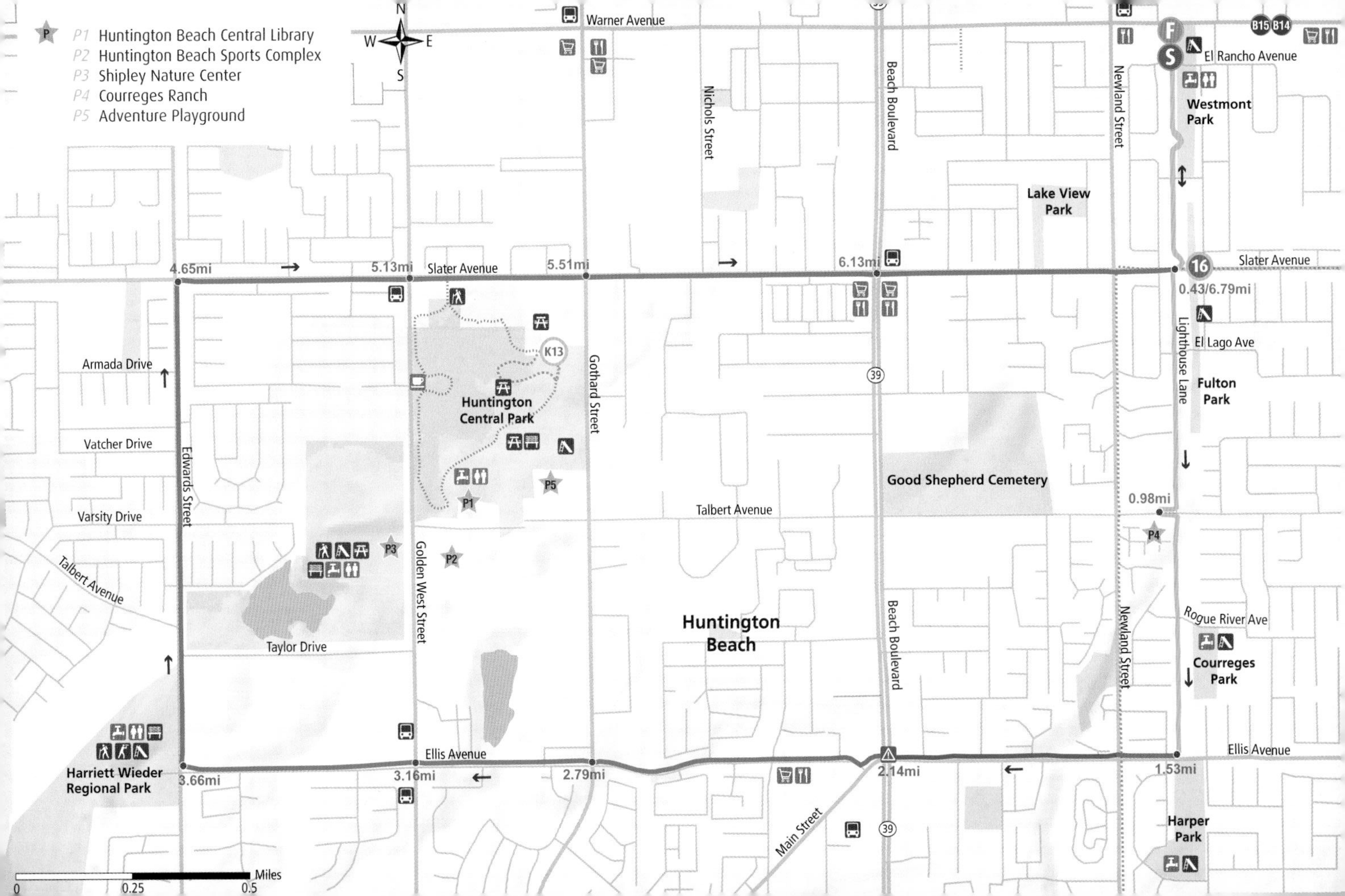
P1 Huntington Beach Central Library
P2 Huntington Beach Sports Complex
P3 Shipley Nature Center
P4 Courreges Ranch
P5 Adventure Playground
N
W
E
S
Warner Avenue
El Rancho Avenue
B15
B14
F
S
Westmont Park
Nichols Street
Beach Boulevard
Newland Street
Lake View Park
4.65mi
5.13mi
Slater Avenue
5.51mi
6.13mi
16
Slater Avenue
0.43/6.79mi
Lighthouse Lane
El Lago Ave
Fulton Park
K13
Armada Drive
Huntington Central Park
Gothard Street
39
Vatcher Drive
Edwards Street
Good Shepherd Cemetery
P5
P1
0.98mi
Varsity Drive
Talbert Avenue
P4
P3
P2
Golden West Street
Talbert Avenue
Huntington Beach
Newland Street
Rogue River Ave
Courreges Park
Beach Boulevard
Taylor Drive
Ellis Avenue
Ellis Avenue
Harriett Wieder Regional Park
3.66mi
3.16mi
2.79mi
2.14mi
1.53mi
Main Street
Harper Park
Miles
0
0.25
0.5

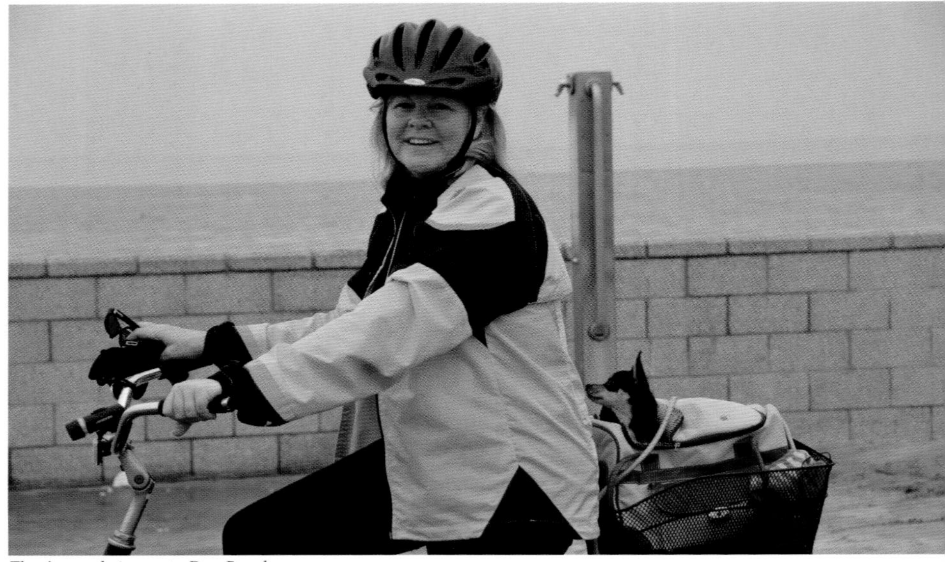

They're on their way to Dog Beach.

At a Glance

Distance 16.85 miles **Elevation Gain** 185′

Terrain

Car-free, paved bike path for the entire ride.

Traffic

None, other than pedestrian.

How to Get There

By bus, there are a number of buses that intersect this route. At its beginning are OCTA routes, 1, 21, 70 and 72. Along the way, there are buses: 25, 29, 33, 35, 170, 172.

By car, take Pacific Coast Highway (Route 1) to Bolsa Chica State Beach, cost to park all day is $10. Upon entering, turn right and drive to the last parking lot.

Food and Drink

Along the ride there are a number of concession stands serving fare you would expect to find at the beach. For a more palatable food selection, stop at the Huntingto Beach Pier at mile 5.25 and head over to Main Street.

Side Trip

Besides a dip in the ocean, there are two notable sid trips along this ride. The first is the Bolsa Chica Eco logical Reserve located across the street from the stat beach entrance. The second is Huntington Beach Mai Street and Pier.

Bikes for Rent

Zack's Pier Plaza, Huntington Pier

Dwight's Beach Concession, 200 yards south of pier.

Links to 14 16 19 31 40 41

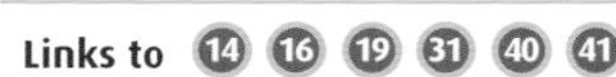

Where to Bike Rating

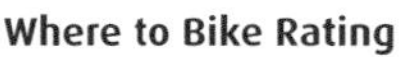

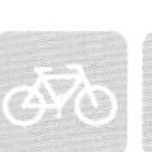

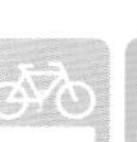

About...

This ride may be the ultimate SoCal recreational ride. Starting at the northern end of Bolsa Chica State Beach, you will travel the entire length on a paved, car-free bike path with a panoramic view of the Pacific Ocean as your constant companion. Consider a stop at Main Street Huntington Beach, aka Surf City. At its southern end you will reach the Santa Ana River Trail and Newport Beach before heading back along the same path to Bolsa Chica.

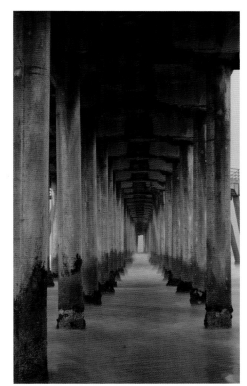

They seemingly go on forever.

'hile this ride is entirely car-free, it is not without ızards. Along with other cyclists, you are certain to ıcounter walkers, joggers, surfers, and beach goers. uring weekend summer months the path can be verrun with pedestrian traffic. If you are interested training or commuting through this part of Orange ounty, your fastest, safest bet is to ride along PCH Ride 19) which parallels this stretch.

Bolsa Chica State Beach has plenty of parking and xpansive beaches so bring a picnic and after the ride, vim and eat. The Ecological Reserve located across e beach entrance is a marvelous side trip. Saved from evelopment after a multi-decade battle, the reserve a combination of dunes and intertidal marsh that home to an amazing variety of wildlife and coastal ants. Over 300 of Orange County's 420 bird species ave been found here, as well schools of fish and matg stingrays.

When you reach the pier, the crush of swimsuit clad odies and the frenetic activity can be dizzying. You ay have to dismount here if you see flashing yellow ghts. A small green space beside the pier is home to acky sack and drum circles and above this, the Pier laza often hosts craft fairs and farmers' markets. Under the pier, lock up your bike and climb the steps to Main Street where surf culture reigns supreme. Over the last decade or so, a great deal of money has been poured into developing and expanding the avenue into a resort style area. There are still plenty of surf and bikini shops, but now you'll also find grand hotels, mega parking structures, and boutique shops. Summer night life here is something to behold. Two old standbys with great eats: the Sugar Shack (breakfast), and the Longboard Restaurant and Pub. Don't forget to take a stroll on the pier.

South of the pier the ride reaches the Santa Ana River and Newport Beach. Here you can catch Ride 31, the Santa Ana River Trail (SART... d back to Bolsa Chica. Keep in mind as you r... e wind picks up in the afternoon and prevai... north-west quarter.

Ride Log

0.0 Ride begins at the northern most parking lot of Bolsa Chica State Beach.
1.37 Main lifeguard headquarters and entrance. Cross PCH here to visit the Bolsa Chica Ecological Reserve.
2.46 Bear left to pass over bridge.
2.5 Leaving Bolsa Chica State Beach.
3.29 Dog Beach begins. Watch for slow, distracted pedestrian traffic and lots of dogs.
4.40 Reach Goldenwest St and path splits, high and low. Stay on the high path as the low is primarily for pedestrian traffic.
5.25 Huntington Pier and Main St. If there are flashing lights, dismount and walk through this section.
5.44 Huntington Beach lifeguard headquarters, trucks passing through, be alert.
6.33 Path bottlenecks, careful. At this point you ca pick up OCTA 35.
8.25 Stay left.
8.26 Bear right
8.40 Take right path to reach Ride 31 Santa Ana River Trai
8.42 Turn around.
9.50 Blind corner.
10.5 Path bottlenecks, be careful.
11.1 Zack's rents bikes.
11.6 Huntington Beach Pier, be prepared to dismour if necessary.
12.0 Path splits. Bear right, uphill.
14.3 Pass over the bridge, then bear left.
15.3 Entrance to Bolsa Chica State Beach.
16.85 End .

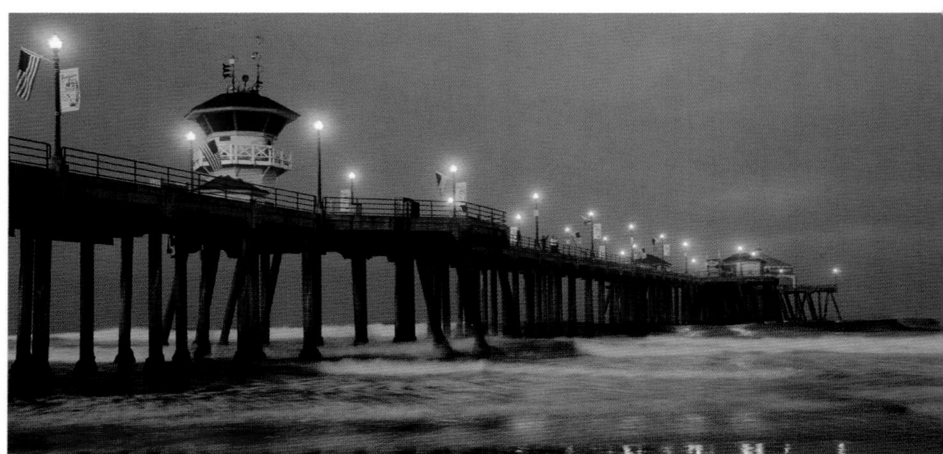

Sunrise at Huntington Beach Pier.

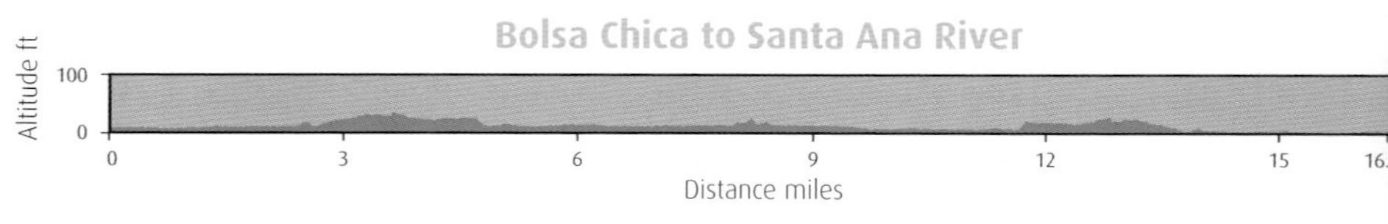

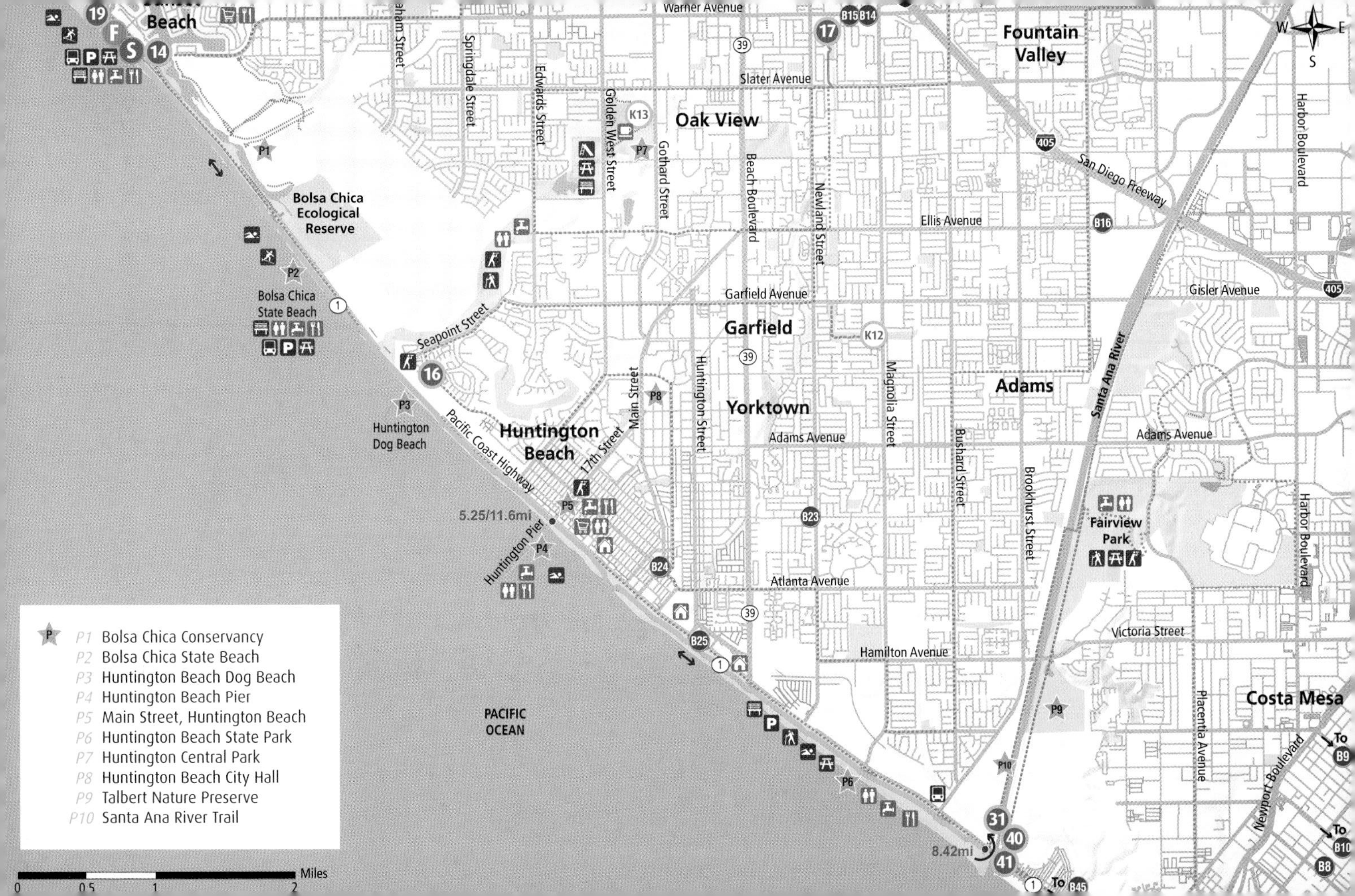

Warner Avenue
Beach
Fountain Valley
Slater Avenue
Springdale Street
Edwards Street
Golden West Street
Gothard Street
Oak View
Beach Boulevard
Newland Street
San Diego Freeway
Harbor Boulevard
Bolsa Chica Ecological Reserve
Ellis Avenue
Bolsa Chica State Beach
Garfield Avenue
Gisler Avenue
Garfield
Seapoint Street
Santa Ana River
Huntington Dog Beach
Huntington Beach
Pacific Coast Highway
17th Street
Main Street
Huntington Street
Yorktown
Magnolia Street
Adams
Adams Avenue
Bushard Street
Brookhurst Street
5.25/11.6mi
Huntington Pier
Fairview Park
Atlanta Avenue
Victoria Street
Hamilton Avenue
PACIFIC OCEAN
Costa Mesa
Placentia Avenue
Newport Boulevard
8.42mi
P1 Bolsa Chica Conservancy
P2 Bolsa Chica State Beach
P3 Huntington Beach Dog Beach
P4 Huntington Beach Pier
P5 Main Street, Huntington Beach
P6 Huntington Beach State Park
P7 Huntington Central Park
P8 Huntington Beach City Hall
P9 Talbert Nature Preserve
P10 Santa Ana River Trail
Miles
0
0.5
1
2

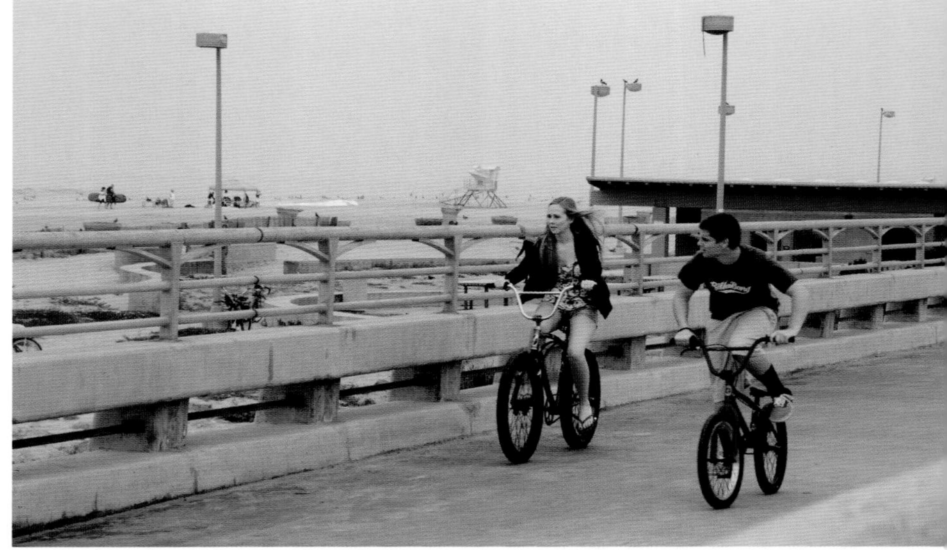

Crossing over the Bolsa Chica Wetlands.

At a Glance

Distance 38.0 miles **Elevation Gain** 351′

Terrain

About a third of this ride travels across well maintained bike paths. The remainder of the route moves along city streets which are mostly smooth with a few stretches of bumpy road. The ride is relatively flat with most of the elevation coming from bridges passing over freeways or bodies of water.

Traffic

Expect traffic along Pacific Coast Highway and Seal Beach Boulevard. Along the Santa Ana River, the route will be busy with cyclists.

How to Get There

By bus, OCTA buses 1, 21, 70 and 72 all make a stop at the ride's beginning.

By car, take Pacific Coast Highway to Bolsa Chica State Beach. After paying, turn right and drive to the very last parking lot.

Food and Drink

One of the best places to fuel up is the Secret Spo a health-minded restaurant located at the intersec tion of Warner and Pacific Coast Highway, near th ride's start/finish. For more traditional fare, stop in the Harbor House Café in Sunset Beach along Pacifi Coast Highway.

Side Trip

Two vastly different Main Streets, one in Seal Beac and one in Huntington Beach. Also along the way Bolsa Chica Ecological Reserve, home to an incredib amount of biodiversity.

Links to 

Where to Bike Rating 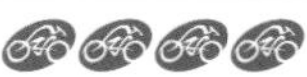

  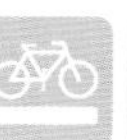  

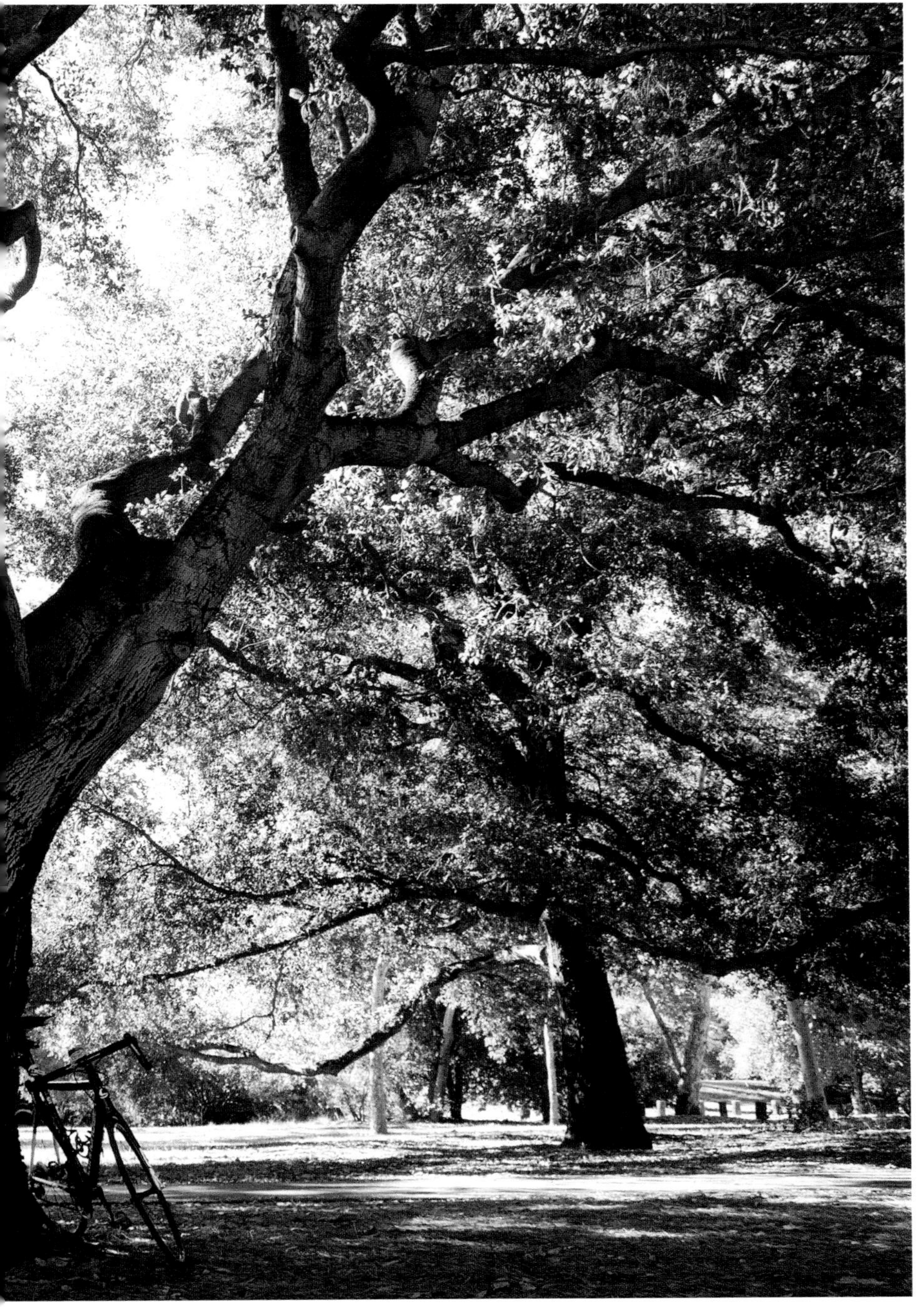

Central Inland

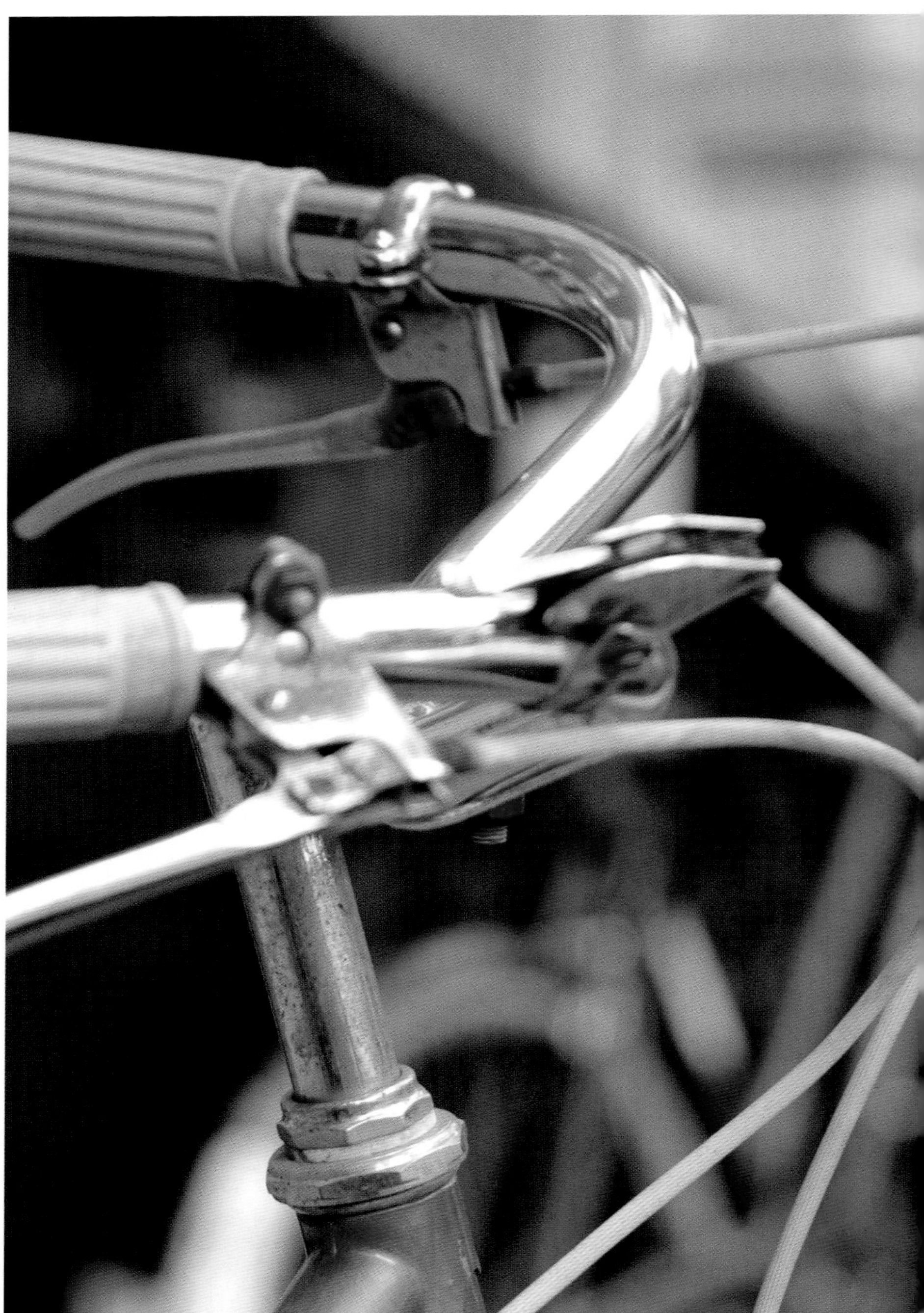

Image Matt Wittmer

Central Inland Overview

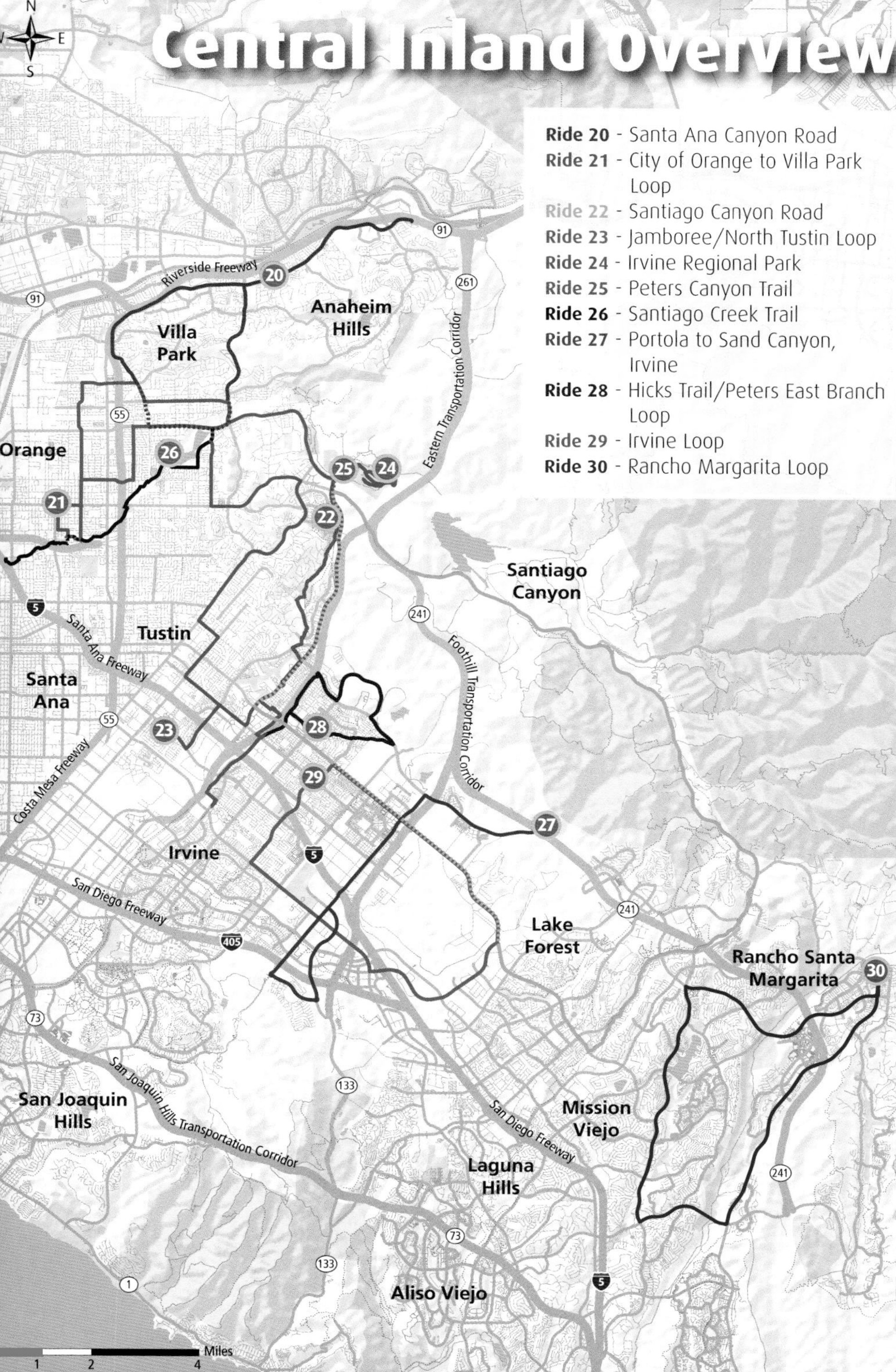

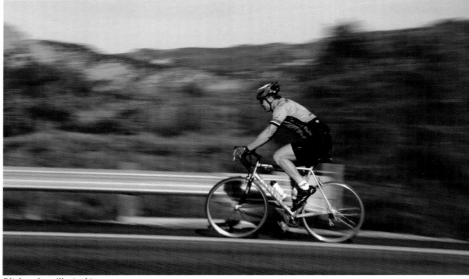

Blink and you'll miss him.

At a Glance

Distance 16.96 miles **Elevation Gain** 1218′

Terrain

This route traverses some of the steepest hills in the Central Inland section.

Traffic

Almost the entire route travels along on-street bike lanes on busy roads.

How to Get There

By bus, OCTA 38 makes stops on the eastern end of the route near Weir Canyon Road.

By car, take exit 36 Imperial Highway southbound off the 91 Freeway. Take the first left onto Santa Ana Canyon Road and travel for one mile, Eucalyptus Park will be on your left.

Food and Drink

The Canyon Plaza is a shopping center near the ride's beginning located at the corner of Santa Ana Canyon Road and Imperial Highway. There are a number of places to eat here including a juice shop, coffee shop and restaurants. Flappy Jacks Pancake House is a excellent breakfast or brunch option, located at 3.9 miles from the start.

Side Trips

Also located in the Canyon Plaza is Rock N' Road Cyclery with a helpful staff and everything you need to get on the road, or on the mountain. For those who love to climb, consider turning right at Weir Canyon Road for another challenging ascent.

Links to 1 21 23 26 31

Where to Bike Rating 

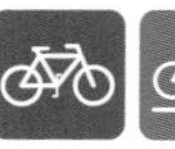   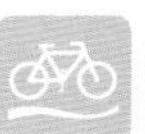 

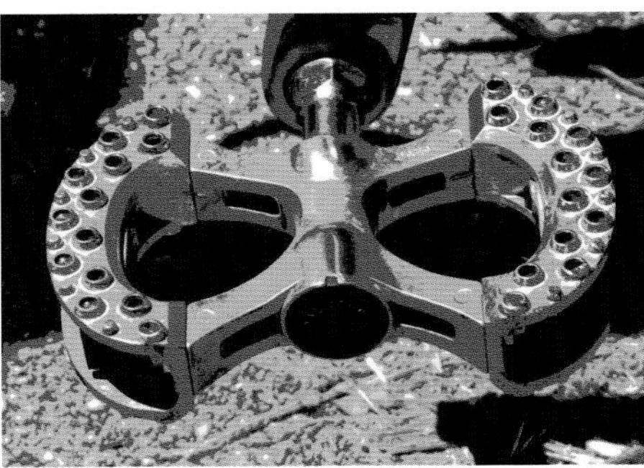

You'll need some pedal power on this ride.

About...

3efore the 91 Freeway, Santa Ana Canyon Road was the primary artery that passed through hese mountains, connecting Anaheim to the :ities of the Inland Empire. Although the ride has ı Where to Bike Rating of 3, even experienced iders will find this route a hearty challenge. For local cyclists, this ride is the backbone of a ıumber of longer and even more challenging raining rides.

arting at Eucalyptus Park, you will head westward, sentially running parallel to the 91 Freeway and later e 55 Freeway. This is a busy stretch that can be heavy th traffic, however the roads are wide and the on-eet bike lanes are well marked. Where the ride be-ns to bend southward, the route narrows and some of e bike lanes become ridiculously pinched and worn; ution should be exercised through here, especially at e entrance and exit of the 55 Freeway.

After this section you will find yourself passing rough the Cities of Orange and Villa Park and the roads iden, traffic is placid and the bike lanes ever-present. lso worth noting is that the road changes names a couple times as indicated in the ride log. At Meats Avenue you ill intersect with Ride 21 and once the route turns left on illa Park Road it intersects with Ride 23.

Without a doubt the toughest part of this ride is the imb up Cannon Street. As you begin this ascent it starts ıt deceptively flat with its peak bending out of sight. nce you reach Serrano Avenue the climbing begins earnest. The steepest stretch is a 7.5 percent grade hich puts this climb, at least over the short distance, in e Tour de France category. At one point I was moving) slowly I was passed by a jogger. It's that steep.

The reward for such a climb is, of course, the de-cent. It is no exaggeration to say that breaking the

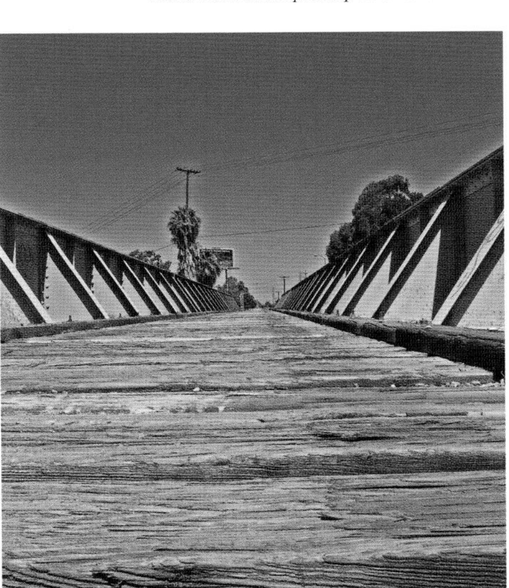

The rail bridge to nowhere.

speed limit is possible, though not advised as you white-knuckle-it down the road. As steep as the climb is, the descent is at a 12 percent grade.

At 13.72 miles the route crosses over Weir Canyon Road and for those who need another challenge, turn right and climb 1.6 miles to the road's end. For those with rubbery legs, continue across Weir Canyon until the turn around point at 14.22 miles. Santa Ana Canyon Road continues for another 1.5 miles, however there is no bike lane and the road narrows here to a dangerous degree, with little shoulder and sharp drops. Many clubs do ride to the end, but it is not recommended in this ride.

Ride Log

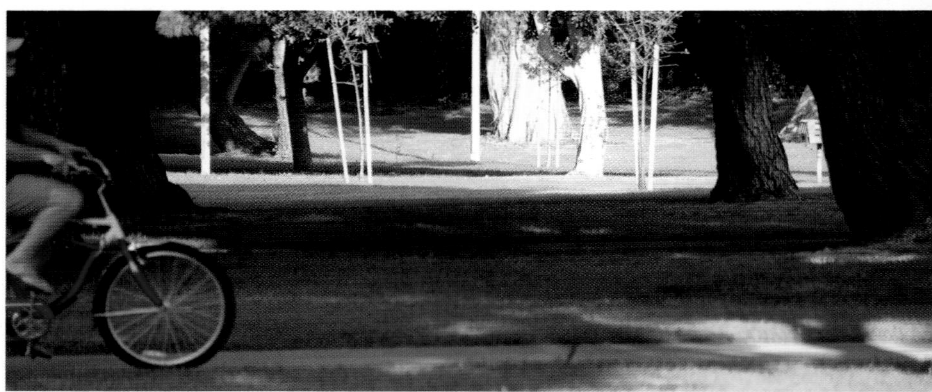

Eucalyptus Park is a pleasant place to let your weary legs recover from the Cannon Street climb.

P1 Santa Ana River Trail
P2 Featherly Regional Park

0.0 Begin ride on Santa Ana Canyon Rd, in front of Eucalyptus Park.
0.31 Cross Anaheim Hills Dr.
1.0 Cross Imperial Hwy.
1.66 Cross Royal Oak Rd.
2.34 Cross Lakeview Dr.
3.50 Santa Ana Canyon Rd changes name to Santiago Blvd.
3.92 Flappy Jacks Restaurant on your right.
4.10 Cross Lincoln Ave.
5.02 Cross Meats Ave.
5.44 Cross Taft Ave.
5.70 Santiago Blvd now becomes Wanda Rd.
5.96 Turn left onto Villa Park Rd.
6.47 Cross Center Dr.
7.17 Cross Hewes St.
7.50 Turn left onto Cannon St.
7.96 Cross Taft Ave.
8.13 Cross Serrano Ave.
9.26 Reach the peak just before Via Escola.
9.98 Cross Nohl Ranch Rd.
10.51 Turn right onto Santa Ana Canyon Rd.
11.52 On your left, Eucalyptus Park.
11.75 Cross Fairmont Blvd.
13.72 Cross Weir Canyon Rd.
14.22 At Woodcreek Rd the on-road bike lane end cross to other side of road and turn back.
14.73 Cross Weir Canyon Rd.
16.71 Cross Fairmont Blvd.
16.96 End.

Santa Ana Canyon Road

Please note: the profile for Ride 20 is depicted in 200ft vertical increments due to unusually high elevation.

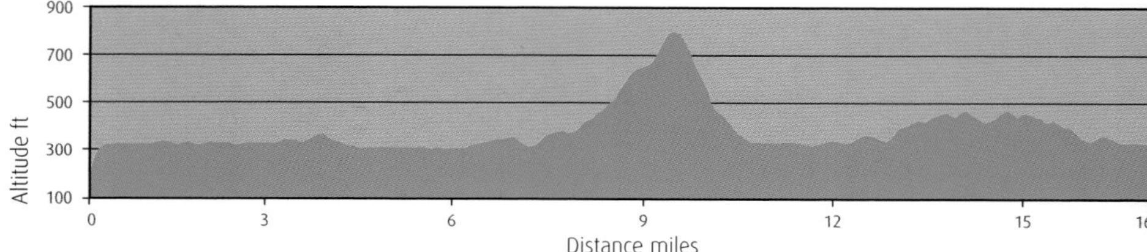

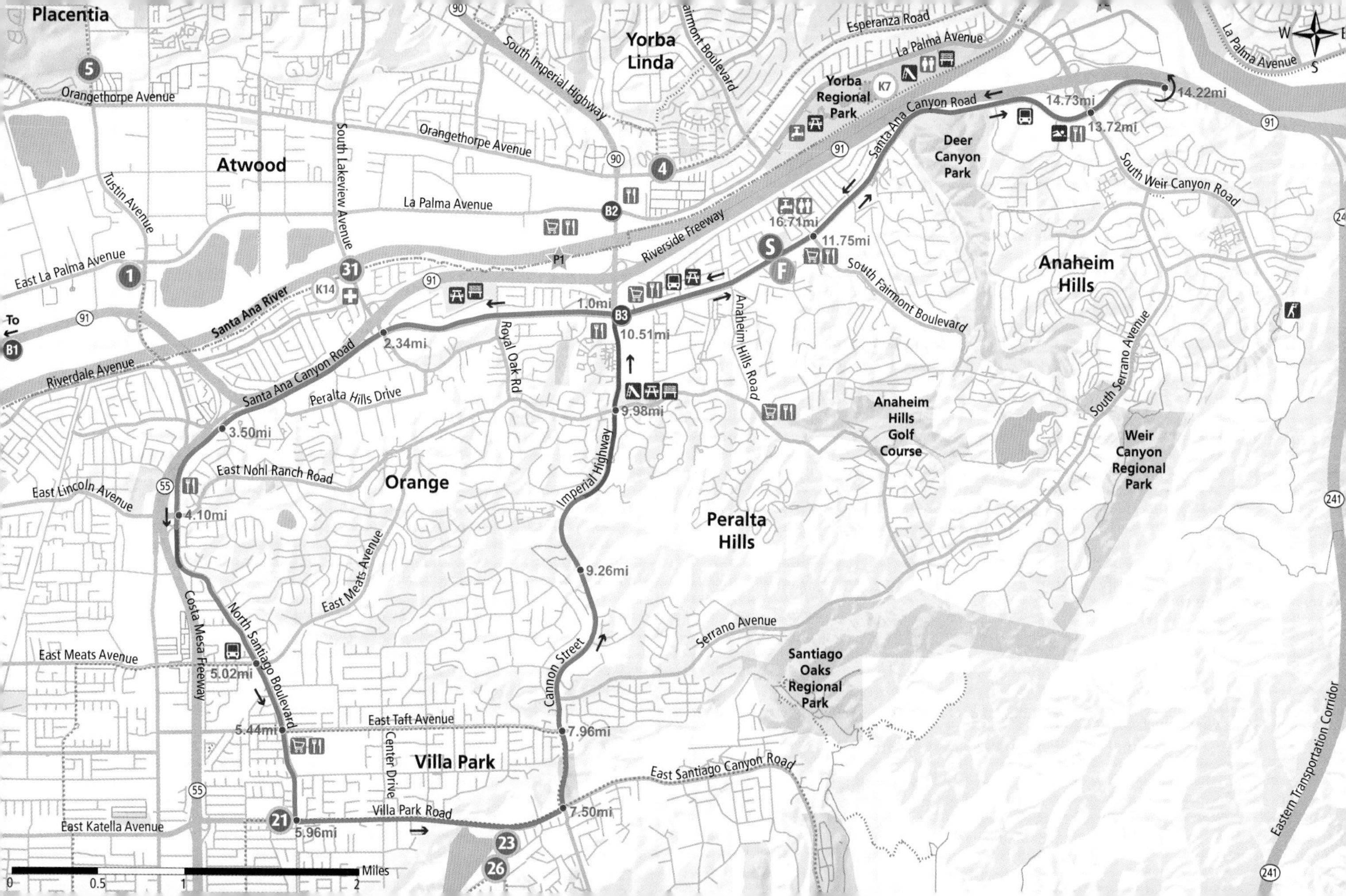

Placentia
Yorba Linda
Atwood
Orange
Villa Park
Anaheim Hills
Peralta Hills
Yorba Regional Park
Deer Canyon Park
Anaheim Hills Golf Course
Weir Canyon Regional Park
Santiago Oaks Regional Park
Santa Ana River
Orangethorpe Avenue
South Imperial Highway
Esperanza Road
Fairmont Boulevard
La Palma Avenue
Tustin Avenue
South Lakeview Avenue
East La Palma Avenue
Riverside Freeway
Riverdale Avenue
Santa Ana Canyon Road
Royal Oak Rd
Peralta Hills Drive
Anaheim Hills Road
South Fairmont Boulevard
South Weir Canyon Road
South Serrano Avenue
Imperial Highway
East Nohl Ranch Road
East Lincoln Avenue
East Meats Avenue
North Santiago Boulevard
Costa Mesa Freeway
Cannon Street
Serrano Avenue
East Taft Avenue
Center Drive
East Santiago Canyon Road
Villa Park Road
East Katella Avenue
Eastern Transportation Corridor
To B1
1.0mi
2.34mi
3.50mi
4.10mi
5.02mi
5.44mi
5.96mi
7.50mi
7.96mi
9.26mi
9.98mi
10.51mi
11.75mi
13.72mi
14.22mi
14.73mi
16.71mi
Miles
0
0.5
1
2

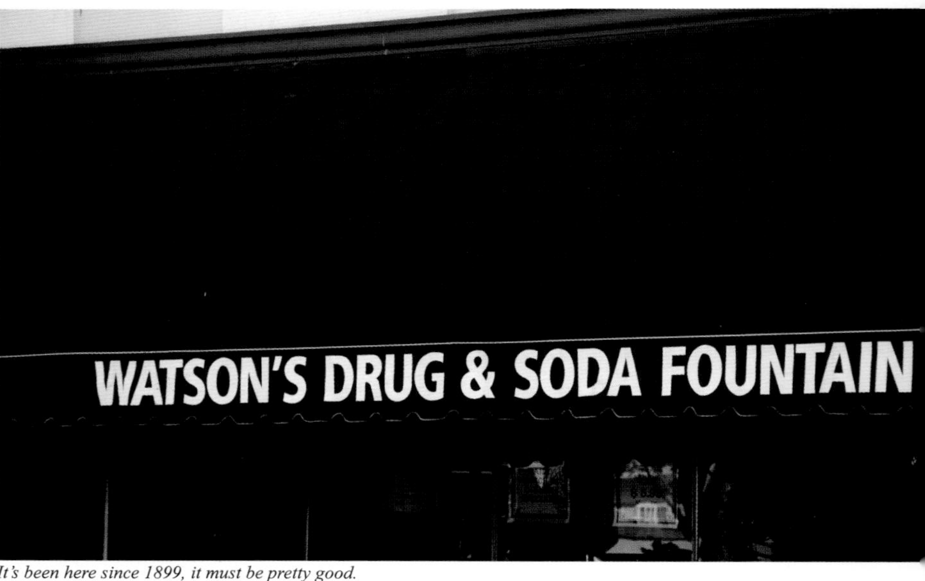

It's been here since 1899, it must be pretty good.

At a Glance

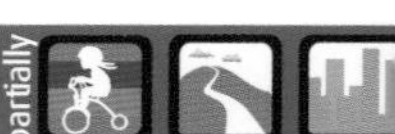

Distance 12.64 miles **Elevation Gain** 390′

Terrain

This ride is mostly flat with a few gentle climbs along well maintained roads.

Traffic

Overall traffic is light, however near the ride's start and finish is Orange's plaza and traffic can be heavier here.

How to Get There

By bus, OCTA routes 54, 56 and 59 make stops close to the start.

By car, take CA-22 to exit 16, Glassell/Grand. Turn north onto Glassell Street and travel for 0.8 miles until you reach the roundabout. Turn right at the first exit onto Chapman Avenue, then a quick right onto Orange Street. Public parking is available here.

By train, Amtrak and Metrolink lines stop at the nearby train depot, located on the opposite side of the roundabout from the ride's start.

Food and Drink

When the ride comes to an end, you will have to ma some tough decisions concerning where to dine there is an almost endless selection in Orange's h toric district.

Side Trip

Antiquing in the historic district is serious business a there are plenty of shops to peruse, be prepared to pa with your money. North of the start is Chapman Ur versity which has a beautiful campus worthy of a stro

Links to    K19

Where to Bike Rating 

About...

This is a challenging training ride that will test the mettle of even experienced riders. Jumping off from Peters Canyon Regional Park, you will immediately find yourself riding away from civilization and into the wilderness. The first 11.5 miles consists of steady, undulating climbs, followed by nearly 16 miles of steady descent. Finally the ride finishes with nearly 500 feet of climbing over four miles. This is a ride of extremes.

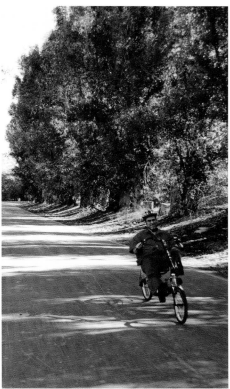

A recumbent rider cruising along Aliso Creek Trail.

antiago Canyon Road is a thin ribbon of asphalt in a ıst, empty wilderness. As you travel this road, Whitıg Ranch Wilderness Park will be on your right and leveland National Forest on your left. This is a ride əst done with friends and preferably on a well-mainined bike. Before setting out make certain you have ıough water and the tools needed to make basic reairs. You do not want to be stranded along this stretch.

At 5.92 miles you will find yourself passing Irvine ake a scenic, 750 acre reservoir that is primarily a shing and camping area. Created in 1931when Sanago Creek was dammed, the lake is operated by the errano Water District and provides the cities of Villa ark and Orange with drinking water. Fishing licenses e not required and all-day passes costs $22 per adult.

At about 11.5 miles the route reaches its highest oint and a well-earned, long descent begins with the rst couple of miles being the steepest. At 12.97 the oad intersects with Live Oak Canyon Road and this where you will find the famous Cook's Corner, the ther kind of "biker" bar, as in motorcycles. You are robably not going to want to visit this place in your oandex.

At 13.27 miles the ride continues along Aliso Creek Trail which is also part of Ride 43. This upper section of the trail runs along a natural bottomed creek overshadowed by giant sycamores and eucalyptus. After the stark stretch of Santiago Canyon, this part of the ride will seem wonderfully lush and green. Sadly, at 18.31 miles the route leaves the trail and turns right onto Trabuco Road for the return leg. It is important to note that there are absolutely no signs here to indicate exits off the river trail so pay attention to your mileage or you will fly past this turn.

Trabuco Road, which turns into Irvine Boulevard at 22.39 miles, has on-road bike paths with a moderate amount of traffic. It will carry you through the northern section of Irvine to Jamboree Road and the final climb of the ride. This climb is a long, low grade ascent, 460 feet over 3.71 miles.

Ride Log

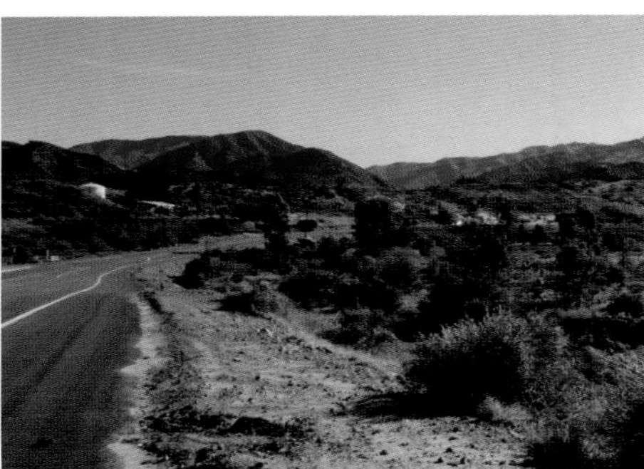
Stark and lonely, Santiago Canyon has a rugged beauty.

0.0 Begin ride at Peters Canyon Regional Park parking, off of Canyon View Ave.
0.14 Turn left onto Jamboree Rd.
0.67 Turn right onto Santiago Canyon Rd.
1.72 Bear left and watch for traffic entering Hwy 241.
4.1 Irvine Lake on your left.
12.97 Bear right, Cook's Corner restaurant on your left.
13.08 Cross Ridgeline Rd.
13.27 Bear right onto Aliso Creek Bikeway.
13.90 Bear right.
17.12 Bear right and pass under bridge.
17.21 Turn right.
17.30 Pass Sundowner's Park. No restrooms, but water is available here.
18.28 Bear left off of Aliso Creek Bikeway, head towards Trabuco Rd. There are no street signs here.
18.31 Turn right onto Trabuco Rd.
18.65 Cross El Toro Rd.
19.43 Cross Lake Forest Dr.
22.39 Cross Bake Pkwy. Trabuco turns into Irvi Blvd here.
22.93 Cross Alton Pkwy.
24.25 Cross over Hwy 133, watch for traffic exiti and entering.
24.43 Cross Sand Canyon Rd.
25.41 Cross Jeffrey Rd.
26.13 Cross Yale Ave.
26.90 Cross Culver Dr.
27.75 Cross Marketplace Rd.
28.02 Turn right onto Jamboree Rd.
28.38 Cross Robinson Dr.
29.02 Cross Champion Way.
29.32 Cross Portola Pkwy.
31.22 Cross Pioneer Way.
32.38 Turn left onto Canyon View Ave.
32.55 End.

P
P1 Peters Canyon Reservoir and Regional Park
P2 Irvine Regional Park
P3 Orange County Zoo
P4 Great Park Balloon Ride
P5 Tustin Sports Park
P6 O'Neill Regional Park
P7 Modjeska Canyon
P8 Irvine Spectrum Center

Santiago Canyon Road

Please note: the profile for Ride 22 is depicted in 500ft vertical increments due to unusually high elevation.

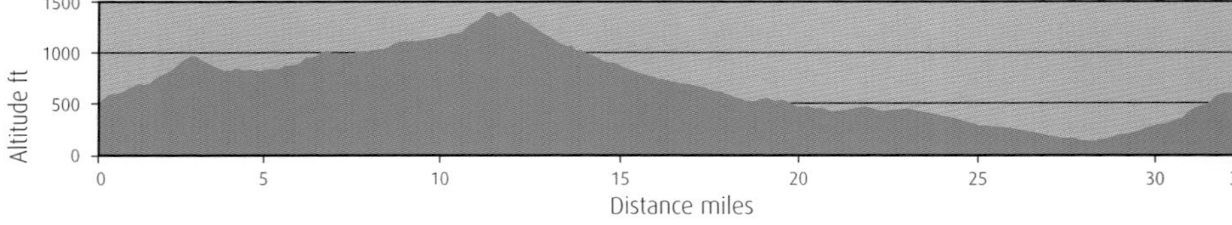

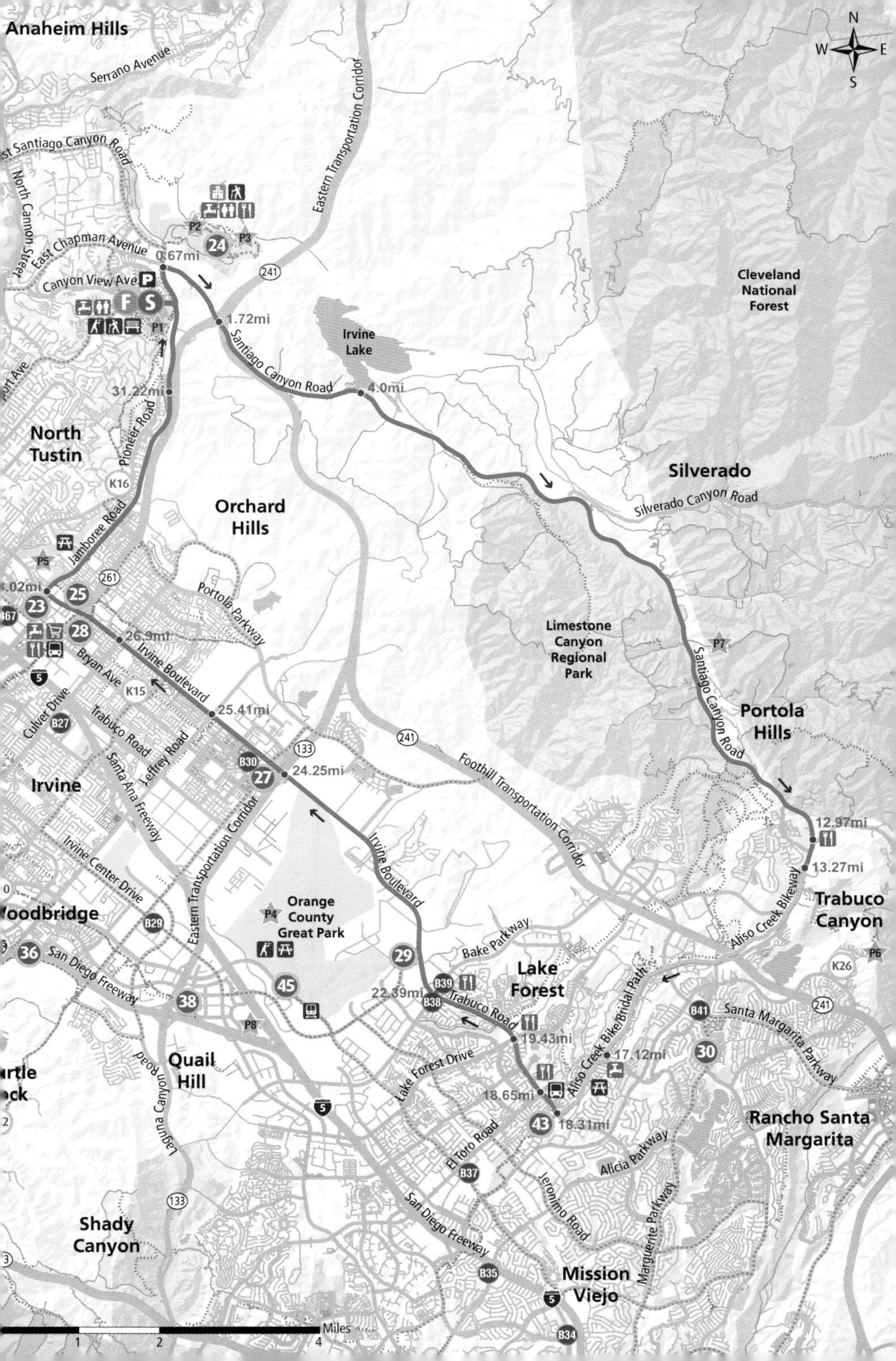

Anaheim Hills
Serrano Avenue
Eastern Transportation Corridor
East Santiago Canyon Road
North Cannon Street
East Chapman Avenue
0.67mi
Canyon View Ave
1.72mi
Santiago Canyon Road
Irvine Lake
4.0mi
31.22mi
Pioneer Road
North Tustin
K16
Jamboree Road
Orchard Hills
Cleveland National Forest
Silverado
Silverado Canyon Road
Portola Parkway
Limestone Canyon Regional Park
26.9mi
Irvine Boulevard
Bryan Ave
K15
Culver Drive
Trabuco Road
Jeffrey Road
25.41mi
24.25mi
Santa Ana Freeway
Irvine
Foothill Transportation Corridor
Portola Hills
12.97mi
13.27mi
Aliso Creek Bikeway
Trabuco Canyon
Irvine Center Drive
Eastern Transportation Corridor
Orange County Great Park
Woodbridge
San Diego Freeway
Bake Parkway
Lake Forest
22.39mi
Trabuco Road
19.43mi
Aliso Creek Bike/Bridal Path
17.12mi
Santa Margarita Parkway
Quail Hill
Lake Forest Drive
18.65mi
18.31mi
Laguna Canyon Road
El Toro Road
Alicia Parkway
Jeronimo Road
Marguerite Parkway
Rancho Santa Margarita
Shady Canyon
San Diego Freeway
Mission Viejo
Miles
1
2
4

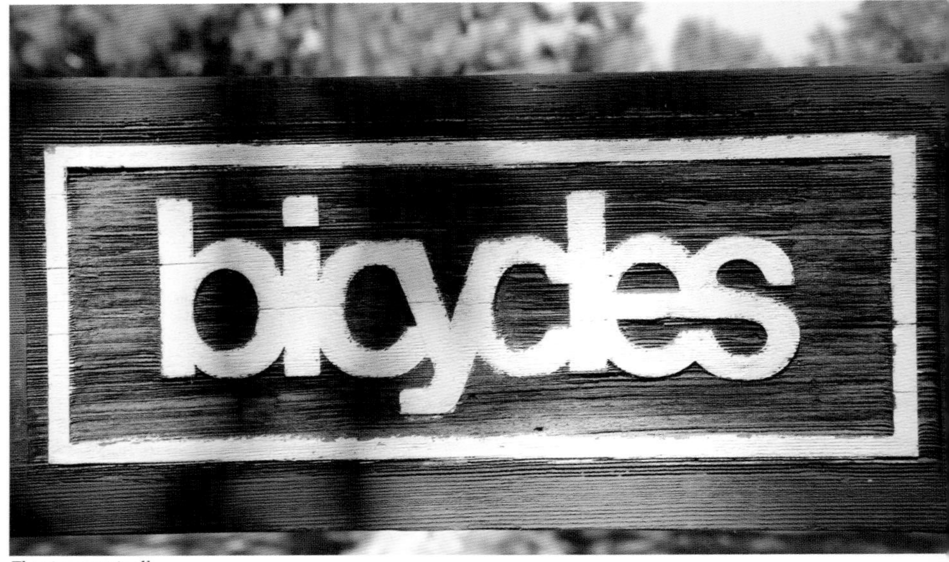

The sign says it all.

At a Glance

Distance 23.34 miles **Elevation Gain** 1294′

Terrain

This route is full of climbs with one especially long, moderately steep section along Jamboree Avenue, and a very steep but shorter section along Chapman Avenue. The entire ride travels along on-street bike lanes.

Traffic

Although roads and bike lanes are wide along this route, be prepared for heavy traffic at times.

How to Get There

By bus, there are no bus routes to the ride's start, however, OCTA 54 intersects with Chapman Avenue near the halfway point.

By car, take exit 101 Red Hill Road, southbound, off of Interstate 5. After 0.5 miles turn left onto Walnut Avenue, followed by a right onto Oxford Avenue at 0.3 miles. Turn left onto Roanoke Avenue, the Centennial Park parking lot will be on your right.

Food and Drink

After the steep climb up Chapman, you may be looking for a friendly place to stop. Consider the nondescript shopping center at Chapman Avenue and Newport Boulevard.

Side Trip

Peters Canyon and Irvine Regional Park are both beautiful places to spend a few hours exploring. At the intersection of Bryan Avenue and Jamboree Road you will find the sprawling Irvine Marketplace with plenty of shopping opportunities.

Links to 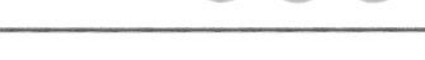 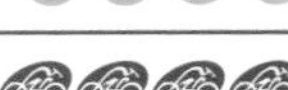

20 21 22 24 25 26 28 K16 K18

Where to Bike Rating

  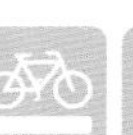 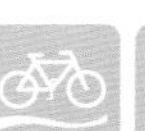 

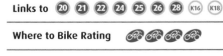

About...

This route is a challenging training ride used by top cyclists, clubs and recreationalists throughout the area. It is a rare day when you ride this route and don't at some point find yourself traveling with a peloton of riders. Two memorable climbs make up this ride, the first a low grade, five mile slog up Jamboree. The second hill that is sure to stick in your mind is the shorter but steeper climb up Chapman Avenue.

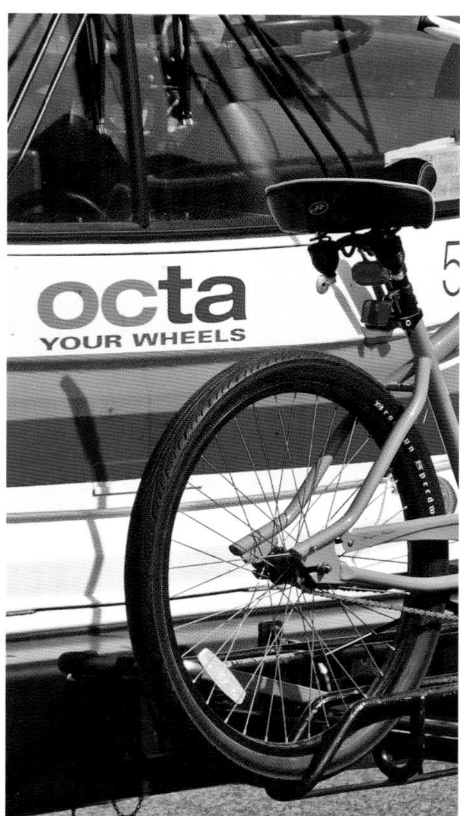

This is the smart way to tackle those hills.

This ride begins at Centennial Park in Tustin, site of Kids' Ride 18. The first few miles are pleasantly flat before you turn onto Jamboree Road at 2.66 miles. Here you will begin the first ascent, with this lower section of such a low grade you may not even notice you are going uphill. This is also where the route passes the Irvine Marketplace, a sprawling shopping center. Watch for traffic exiting and entering parking lots, especially on weekends.

At 7.43 miles you will find yourself passing Peters Canyon Regional Park and if you are looking for a place to break and picnic, you could do worse than stopping here. This beautiful park is home to mule deer, raccoons, hawks, water fowl and a large reservoir. Mountain bikers will find enough trails to keep them trekking all day. Jamboree ends at Irvine Regional Park, an equally beautiful open space that is worthy of a day's exploration, as well as home to Ride 24.

On Chapman Avenue you will find yourself staring up a mountain. Steep, but thankfully short. After the long, slow climb of Jamboree at least this hill is surmounted relatively quickly. At the intersection of Chapman and Newport Boulevard, on your right, you will find a non-descript shopping center where a number of restaurants reside. Try Cyrano's Caffe, a breakfast and lunch place and treat yourself to a stack of pancakes or try the eggs Florentine. Also located here is a taco shop, pizzeria and the upscale Fish House Market and Grill.

Once on Newport Boulevard there is one more relatively small hill to climb, but after the other hills, you are going to really feel these last 125 feet. From here it is literally all downhill, an exhilarating, well-earned descent from the top of Newport until it becomes a gentle slope near La Colina Drive. Worth noting is the fact that La Colina is a smaller street and you could easily zip right past it if you are not looking for it at 18.94 miles.

Ride Log

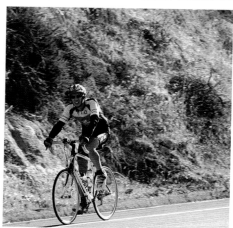
He looks like he's in pain, doesn't he?

P1 Peters Canyon Reservoir
P2 Orange County Zoo
P3 Irvine Park Railroad
P4 Santiago Canyon College
P5 Tustin Sports Park
P6 Irvine Marketplace

0.0 Begin ride at Centennial Park parking lot, near the intersection of Sycamore Ave and Canterbury Ave.
0.28 Turn right on Oxford Ave.
0.36 Turn right on Walnut Ave.
0.96 Turn left onto Tustin Ranch Rd.
2.05 Turn right on Bryan Ave.
2.66 Turn left onto Jamboree Rd, Irvine Marketplace on the right.
3.10 Cross Irvine Blvd.
3.29 Riding parallel to Ride 25, Peters Canyon Trail.
3.46 Cross Robinson Dr.
3.76 Cross Trevino Dr.
4.12 Cross Champion Way.
4.41 Cross Portola Pkwy.
7.43 Cross Canyon View Ave. A left here will take you into Peters Canyon Regional Park.
7.98 Cross Chapman Ave.
8.21 Turn left onto Santiago Canyon Rd.
11.19 Cross Cannon St.
11.52 Turn left onto Hewes St.
11.78 Turn left onto Rancho Santiago Blvd.
13.09 Turn left onto Chapman Ave.
13.41 Cross Crawford Canyon Rd.
15.06 Turn right onto Newport Blvd.
15.61 Cross Canyon View Ave, Peters Canyon Park on your left.
17.93 Cross Foothill Blvd.
18.61 Cross 17th St.
18.94 Turn left onto La Colina Dr.
19.43 Turn right onto Red Hill Ave.
19.92 Cross Irvine Blvd.
20.42 Turn left onto Bryan Ave.
21.28 Right on Tustin Ranch Rd.
21.67 Entrance/exit to Interstate 5, watch for traffic.
22.41 Turn right onto Walnut Ave.
22.94 Left onto Oxford Ave.
23.03 Turn left onto Roanoke Ave.
23.34 End.

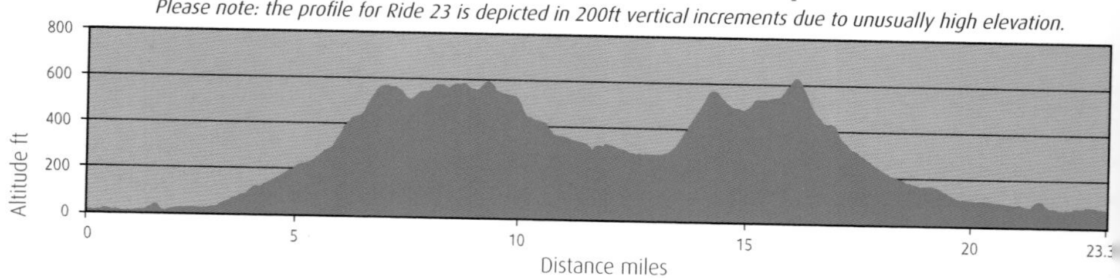

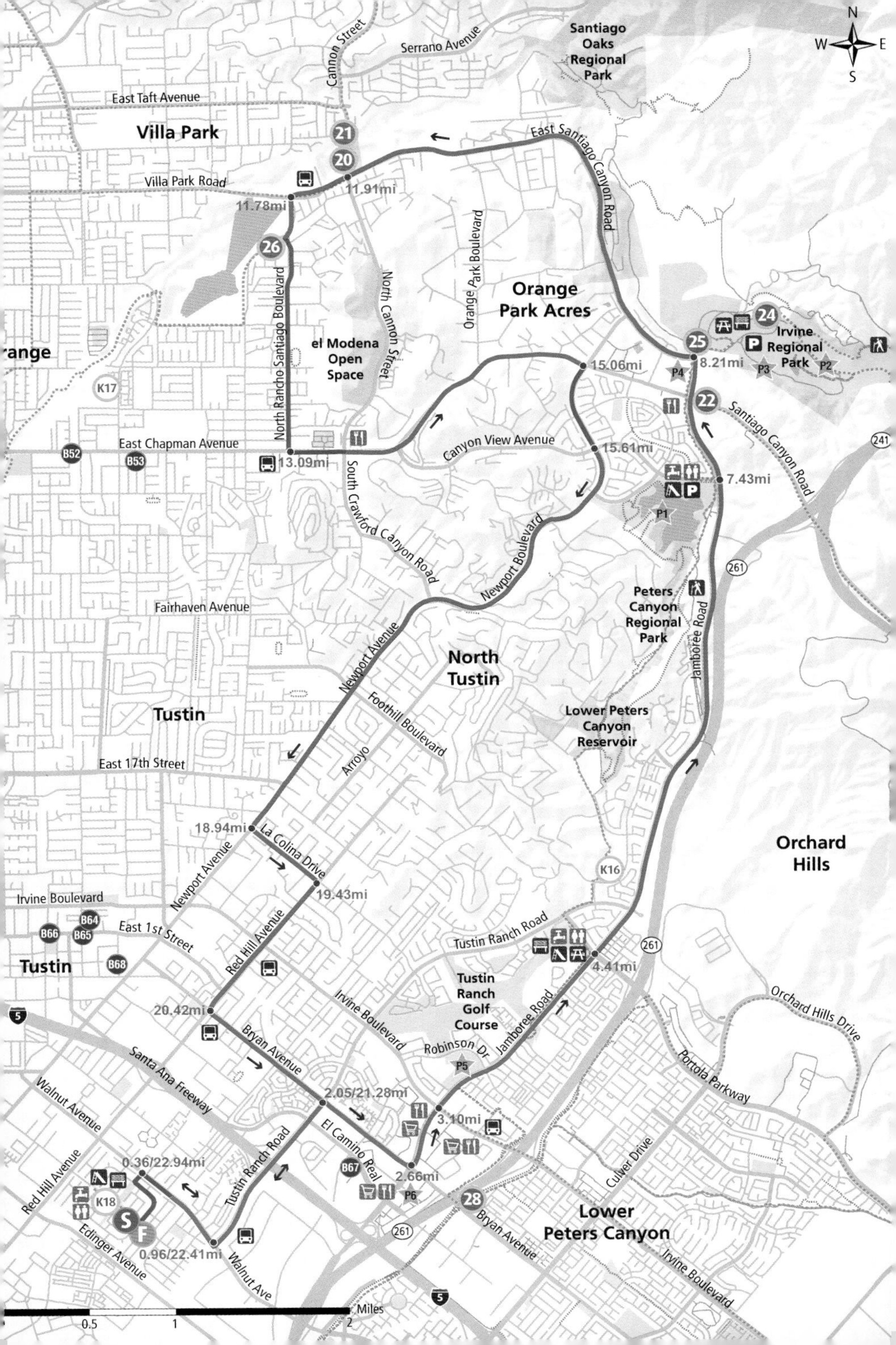
Santiago Oaks Regional Park
Serrano Avenue
Cannon Street
East Taft Avenue
Villa Park
21
20
East Santiago Canyon Road
Villa Park Road
11.91mi
11.78mi
26
North Rancho Santiago Boulevard
North Cannon Street
Orange Park Boulevard
Orange Park Acres
el Modena Open Space
24
25
Irvine Regional Park
8.21mi
P4
P3
P2
15.06mi
22
Santiago Canyon Road
K17
East Chapman Avenue
Canyon View Avenue
15.61mi
B52
B53
13.09mi
7.43mi
241
South Crawford Canyon Road
P1
Newport Boulevard
261
Fairhaven Avenue
Peters Canyon Regional Park
Jamboree Road
Newport Avenue
North Tustin
Foothill Boulevard
Tustin
Lower Peters Canyon Reservoir
Arroyo
East 17th Street
18.94mi
La Colina Drive
Orchard Hills
Newport Avenue
K16
19.43mi
Irvine Boulevard
B64
East 1st Street
Red Hill Avenue
Tustin Ranch Road
B66
B65
261
Tustin
B68
4.41mi
Tustin Ranch Golf Course
Irvine Boulevard
Jamboree Road
Orchard Hills Drive
5
20.42mi
Bryan Avenue
Robinson Dr
Santa Ana Freeway
P5
Portola Parkway
2.05/21.28mi
Walnut Avenue
3.10mi
El Camino Real
Culver Drive
0.36/22.94mi
Tustin Ranch Road
B67
2.66mi
Red Hill Avenue
K18
P6
28
Lower Peters Canyon
S
F
261
Bryan Avenue
Edinger Avenue
0.96/22.41mi
Walnut Ave
Irvine Boulevard
5
0.5
1
2
Miles
N
W
E
S

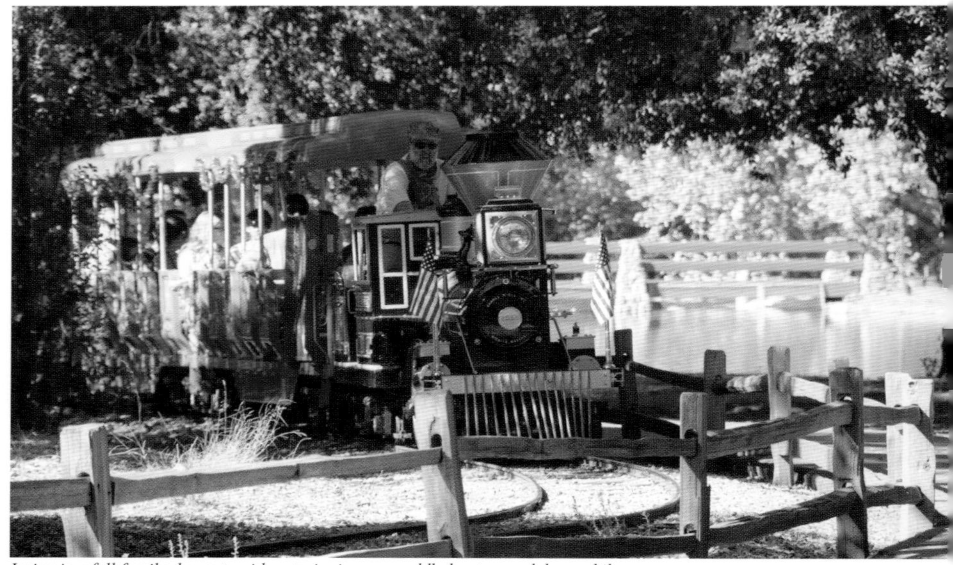
Irvine is a full family day out - ride a train, jump a paddle boat or pedal your bike.

At a Glance

Distance 2.95 miles **Elevation Gain** 85′

Terrain

Flat bike path with a few bumpy sections.

Traffic

This is a car-free ride. Expect a lot of pedestrian traffic on weekends.

How to Get There

By bus, OCTA bus 54 makes a stop on Santiago Canyon Road. From there the park is a 0.2 miles ride.

By car, exit the 55 Freeway at exit 14, Chapman Avenue heading eastbound. After 4.1 miles turn left onto Jamboree Road, then right onto Irvine Park Road after 0.2 miles. This road takes you right into the park. Admission is $3 weekdays, $5 weekends.

Food and Drink

There are two snack bars located in the park, one near the train station and the other by the lake across from the zoo. There are also numerous picnic tables and barbecues

Side Trip

There is a full day's worth of things to do during this ride. Orange County Zoo is located here as is a nature center, an outdoor bandstand and a lake. Pony rides are available for the little ones and for the bigger kids, hiking and mountain biking trails beckon.

Bike Hire

At the ride's start, beside the snack bar, a variety of bikes are available for rent including quads, cruisers and kid's bikes.

Links to 22 23 25

Where to Bike Rating 

  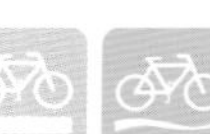 

About...

Once part of the enormous Irvine Company ıoldings, this park came into existence when ames Irvine, Jr. donated the first 160 acres, ncluding the oak grove and rancho, in 1876. Over the years it grew to include the Orange County Zoo, a lake, a train line, equestrian facilities and hiking trails all contained within 477 acres. On this family oriented ride, there are enough outdoor activities that you will be happy to visit this park again and again.

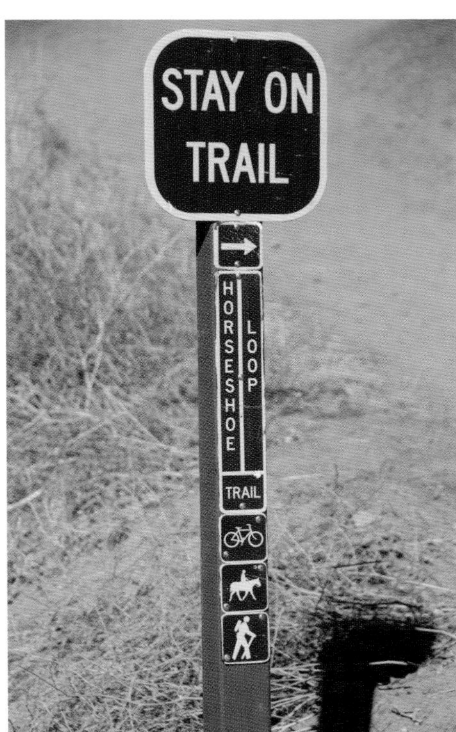

The many trails to explore in this park will keep you coming back for more and more.

t the heart of the park, where the ride begins, you will ıd a beautiful, peaceful grove of Coast Live Oaks, e only native oak that thrives in coastal California. tting under these ancient giants, some over 250 years d and four feet in diameter, it is easy to forget the istering desert surrounding you. This was James Irne's "garden". Here you will find the nature center ıd bandstand and nearby the zoo. As you enjoy the ıade and watch the free-roaming peacocks, you are ıre to catch the busy staccato of woodpeckers overead hard at work.

The Orange County Zoo grew out of a 1905 colction of red foxes, that later included mule deer and ligators. Today its focus is largely on plants and aniıals native to the southwest. Among the animals you ill see are black bears, mountain lions, bald eagles ıd red tail hawks. There is also a section dedicated to omesticated animals including pot belly pigs, goats ıd sheep. Admission to the zoo is $2 for ages three ıd over and free to kids two and under.

The Irvine Park Railroad is a 1/3 scale train that kes visitors on a loop alongside the lake. Located ext to the train, are pony rides and an equestrian cent- where you can rent horses to ride the trails. Paddle boats are also available, located near the bike rentals. Visit www.irvineparkrailroad.com to find schedules and prices for all these activities.

Once you leave the oak grove area, the ride travels a path across Santiago Creek and right up against foothills on the opposite side. Here you will find mountain bike trails and woodlands to ride and hike. Keep in mind that these foothills lead into the Santa Ana Mountains, a wilderness area that is home to mountain lions, coyotes and rattlesnakes. Exercise caution as you explore and always travel with a buddy.

As a family-oriented ride, this route avoids all roads except a single road crossing. For those interested in a longer ride, explore the peaceful roadways that wander the park, including a giant looping route that connects the park's oldest and newest sections, located just to your left as you enter the park.

Ride Log

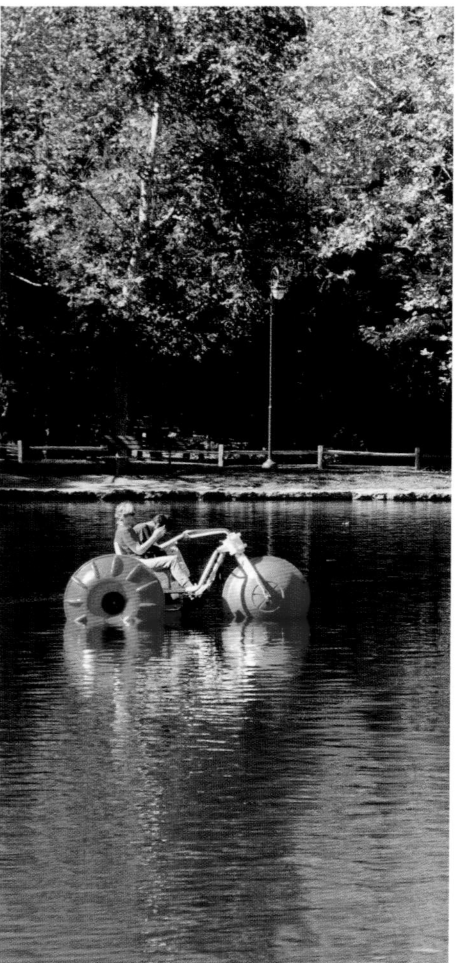

They look lonely out there.

P1 Orange County Zoo
P2 Irvine Park Railroad
P3 Pony rides
P4 Santiago Canyon College
P5 The Irvine Ranch Outdoor Education Center

0.0 Begin ride in front of the Orange County Zoo e trance.

0.02 Turn left. Bike rentals on your right.

0.06 Turn left.

0.14 Continue straight on path.

0.33 Cross park road.

0.44 Turn right.

0.69 Turn left.

1.06 Horseshoe Loop trailhead on your right.

1.55 Turn right.

1.82 Turn around and return in direction you ju came.

2.09 Continue straight on path.

2.46 Bear right.

2.49 Turn right.

2.59 Cross park road.

2.78 Continue straight.

2.86 Bear right.

2.92 Bear right.

2.95 End.

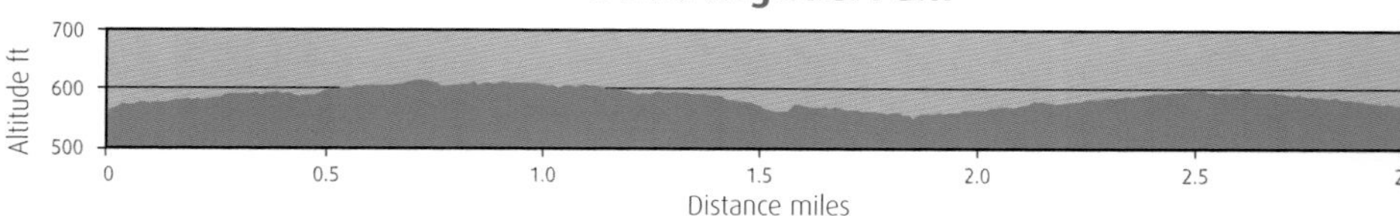

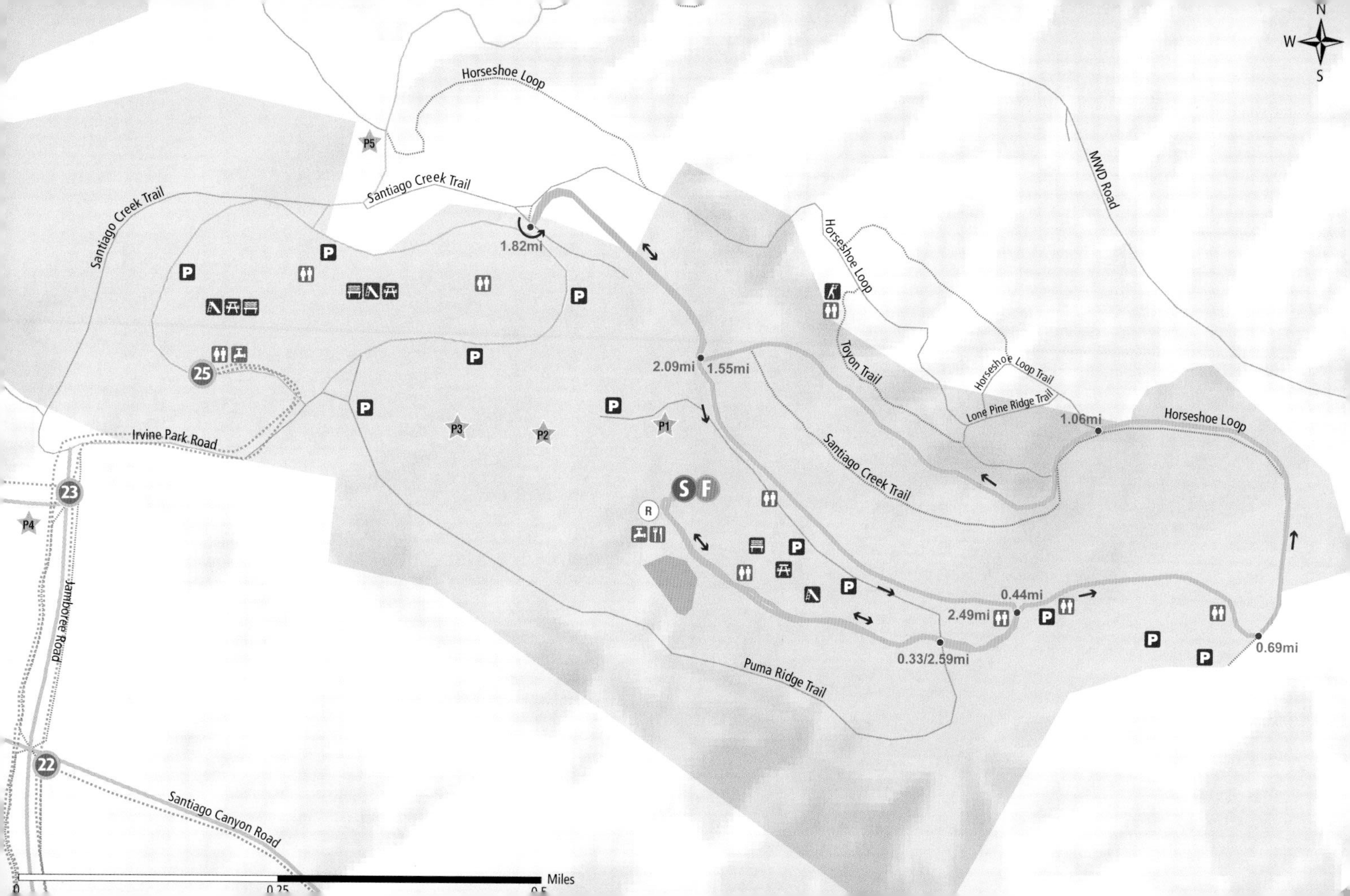
N
W
S
Horseshoe Loop
P5
Santiago Creek Trail
Santiago Creek Trail
1.82mi
MWD Road
Horseshoe Loop
25
2.09mi
1.55mi
Toyon Trail
Horseshoe Loop Trail
Lone Pine Ridge Trail
1.06mi
Horseshoe Loop
P3
P2
P1
Irvine Park Road
Santiago Creek Trail
23
S
F
R
P4
0.44mi
2.49mi
0.33/2.59mi
0.69mi
Jamboree Road
Puma Ridge Trail
22
Santiago Canyon Road
0
0.25
Miles

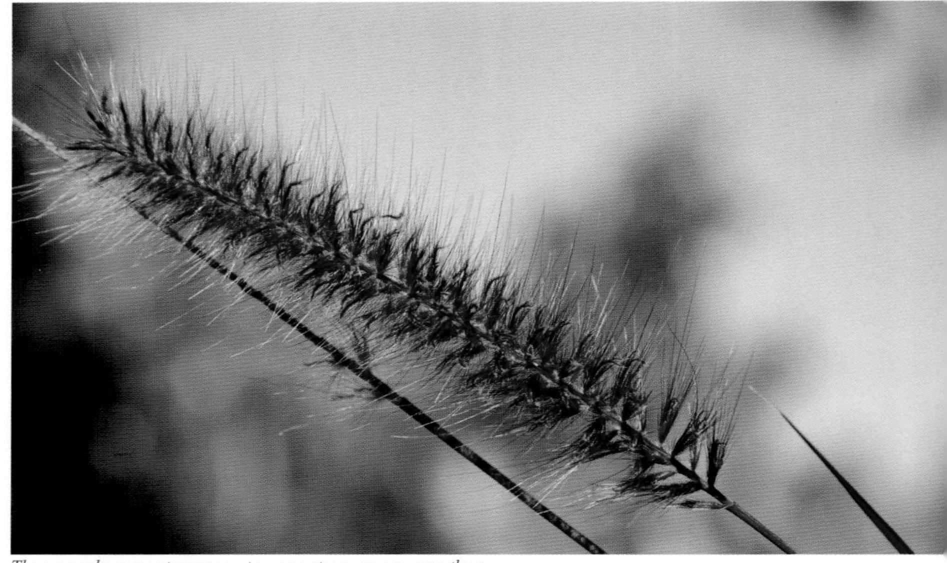

These purple grass stems seem to wave at you as you pass them.

At a Glance

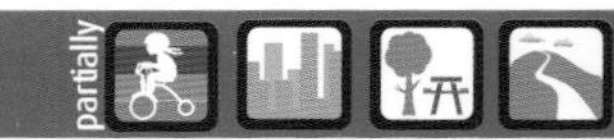

Distance 18.27 miles **Elevation Gain** 987′

Terrain

This route travels almost its entire length across bike paths. There is some steep terrain at the beginning and end through Peters Canyon Park which travels over dirt road.

Traffic

This is virtually a car-free ride. Pedestrian traffic is heavy through Peters Canyon Park, especially on the weekends.

How to Get There

By bus, OCTA bus 54 makes a stop on Santiago Canyon Road. From there the park is a 0.2 miles ride.

By car, exit the 55 Freeway at exit 14, Chapman Avenue heading eastbound. After 4.1 miles turn left onto Jamboree Road, then right onto Irvine Park Road after 0.2 miles. Admission is $3 weekdays, $5 weekends.

Food and Drink

Oddly enough, for all the miles you will cover on thi ride, there are few dining options. Near the beginnin is a shopping center at Jamboree and Chapman Avenu with a couple of fast food options. Also located in th center is John's Place, a friendly diner with tasty ome lets and a well-stocked salad bar.

Side Trip

In addition to the possibility of linking to nine othe rides, you will have the opportunity to explore two re gional parks and picnic at Incredible Edible Park at th halfway mark.

Links to 22 23 24 28 35 K16

Where to Bike Rating 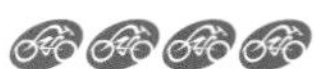

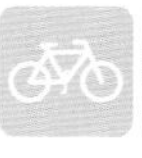  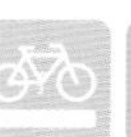  

About...

This is a blissful, car-free ride that meanders through the cities of Tustin and Irvine. Billed as the Mountains to the Sea Trail, this ride starts at Irvine Regional Park and after a steep section in Peters Canyon, heads gently downhill until it turns around at Incredible Edible Park. An amazing amount of planning, landscaping and thought went into this trail and it is simply a beautiful example of what a bike path can be.

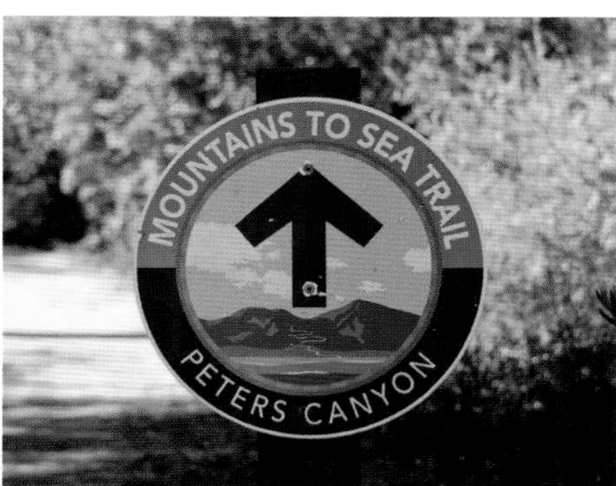

Almost this entire ride is car-free.

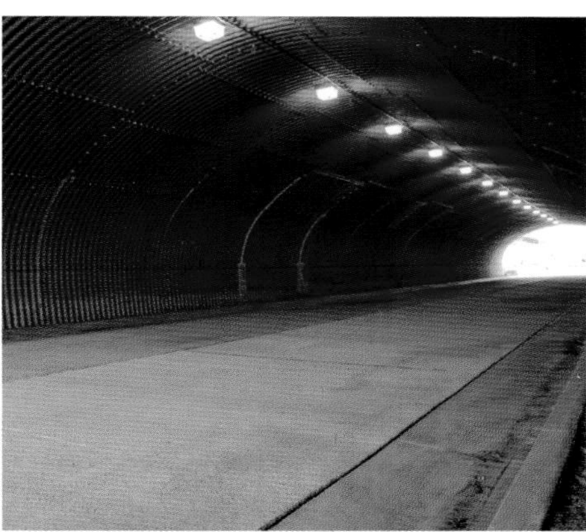

The coolest space-age bike tunnel.

fter leaving Irvine Park, site of Ride 24, you will soon nd yourself traveling through Peters Canyon Region- Park. Encompassing 354 acres, this open space is the ome to mule deer, opossums, raccoons and a huge va- ety of water fowl. Seasonal streams and a freshwater arsh give rise to beautiful glades sprinkled with lush illows and cottonwoods. Mountain bike trails criss- ross the entire park and you could very well spend all ay exploring this canyon. For this route, stick to the ard packed dirt road, and if in doubt of which trail to de, follow the Mountain to the Seas trail signs. Al- ough this trail is navigable by skinny-tire bikes, if ding on dirt isn't your thing, consider traveling along amboree Road when this route enters Peters Canyon ark. At 1.2 miles, turn right onto Pioneer Road and fter 1.4 miles turn right again onto Pioneer Way which ill rejoin this route on bike paths.

Once this route leaves the park, it meanders through vine and Tustin. The paths are wide, beautifully land- caped and well maintained as they weave through oughtfully designed neighborhoods. As I rode I ound myself daydreaming an entire world without ars, with housing and commerce organized around e bike. Bike nirvana!

The turnaround point for this ride is Incredible Edible Park, a unique place with bike paths throughout and a connecting point with Ride 35. The park is an operational farm that is run by Second Harvest Food Bank with the food grown here helping feed 200,000 people each month. Have a picnic and tour the park; you will see broccoli, beans, lettuce and carrots being grown as well as over 80 citrus trees.

For those looking to complete the Mountain to the Sea route in its entirety, continue along the Harvard Side Path which begins in Incredible Edible Park. From there you will connect to San Diego Creek Trail and follow it to the ocean. That part of the trail is covered in the Central Coast section during Ride 38. One-way, the route is about 22 miles.

Ride Log

P1 Orange County Zoo
P2 Irvine Park Railroad
P3 Peters Canyon Reservoir
P4 Tustin Ranch Golf Course
P5 Harvard Athletic Park
P6 Tustin Sports Park
P7 Harvard Side Path

0.0 Begin ride at Irvine Regional Park, in the parking lot closest to the entrance.

0.11 Turn right and head towards park exit. This road turns into Jamboree Rd.

0.40 Cross Santiago Canyon Rd and move onto the path that runs parallel to Jamboree Rd.

0.63 Cross Chapman Ave.

1.19 Cross Canyon View Ave and ride into Peters Canyon Regional Park.

1.35 Bear right.

1.78 Bear right.

3.08 Turn right, following the Mountains to the Sea signs.

3.25 Turn left onto paved trail.

3.45 Cross Silverado Terrace Rd.

4.09 Cross Pioneer Rd.

4.41 Cross Tustin Ranch to trail that continues along Portola Pkwy.

4.68 Trail turns right and runs along Jamboree Rd.

7.05 Trail turns left at Bryan Ave and crosses over two bridges.

7.13 Continue straight, do not turn left.

7.17 Turn left onto path.

7.20 Double back under bridge.

8.36 Continue straight under El Camino Real.

8.97 Turn right, cross train tracks.

9.01 Cross Harvard Ave and ride into Incredible Edible Park.

9.04 Bear right.

9.16 Turn around.

9.28 Turn left.

9.30 Turn right.

9.33 Cross Harvard Ave and return to trail.

9.90 Bear left and pass under Edinger Ave.

10.47 Bear left and pass under Harvard Ave.

10.74 Bear left and pass under El Camino Real.

11.03 Bear left and pass under Bryan Ave.

11.12 Sharp right towards bridge.

11.16 Turn right and cross over bridges.

11.19 Continue straight.

11.27 Turn right back onto trail.

12.95 In Valencia Park, bear left.

13.61 Path turns right alongside Portola Pkwy.

13.84 Cross Tustin Ranch and continue on path.

14.06 Path turns left.

14.17 Cross Pioneer Rd.

15.01 Turn right off of paved path and into Peters Canyon Park.

15.19 Trail T's, turn left.

17.04 Exit park and cross Canyon View Ave onto trail traveling alongside Jamboree Rd.

17.61 Cross Chapman Ave.

17.83 Cross Santiago Canyon Rd.

18.12 Re-enter Irvine Park.

18.14 Turn left at first street.

18.27 End.

Peters Canyon Trail

Please note: the profile for Ride 25 is depicted in 200ft vertical increments due to unusually high elevation.

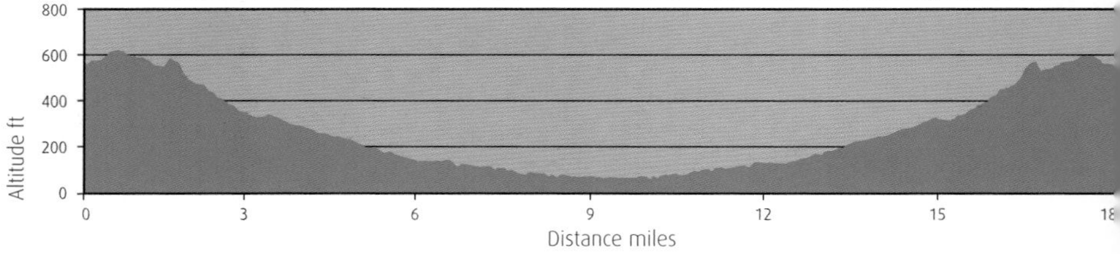

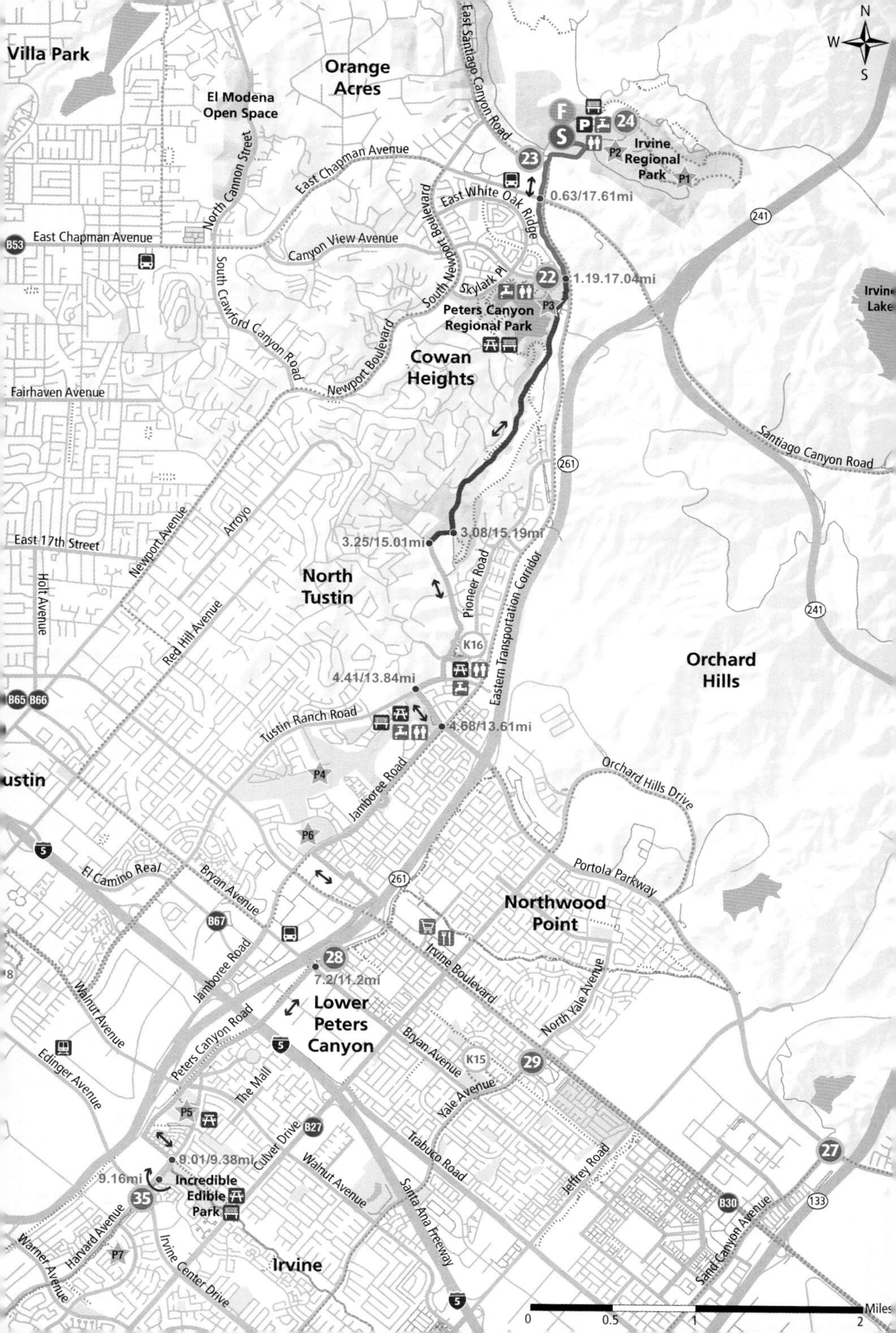
Villa Park
Orange Acres
El Modena Open Space
North Cannon Street
East Santiago Canyon Road
East Chapman Avenue
East White Oak Ridge
0.63/17.61mi
Irvine Regional Park
P1
P2
23
24
F
S
P
241
East Chapman Avenue
B53
Canyon View Avenue
South Newport Boulevard
South Crawford Canyon Road
Skylark Pl
22
1.19.17.04mi
P3
Peters Canyon Regional Park
Irvine Lake
Newport Boulevard
Cowan Heights
Fairhaven Avenue
Santiago Canyon Road
261
Arroyo
Newport Avenue
East 17th Street
3.08/15.19mi
3.25/15.01mi
North Tustin
Pioneer Road
Eastern Transportation Corridor
Holt Avenue
Red Hill Avenue
241
K16
Orchard Hills
4.41/13.84mi
B65
B66
Tustin Ranch Road
4.68/13.61mi
P4
Jamboree Road
Orchard Hills Drive
Tustin
P6
5
Portola Parkway
El Camino Real
Bryan Avenue
261
Northwood Point
B67
Irvine Boulevard
28
7.2/11.2mi
Jamboree Road
Walnut Avenue
Lower Peters Canyon
Peters Canyon Road
North Yale Avenue
Edinger Avenue
5
Bryan Avenue
K15
29
The Mall
Yale Avenue
P5
Culver Drive
B27
27
9.01/9.38mi
Walnut Avenue
Trabuco Road
Jeffrey Road
9.16mi
Incredible Edible Park
35
Santa Ana Freeway
B30
133
Harvard Avenue
Sand Canyon Avenue
Warner Avenue
P7
Irvine Center Drive
Irvine
5
0
0.5
1
2
Miles
N
W
S

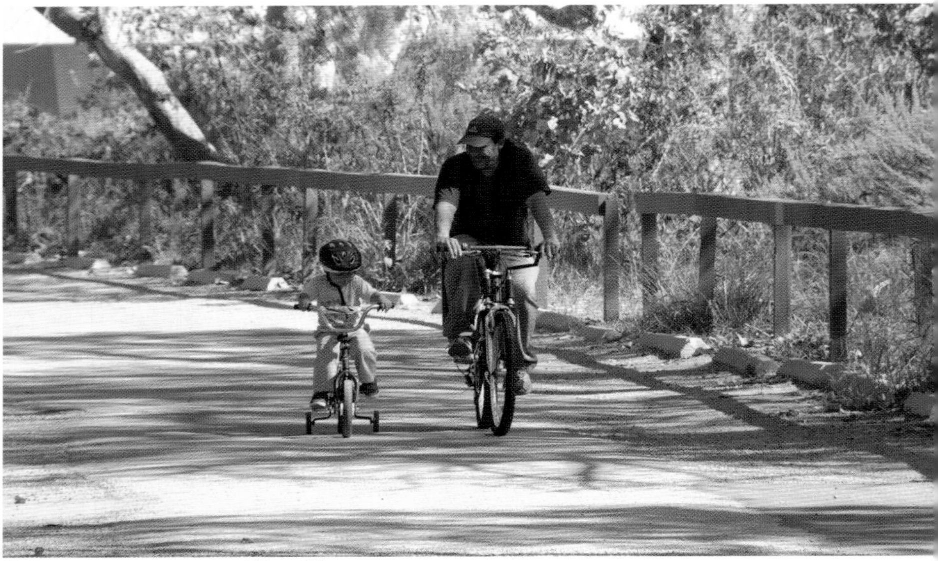

You're never too young to start riding a bike.

At a Glance

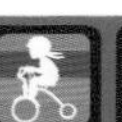
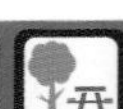

Distance 12.53 miles **Elevation Gain** 459′

Terrain

This ride is mostly flat and travels along a well-maintained bike path, occasionally crossing streets.

Traffic

Virtually car-free, on weekends this route is busy with pedestrians.

How to Get There

By bus, take OCTA 54 to the intersection of Chapman Avenue and Prospect Street. Grijalva Community Park is 0.3 miles to north of bus stop off Prospect Street.

By car, take exit 14, Chapman Avenue, off of California Highway 55. Travel east on Chapman for 0.6 miles then turn left onto Prospect Street. Grijalva Community Park will be on your left.

Food and Drink

The ride turns around at Mainplace Shopping Center which has a number of eateries located within. Th Discovery Science Center has two fast food restauran inside if you plan on visiting. Otherwise, pack a lunc and stop at one of the many parks to enjoy a picnic.

Side Trips

In addition to four distinctly different parks to explor this ride passes through the Santiago Park Nature Pr serve, past the Bowers Museum and the Discovery Sc ence Center, as well as having a turnaround point at th Mainplace Shopping Center in Santa Ana.

Links to 20 21 23 K17 K19    

Where to Bike Rating 

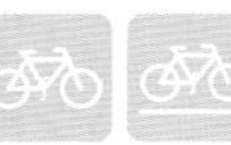  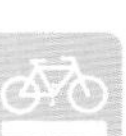  

About...

'he Santiago Creek Trail is a smooth bike path :hat meanders through the Cities of Orange ınd Santa Ana following the creek bed. At imes it passes through wild natural spaces hen manicured, green parks, until ultimately lelivering you to a gigantic shopping center. \long the way there are plenty of diversions on this family ride including two museums, ı number of playgrounds and two long, old-ashioned steel slides the kids will love to zoom lown. You just might be tempted too!

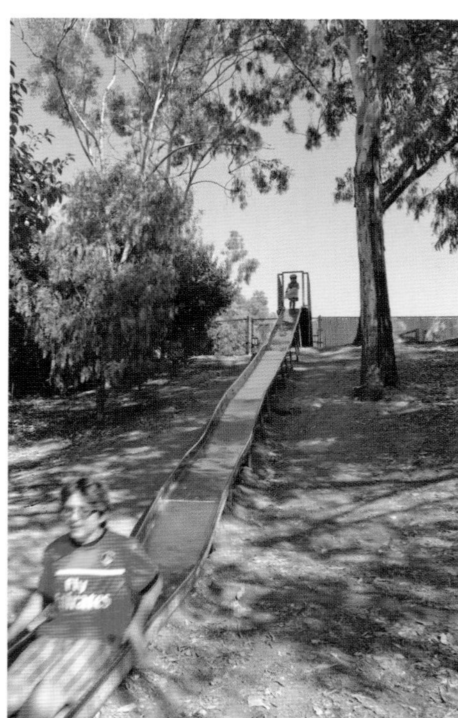

Have you ever seen a slide that long?!

ginning at Grijalva Community Park at one end of : Santiago Creek Trail, this is also the site of Kids' de 17. Even as I write, this trail is expanding north o Villa Park, with the newly completed construction an underpass that comes out alongside Collins Av-ue. From there the route will travel alongside San-go Reservoir and then into the City of Villa Park, atly extending this car-free ride.

After passing through Hart Park, site of Kids' Ride , Santiago Creek enters a wild phase with a natu- stream bed teeming with sycamores, live oaks and ısh. This is the Santiago Creek Nature Preserve and :e you will find a nature center where hikes are or-ıized and interpretive displays provide information out the flora and fauna of the area. Before reaching nature center there are two steel slides almost hid-ı in the hillside. Pick up a patch of rug, sit down and d on tight as you zoom down at high speeds.

The ride's highlights are the two museums located ır the turnaround point. On your left before you ss under Main Street will be the Bowers Museum. e permanent collections here focus on art of Native ıerica, Africa and the Asian Pacific among others 1 the museum has a reputation of offering highly interesting special exhibits. Also at the Bowers is the Kidseum which offers multi-faceted art and cultural experiences for children.

On the other side of Main Street is the popular Discovery Center Museum complete with the giant black cube that towers over it, the cockpit of the Endeavour Space Shuttle, lift rockets and space capsules. Inside the center, kids of all ages will wander through the giant digestive system of a dinosaur, learn how weather systems function, what happens to buildings during earthquakes and how water can reshape mountains. The Discovery Theater offers fun educational movies as well.

And finally, if shopping is your thing, Santiago Creek Trail ends at Mainplace Shopping Center. At this point you will find yourself on busy city streets, passing through a crowded parking lot so exercise caution here.

Ride Log

0.0 Begin where path starts beside the sports center.

0.02 Turn right; do not cross pedestrian bridge yet.

0.63 Bear right.

0.75 Bear left.

0.93 Bear left.

1.43 Follow path as it turns left alongside Hewes St.

2.33 Turn around and return.

3.73 Turn right as path travels alongside Prospect St.

4.03 Bear left.

4.64 Return to start, turn right across pedestrian bridge.

4.66 Turn left onto path. DO NOT turn right.

5.01 Continue straight.

5.37 Follow trail as it crosses pedestrian bridge.

6.06 Continue straight and pass under Tustin St.

6.60 Bear right and pass under Cambridge St.

6.97 Continue straight.

7.06 Turn right. DO NOT continue straight here.

7.21 Continue straight.

7.31 Cross park entrance road, motor traffic has right of way.

7.35 Turn right and cross pedestrian bridge.

7.36 Turn left back onto path.

7.76 Bear left, nature center is located here.

8.04 Cross Lawson Way.

8.15 Cross pedestrian bridge.

8.20 Turn right.

8.33 Bear right and pass under Main St. Bowers Museum on your left.

8.40 Discovery Science Center on your left.

8.52 Continue straight. Do not turn left, unsafe p under bridges.

8.57 Path ends at Mainplace Dr, across the street fr Mainplace Shopping Center. Turn around.

8.93 Bear left and cross bridge.

9.09 Cross Lawson Way.

9.46 In Santiago Park, visit the long slides.

9.76 Turn right, cross pedestrian bridge.

9.82 Cross park entrance.

10.07 Turn left.

10.16 Bear right.

10.44 Bear left under bridge.

10.93 Bear left and pass under bridges.

11.07 Continue straight, watch for blind corner.

11.71 Turn left and cross pedestrian bridge.

12.48 Turn right and cross pedestrian bridge.

12.49 Continue straight.

12.53 End.

P

P1 Discovery Science Center
P2 Bowers Museum
P3 Main Place Mall
P4 Chapman Historic District
P5 Chapman University
P6 Angel Stadium
P7 Santiago Creek Wildlife & Watershed Center, Santiago Park Nature Reserve
P8 Honda Center

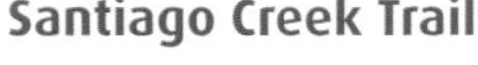

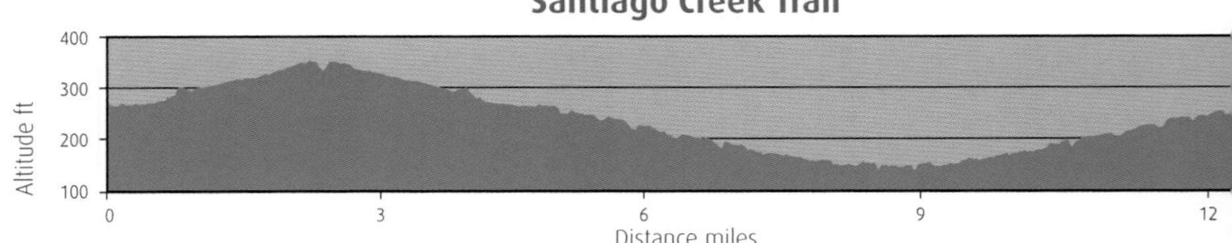

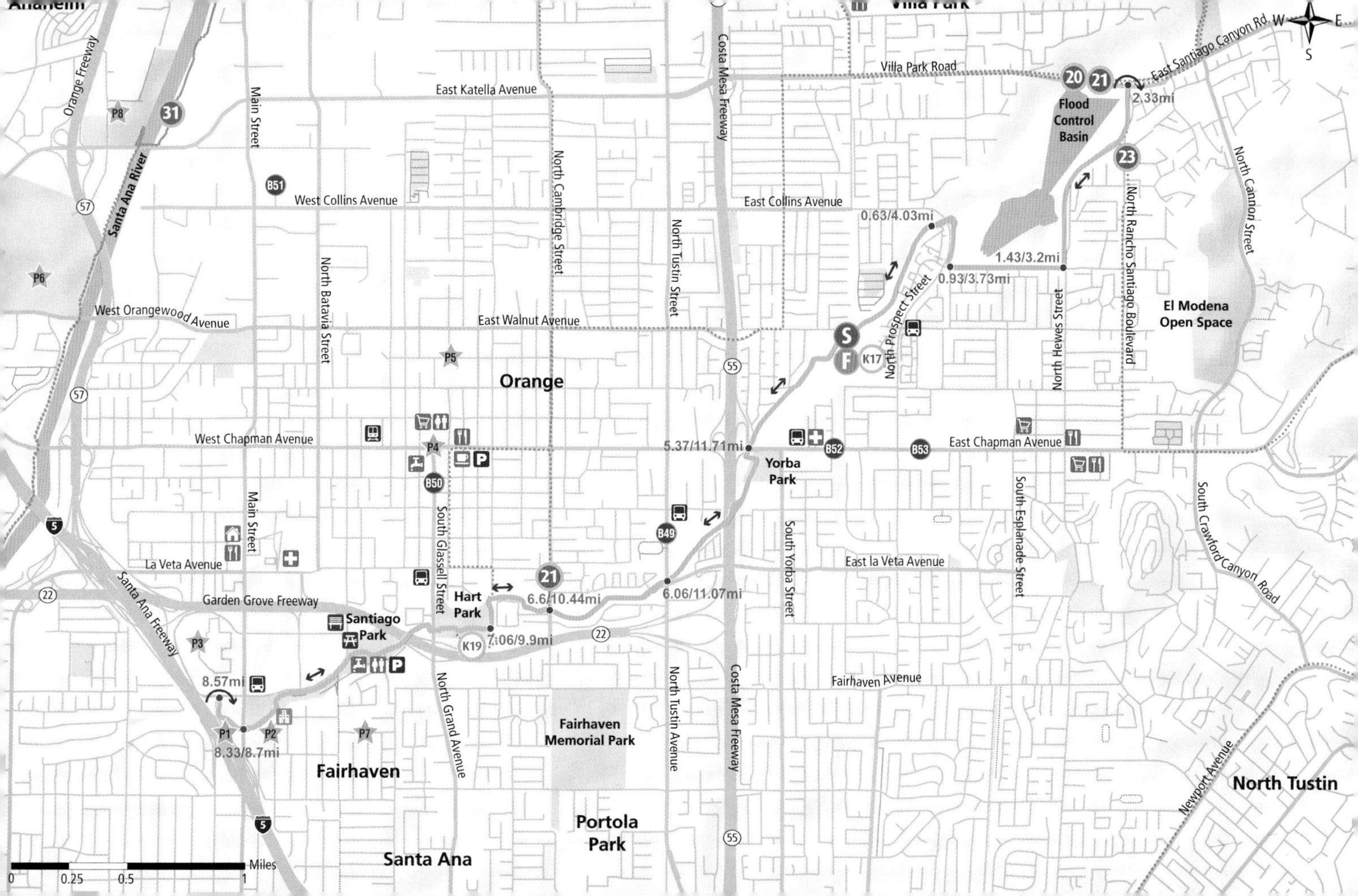

Villa Park Road
East Santiago Canyon Rd.
20
21
2.33mi
Flood Control Basin
23
East Katella Avenue
Orange Freeway
P8
31
Main Street
North Cambridge Street
Costa Mesa Freeway
North Cannon Street
B51
West Collins Avenue
East Collins Avenue
57
Santa Ana River
0.63/4.03mi
North Tustin Street
North Batavia Street
1.43/3.2mi
0.93/3.73mi
North Rancho Santiago Boulevard
P6
West Orangewood Avenue
East Walnut Avenue
North Prospect Street
El Modena Open Space
S
F
K17
North Hewes Street
P5
Orange
55
West Chapman Avenue
P4
5.37/11.71mi
B52
B53
East Chapman Avenue
Yorba Park
B50
South Glassell Street
South Esplanade Street
South Crawford Canyon Road
5
B49
South Yorba Street
La Veta Avenue
East la Veta Avenue
22
Santa Ana Freeway
Garden Grove Freeway
Hart Park
6.6/10.44mi
6.06/11.07mi
Santiago Park
P3
K19
7.06/9.9mi
8.57mi
Fairhaven Avenue
North Grand Avenue
North Tustin Avenue
P1
P2
P7
8.33/8.7mi
Fairhaven Memorial Park
Fairhaven
Newport Avenue
North Tustin
Portola Park
Santa Ana
Miles
0
0.25
0.5
1

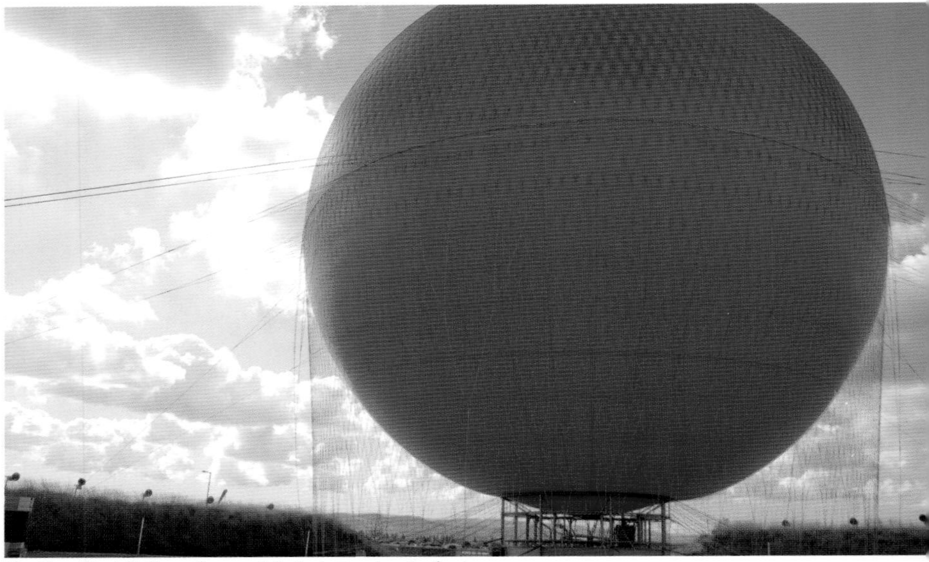
The Great Park Balloon. You won't find a better view for free!

At a Glance

Distance 15.85 miles **Elevation Gain** 762′

Terrain

This ride travels a combination of bike paths and on-road bike lanes, starting with a long downhill and ending with a moderate climb back to the start.

Traffic

This region of Orange County is not heavily populated and traffic is relatively light. The intersections with Interstates 5 and 405 are the exceptions and traffic can be high here.

How to Get There

By car, take exit 25 off of CA-241, a toll road. Head north 0.1 miles and park in the Portola staging area.

Food and Drink

Your best dining options are in the Quail Hill Village Center which has a number of dining options, located at 7.0 miles. Try Lucca Café, a deli that focuses on organic produce and meats or Thai Bamboo is an exc lent choice. Quail Hill Community Park is an attracti park to picnic with a view.

Side Trip

The ride's start is at the edge of Limestone Canyon a Whiting Ranch Parks, two contiguous wildernes that cover a combined 4,300 acres. The Orange Cou Great Park is a short detour off the middle section the ride and at the other end, park the bikes and h the Quail Hill Loop.

Links to 

Where to Bike Rating 

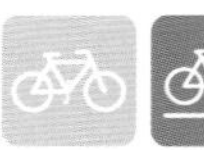    

About...

This is a big connecting ride that runs through the heart of northern Irvine. There are so many on-street bike paths through this region that the variations of this route are endless. For those looking for a mostly flat loop along well-maintained, wide bike paths, this fits the bill nicely. As new neighborhoods are developed along these roads, look for more cycling opportunities to appear.

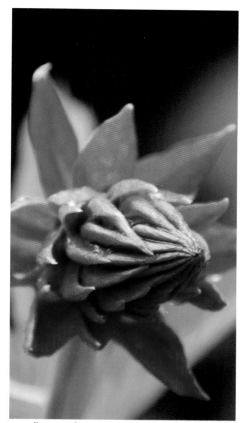

Fearsome flowers can be found in Jeffrey Open Space.

The ride starts at Northwood Community Park, site of the Kids' Ride 15 and from here makes its way to Irvine Boulevard. At 1.21 miles the trailhead for Jeffrey Open Space Trail will be on your right. Although only a bit longer than a mile, riders who visit this trail can get a taste of the future. The concept behind this open space corridor is that it will one day be a 20 mile, north-south connector route that starts at Portola Parkway and travels all the way to Quail Hill and eventually from there to Crystal Cove State Park on the coast. Beautifully landscaped, environmentally friendly, this is what bike routes of the not too distant future will look like in Irvine. Take your time to explore the side routes, read the interpretive signs and examine the well thought out design.

After passing Sand Canyon Avenue, you will find yourself navigating a long stretch of emptiness as Irvine Boulevard passes through what was once El Toro Marine Corp Base, and in the future is to become the Orange County Great Park. The landscape along this section seems to be in transition, caught somewhere between civilization and ruin, development and wilderness. What this means for the cyclist is wide open roads with few stoppages and almost no traffic. Keep in mind that once you cross Sand Canyon Avenue, there are no parks, water sources or restrooms. Make sure everything is in order before setting out.

At 6.97 miles this route interlocks with Ride 34 of the Central Coast section, a looping ride through the well-developed heart of the City of Irvine. By connecting here you could ride a 31 mile, grand tour of the city, extensively exploring the cycling portion of Irvine's transit system.

At 11.05 miles the route crosses Jeffrey Road again, and on your right is the Irvine Village Center where you will find Paradise Perks Coffee and Teas, a quirky, comfortable place to fuel up. Also in this center are Thai, Indian and Japanese restaurants.

Ride Log

P1 Jeffrey Open Space Trail
P2 Great Park Balloon Ride
P3 Irvine Spectrum Center
P4 North Lake
P5 South Lake
P6 Irvine Fine Arts Center
P7 Quail Hill trailhead
P8 Irvine Valley College

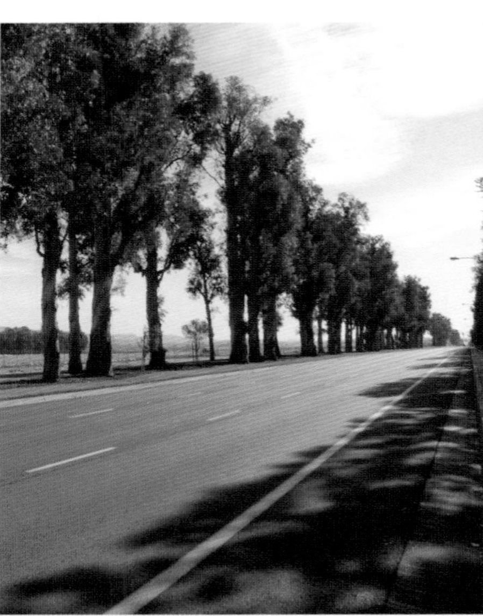

Eucalyptus trees stand at attention along Irvine Boulevard.

0.0 Begin this ride at the corner of Yale and Bryan av-enues, across the street from Northwood Communit[y] Park.

0.48 Turn right onto Irvine Blvd.

1.21 Cross Jeffrey Rd, Jeffrey Open Space Trail en-trance on the right.

2.16 Cross Sand Canyon Ave.

2.33 Cross over Hwy 133, watch for traffic.

5.39 Turn right onto Alton Pkwy.

6.97 Cross Barranca Pkwy.

7.97 Coffee and bagel shops located in shopping cen-er to the left.

8.16 Bike path intersects with Interstate 5 entrance watch for traffic.

8.61 Turn right onto Irvine Center Dr.

8.88 Cross Barranca Pkwy.

9.93 Sand Canyon Cyclery on your left.

10.05 Cross Sand Canyon Ave.

10.29 Cross Valley Oak Dr.

11.05 Cross Jeffrey Rd.

11.77 Turn right onto Yale Ave.

12.77 Cross Walnut Ave.

13.29 Cross Trabuco Rd.

13.57 Cross Southwood Rd.

13.82 Cross Bryan Ave.

13.85 End.

Irvine Loop - Irvine Boulevard, Alton Parkway, Irvine Center Drive

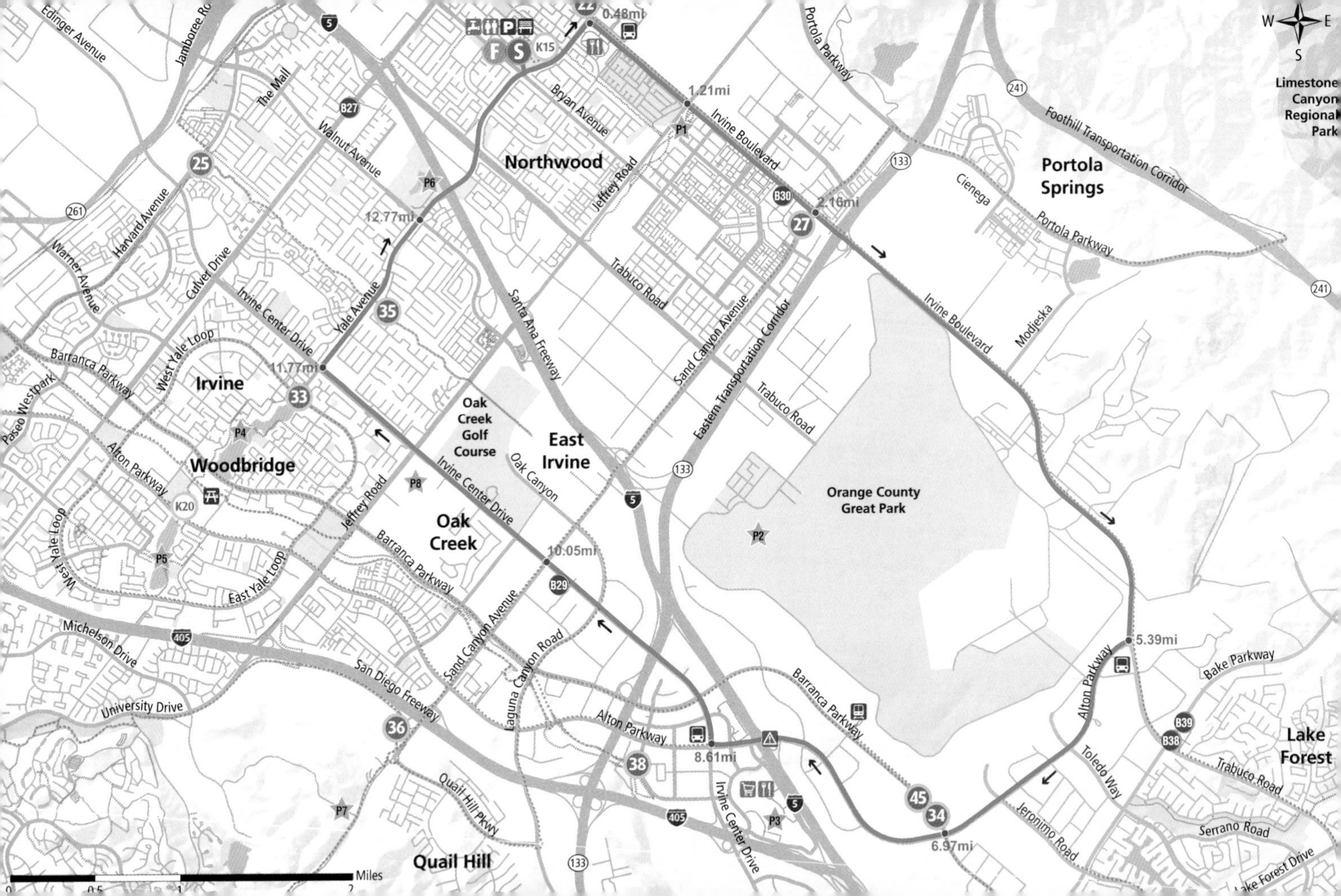

Northwood
Portola Springs
Limestone Canyon Regional Park
Irvine
Woodbridge
East Irvine
Oak Creek
Oak Creek Golf Course
Orange County Great Park
Lake Forest
Quail Hill
Irvine Boulevard
Irvine Center Drive
Alton Parkway
Barranca Parkway
Trabuco Road
Sand Canyon Avenue
Jeffrey Road
Yale Avenue
Walnut Avenue
Bryan Avenue
Culver Drive
Harvard Avenue
Warner Avenue
Edinger Avenue
Jamboree Ro
The Mall
West Yale Loop
East Yale Loop
Paseo Westpark
Michelson Drive
University Drive
San Diego Freeway
Santa Ana Freeway
Eastern Transportation Corridor
Foothill Transportation Corridor
Portola Parkway
Cienega
Modjeska
Oak Canyon
Laguna Canyon Road
Quail Hill Pkwy
Bake Parkway
Toledo Way
Jeronimo Road
Serrano Road
Lake Forest Drive
0.48mi
1.21mi
2.16mi
5.39mi
6.97mi
8.61mi
10.05mi
11.77mi
12.77mi
Miles
0
0.5
1
2

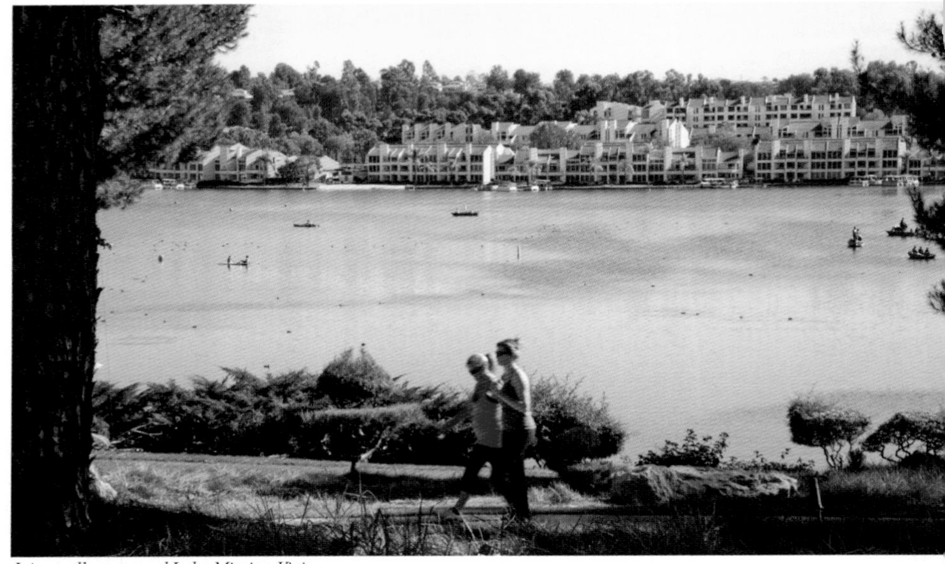

Join strollers around Lake Mission Viejo.

At a Glance

Distance 17.54 miles **Elevation Gain** 1033′

Terrain

This is a hilly ride, at times steep, along on-road bike lanes.

Traffic

There is moderate traffic for most of this ride with heavier traffic around Lake Mission Viejo.

How to Get There

By bus, OCTA 84 makes a stop at the corner of Antonio and Margarita parkways. Begin ride here or head a half mile north along Antonio Parkway to Trabuco Mesa Park.

By car, take exit 19, Santa Margarita Parkway off of toll road CA-241 and head west. After 0.5 miles turn left onto Avenida de las Flores and travel for 1.4 miles, Trabuco Mesa Park will be on your right.

Food and Drink

Located at the corner of Antonio and Santa Margarit parkways is a shopping center with a number of dinin opportunities.

Side Trip

Along this ride you will pass Lake Mission Viej which is a pleasant place to picnic. Near the ride's star is O'Neill Regional Park, a vast green space, much o it in a natural state that offers opportunities to hike an bike throughout.

Links to 22 44 45

Where to Bike Rating 

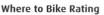

About...

This ride loops through Rancho Santa Margarita, one of Orange County's youngest cities, and Mission Viejo, one of the earliest of the "master planned" communities that Orange County has become known for. The ride is characterized by broad parkways that wind along high ridges before dipping into canyons below. Easy downhills are followed by long steady climbs, all of which make for a modestly challenging, enjoyable ride.

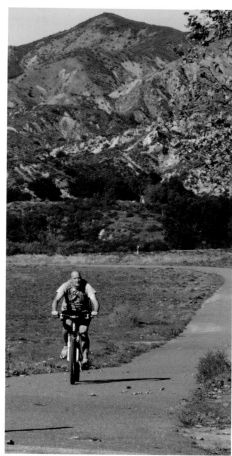

The Live Oak Canyon Trail will allow you to explore O'Neill Regional Park.

he ride begins at Trabuco Mesa Park, an attractive ɔace with many amenities. Located just north of the ark, where Antonio Parkway ends, is the Live Oak anyon Trail, part of Ride 44, which runs alongside ıd into O'Neill Regional Park. Where the trail paral-ls the park it is mostly flat before turning into the can-ɔn along a steeper section. Once in the park, the trail ɔnnects to a number of others, most of which are bet-r suited to hikers, mountain bikers and equestrians. ncompassing 3,358 acres of canyons and hillsides, is park offers much to explore.

The first leg of this ride along Antonio Parkway is eadily downhill. For most of this descent neighbor-ɔods will pass on your right while natural, untouched llsides pass on your left. The road and bike lanes are ide through here and lightly traveled. Near the bot-m, along Oso Parkway, the route is flanked by de-loped hillsides as it crosses over Trabuco Canyon. xpect traffic to pick up through this section.

At 10.92 miles, while traveling along Margeurite ırkway, the route passes Lake Mission Viejo, a man-ade reservoir. Although residency in the city is re-ıired to be on the lake or its beaches, non-members n walk the paths around the lake. At the top of Marguerite Parkway the route turns right onto Santa Margarita Parkway, the steepest section of the ride.

At 16.95 miles, just before reaching Antonio Parkway, the route passes Lago Santa Margarita. This manmade lake stretches over 11.5 acres and is stocked year round with bass, bluegill and catfish and although swimming is not allowed, boating and fishing are. The walk around the lake is a picturesque 1.1 miles. The shopping center next to the Lago has a number of restaurants. Carmelitas offers Mexican fare and Wings Bar and Grill offers casual food with lots of beer choices. Both come with a view of the lake.

Ride Log

P1 Live Oak Canyon Trail
P2 Lago Santa Margarita
P3 Mission Viejo City Hall
P4 Mission Viejo Youth Athletic Park
P5 Aliso Creek Bikeway
P6 Florence Joyner Olympiad Park
P7 Rancho Santa Margarita Hall

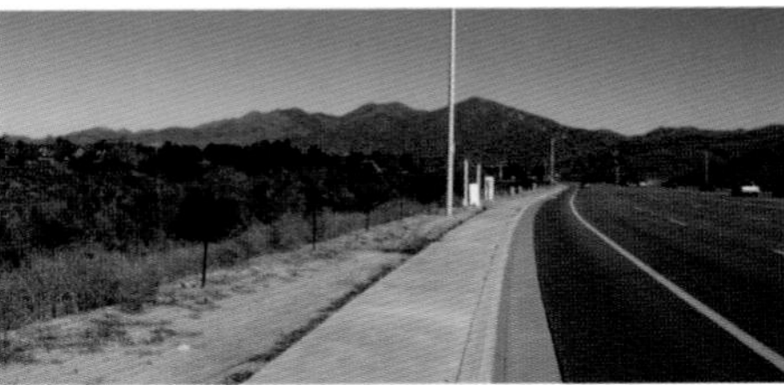

Canyons, mountains and bike lanes make this a picturesque ride.

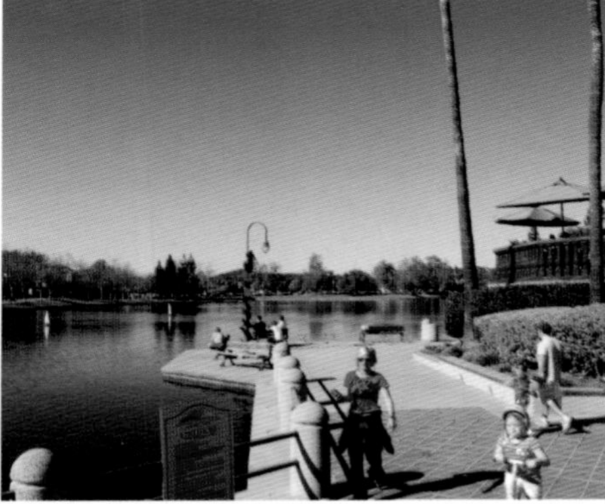

Lago Santa Margarita has lakefront dining options and a 1.1 mile boardwalk tailor made for an after meal walk.

0.0 Begin ride on Antonio Pkwy, across from Trabuc Mesa Park.

0.38 Cross Santa Margarita Pkwy.

1.27 Cross Coto de Caza Dr.

2.10 Crossing over Hwy 241, watch for traffic.

2.44 Cross AvenidaEmpresa.

3.11 Cross Avenida de las Banderas.

5.94 Turn right onto Oso Pkwy.

6.88 Cross Felipe Rd.

7.76 Turn right onto Marguerite Pkwy.

8.67 Cross La Paz Rd.

9.40 Cross Jeronimo Rd.

9.85 Cross Trabuco Rd.

10.92 Cross Alicia Pkwy, Lake Mission Viejo on you right.

11.41 Cross Vista del Lago. Public access to the lak is along this road.

11.94 Cross Olympiad Rd.

12.69 Turn right onto Santa Margarita Pkwy.

13.76 Melinda Park on your right, this is a good plac to break if needed.

13.91 Cross Melinda Way.

14.51 Cross Alicia Pkwy.

15.17 Cross Avenida Impresa.

16.97 Turn left onto Antonio Pkwy.

17.54 End.

Rancho Margarita Loop

Please note: the profile for Ride 30 is depicted in 250ft vertical increments due to unusually high elevation.

Altitude ft: 1250, 1000, 750, 500, 250

Distance miles: 0, 3, 6, 9, 12, 15, 1

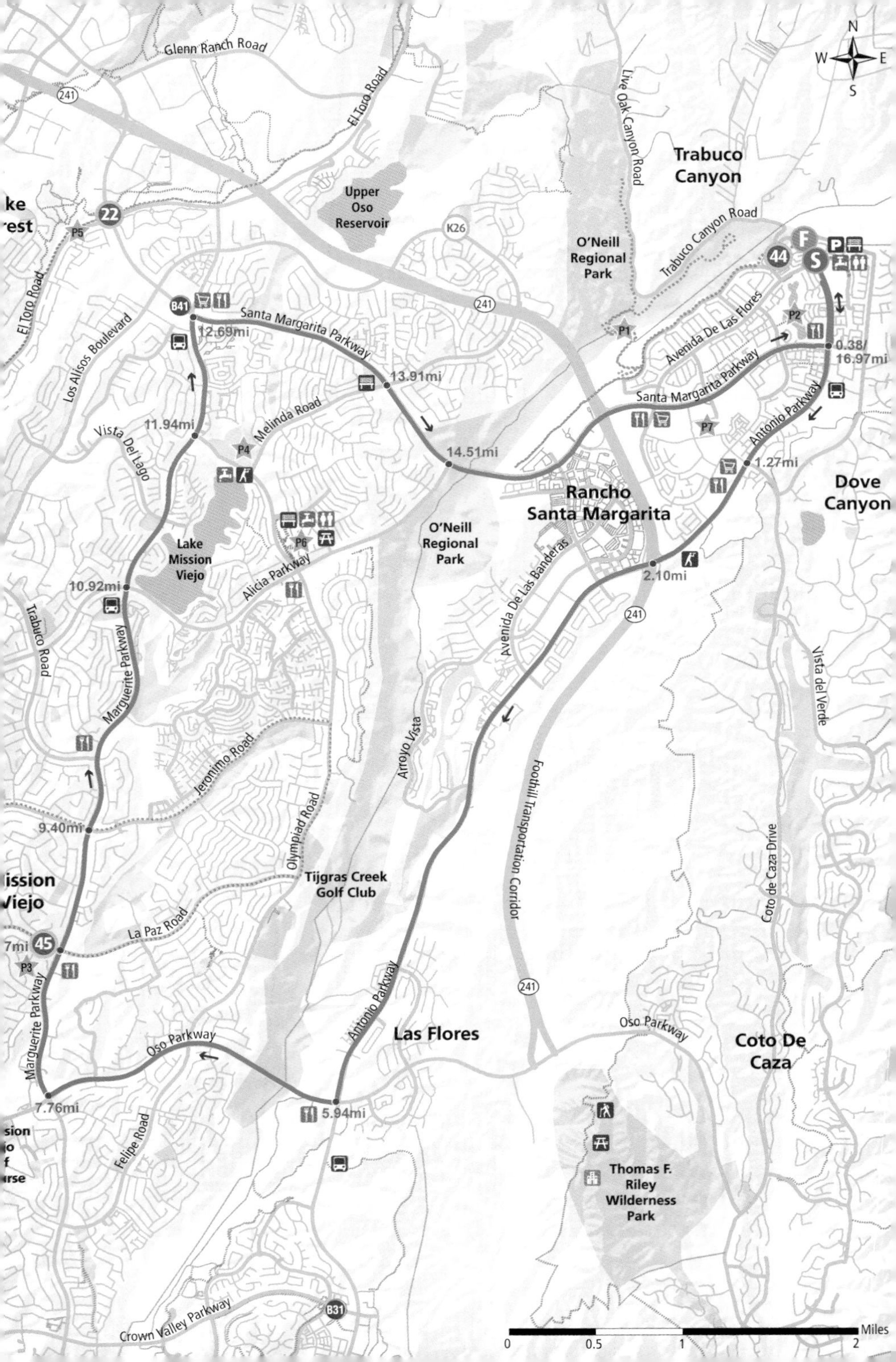

N
W
E
S
Glenn Ranch Road
El Toro Road
Live Oak Canyon Road
Trabuco Canyon
Upper Oso Reservoir
K26
241
22
P5
ke
rest
Trabuco Canyon Road
O'Neill Regional Park
F
S
44
P
B41
12.69mi
Santa Margarita Parkway
P1
P2
Avenida De Las Flores
0.38/
16.97mi
El Toro Road
Los Alisos Boulevard
13.91mi
Melinda Road
Santa Margarita Parkway
11.94mi
Vista Del Lago
P4
14.51mi
Antonio Parkway
P7
1.27mi
Dove Canyon
Rancho Santa Margarita
Lake Mission Viejo
P6
O'Neill Regional Park
Alicia Parkway
Avenida De Las Banderas
2.10mi
10.92mi
Trabuco Road
Marguerite Parkway
Vista del Verde
Jeronimo Road
Arroyo Vista
Olympiad Road
Foothill Transportation Corridor
9.40mi
ission
Viejo
Tijgras Creek Golf Club
Coto de Caza Drive
La Paz Road
7mi
45
P3
Marguerite Parkway
Antonio Parkway
Oso Parkway
Las Flores
Oso Parkway
Coto De Caza
7.76mi
5.94mi
Felipe Road
sion
jo
f
urse
Thomas F. Riley Wilderness Park
Crown Valley Parkway
B31
Miles
0
0.5
1
2

Central Coast

This section is made up of coastal flood plains, rivers and bays with hilly sections to the southeast. Bounded by the Santa Ana River to the west, Interstate 5 to the north and east, this is the part of Orange County made famous by television shows and has often been referred to as the Gold Coast. Affluent seaside neighborhoods edge coastal cliffs and marinas, while inland attractive planned-communities define the California suburban lifestyle. This is probably the most bicycle-friendly part of the county and it shows in the hundreds of miles of bike paths and lanes woven across the landscape.

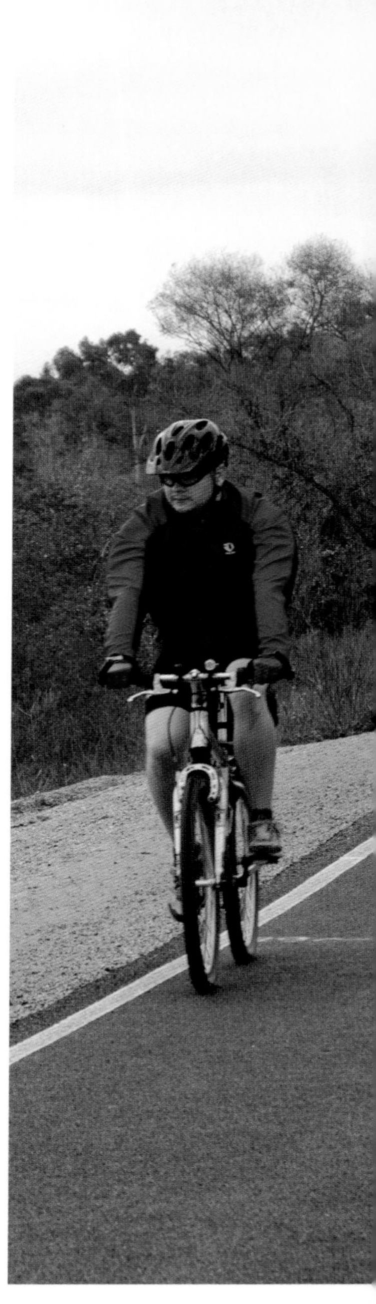

The Santa Ana River is the largest river in Southern California, spanning four counties before spilling into the Pacific Ocean. The Santa Ana River Trail, Ride 31, runs 30 miles along the river and plans are in the works to expand another 40 miles. Whether ridden for recreation, training or commuting, this bustling route has earned its nickname as Orange County's bicycle superhighway.

For those looking for panoramic rides along off-road bikes paths, this section has more than its fair share. Loop around Newport Beach's breathtaking Back Bay on Ride 39, or bring a date and explore Balboa Peninsula on Ride 41. San Diego Creek is the lower portion of the Mountain to the Seas Trail and is an excellent route for riders of all abilities. Shady Canyon Trail, Ride 36, spins nearly 14 miles through parks and wilderness as you climb into the San Joaquin Hills before looping through Irvine and back to William R. Mason Regional Park. For spectacular ocean views and pristine beaches to lounge upon, Ride 42 explores Crystal Cove State Beach, a short ride that will provide all-day fun.

With over 301 miles of bike lanes and paths, the City of Irvine leads the way in bicycling infrastructure; you could plot dozens of safe rides in this city alone. Well planned and maintained, this web of bike lanes allows cyclists to access every nook and cranny of the city. Ride 37 tours the University of California, Irvine campus while connecting the Turtle Rock neighborhood. Take in a giant cross section of the city on Ride 34, a long loop perfect for commuting and training that travels Alton and Barranca parkways. Walnut Bike Trail, Ride 35, is a car-free ride that traverses Incredible Edible Park and is a safe, fun outing for families looking to build up mileage.

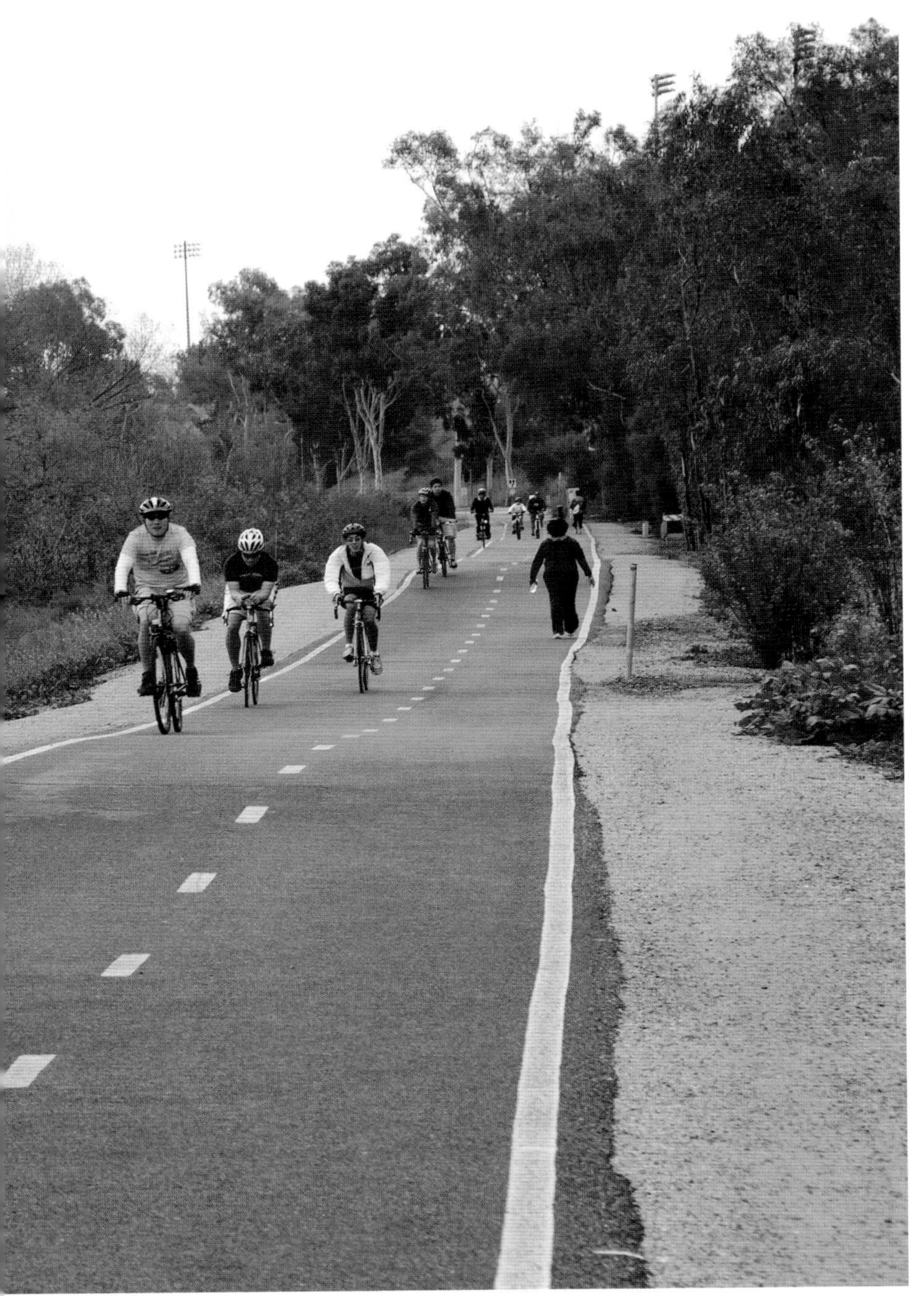

Central Coast

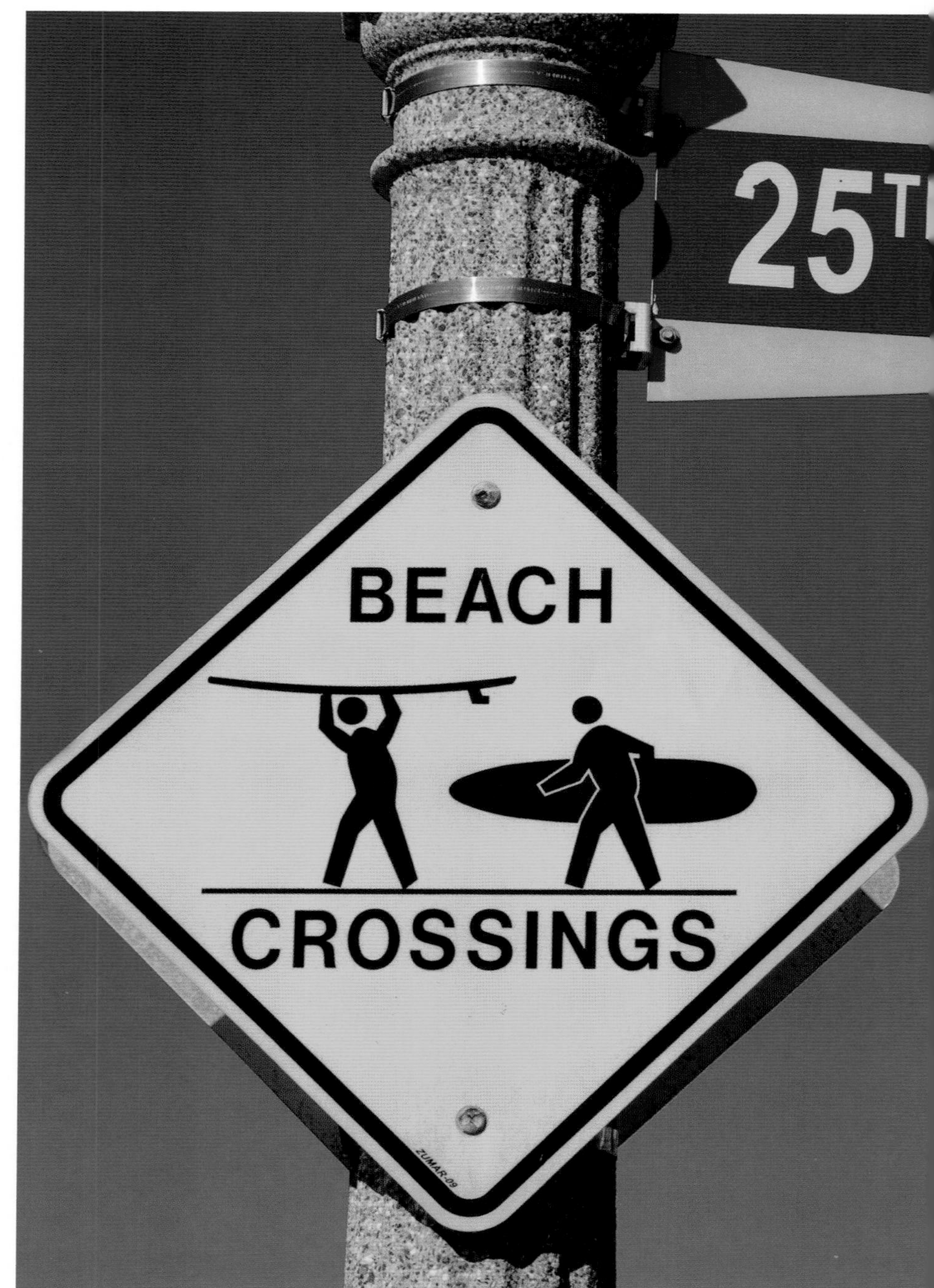
25T
BEACH
CROSSINGS
ZUMAR-09

Central Coast Overview

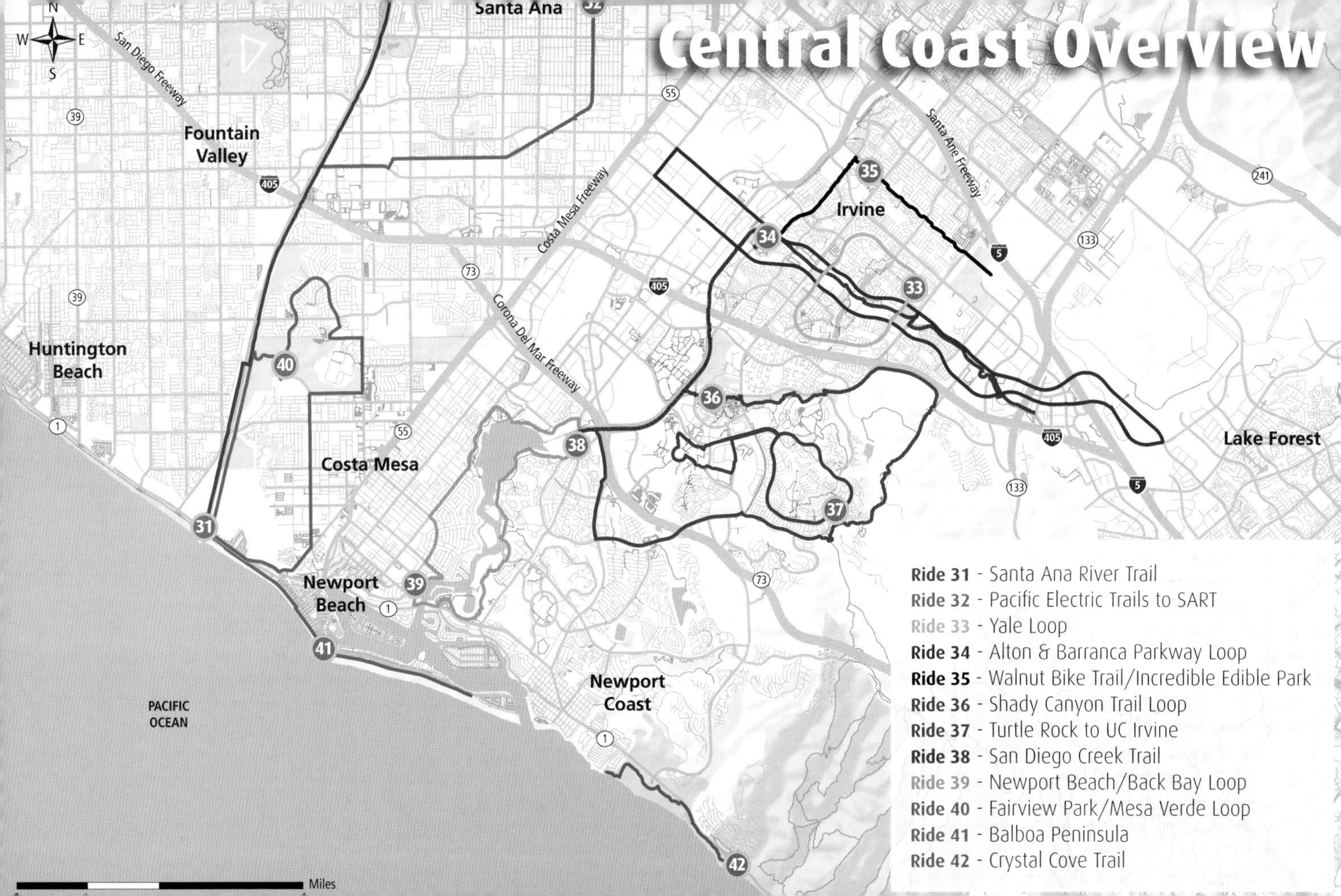

Santa Ana
Fountain Valley
Huntington Beach
Costa Mesa
Newport Beach
Newport Coast
Irvine
Lake Forest
PACIFIC OCEAN
San Diego Freeway
Costa Mesa Freeway
Corona Del Mar Freeway
Santa Ane Freeway
Miles
N
S
E
W
Ride 31 - Santa Ana River Trail
Ride 32 - Pacific Electric Trails to SART
Ride 33 - Yale Loop
Ride 34 - Alton & Barranca Parkway Loop
Ride 35 - Walnut Bike Trail/Incredible Edible Park
Ride 36 - Shady Canyon Trail Loop
Ride 37 - Turtle Rock to UC Irvine
Ride 38 - San Diego Creek Trail
Ride 39 - Newport Beach/Back Bay Loop
Ride 40 - Fairview Park/Mesa Verde Loop
Ride 41 - Balboa Peninsula
Ride 42 - Crystal Cove Trail

No cars, but plenty of pedestrians.

At a Glance

Distance 43.79 miles **Elevation Gain** 1118′

Terrain

This route travels entirely over bike paths. Although there is some climbing, it is mostly long, low-grade elevation.

Traffic

Car-free, this trail is very popular and you will find it carries quite a bit of pedestrian traffic.

How to Get There

By bus, OCTA route 1 and 33 both makes stops at the Huntington Beach State Park, near the start.

By car, take Pacific Coast Highway to the Brookhurst Street and turn into Huntington Beach State Park. Turn left upon entering and drive to the most southerly parking lot.

Food and Drink

While there are a number of parks along the route to re-fill water bottles, there is no easily accessible dinin option. Near the ride's start is colorful Main Street Huntington Beach, and in the other direction you will fin options along Pacific Coast Highway in Newport Beach

Side Trip

This ride travels past Talbert Regional Park which i an attractive nature preserve. At the turnaround poin is Yorba Regional Park with miles of bike paths running around lakes, all shaded by mature pines an sycamores.

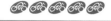

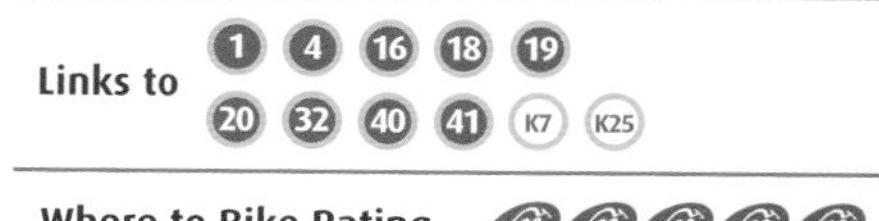

Where to Bike Rating

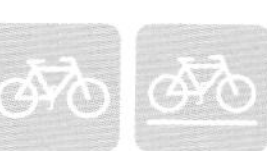

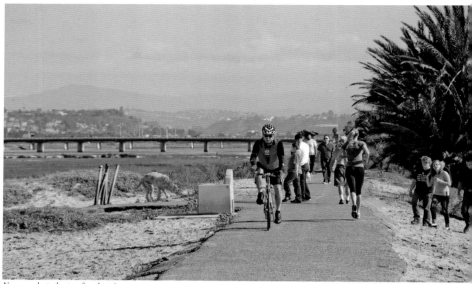
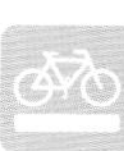

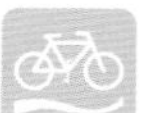

About...

This route, which starts near downtown Santa Ana, whisks you alternately past residential homes, gritty industrial buildings, alongside actual railroad tracks and trains, then through a commercial zone until finally connecting to the Santa Ana River Trail. The Pacific Electric Bicycle Trail is a reminder of the Red Line that once connected Orange County to the distant city of Los Angeles.

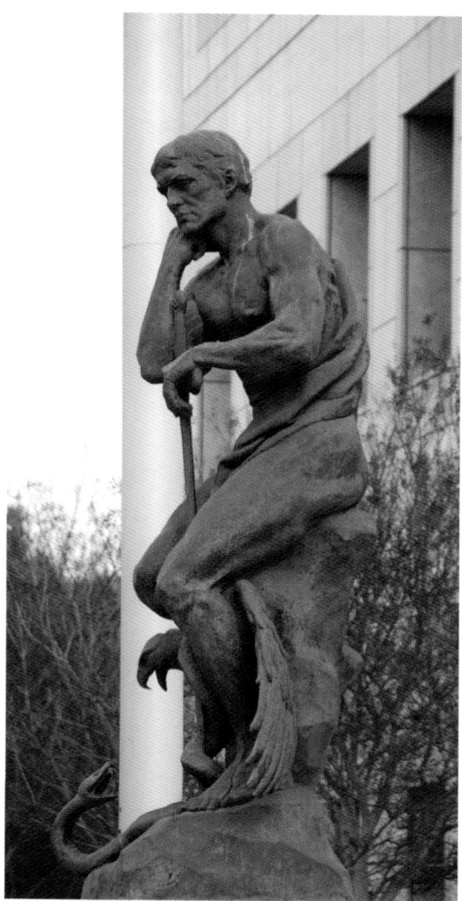

Santa Ana has a vibrant art scene.

'he oldest incorporated city in Orange County, Santa na is also the county seat. Densely populated by com- ercial, retail and residential buildings, downtown anta Ana is home to a vibrant arts and nightlife scene 'ith numerous galleries and dining opportunities. The layground will challenge your taste buds with their astronomic debauchery, located at Fourth and Spur- eon streets. More casual and comfy, the Gypsy Den : 125 North Broadway is located a few blocks away. he promenade along Second Street is the focal point f much of the art scene and in constant flux. There e still a number of buildings that date to the city's ounding. The Howe-Waffle House, a beautiful Victo- an home once owned by prominent physicians, is an xcellent example and is open for tours.

The first 1.8 miles of this route passes through resi- ential neighborhoods and is often crossed by smaller reets. This section can be hazardous as it is not al- ays clear who has the right of way; exercise caution. trollers and joggers also use this path which at times n be rather narrow.

The path quickly passes into a more urban environ- ent as you find yourself traveling alongside com- ercial freight lines. Industry and concrete line the ail. At 2.92 miles the route forks and you will want make certain to turn right and cross the pedestrian bridge. Traveling straight here will leave you stranded at a dangerously busy six lane road without bike lanes.

At 5.16 miles, after traveling along Susan Avenue, the route reaches MacArthur Boulevard. Signs here can be confusing regarding the bike lane. The sidewalk is a designated bike path. Although narrow at first, the sidewalk soon broadens into a more typical bike path. It is not recommended that cyclists travel on the road as there is absolutely no shoulder to ride along. At 6.13 this route intersects with the Santa Ana River Trail and for those looking to add mileage, head south to beach or ride north into the Santa Ana Mountains.

Ride Log

P1 Downtown Santa Ana
P2 Ronald Reagan Federal Building
P3 Old Orange County Courthouse
P4 Santa Ana Zoo
P5 South Coast Plaza
P6 Santa Ana River Trail

0.0 Begin ride at the corner of Maple St and Chestnut Ave.
0.34 Cross Wakeham Ave.
0.61 Cross McFadden Ave.
1.84 Cross Warner Ave.
2.10 At the intersection of Adams and Orange streets cross to the opposite corner.
2.13 Turn right, back onto bike path.
2.26 Turn left and move towards crosswalk.
2.30 Cross Main St and return to bike path.
2.67 Cross Dyer Rd, then bear right to return to path.
2.92 Turn right at pedestrian bridge, do not continue straight.
2.93 Cross Flower St.
3.42 Continue straight, then bear right along Alton Ave.
3.49 Cross Bristol St.
3.87 Cross Bear St.
4.17 Cross Raitt St.
4.55 Cross Greenville St.
4.77 Cross Fairview St.
5.02 Bike path ends, turn left onto Susan St which ha an on-street bike path.
5.16 Turn right onto MacArthur Blvd bike path.
5.54 Cross Harbor Blvd.
6.05 Bear right towards Santa Ana River Trail.
6.13 Turn around.
6.70 Cross Harbor Blvd.
7.09 Turn left onto Susan Ave.
7.24 Turn right back onto bike path that runs besid Alton Ave.
7.47 Cross Fairview St.
7.69 Cross Greenville St.
8.37 Cross Bear St.
8.74 Cross Bristol St.
8.83 Bear left and follow path away from Alton Ave.
9.32 Cross Flower St then cross pedestrian bridge.
9.34 Turn left.
9.54 Bear right and cross Dyer St.
9.58 Bear right back onto trail.
9.93 Cross Main St.
9.96 Turn left then bear right back onto trail.
10.11 Turn left and cross to far corner to resume alon trail.
10.42 Cross Warner Ave.
11.17 Cross Edinger Ave.
11.63 Cross McFadden Ave.
12.25 End.

Pacific Electric Trails to SART

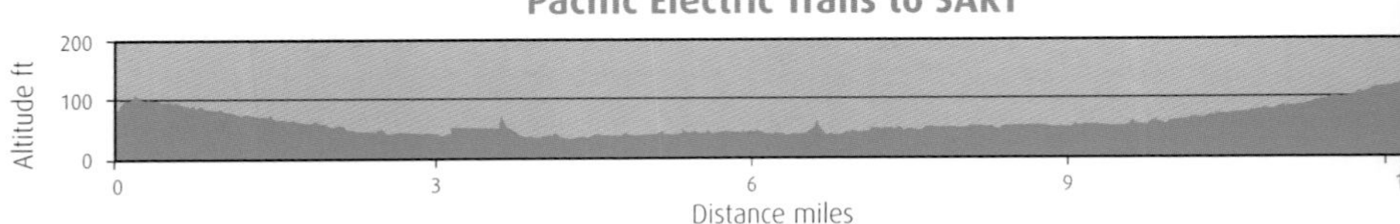

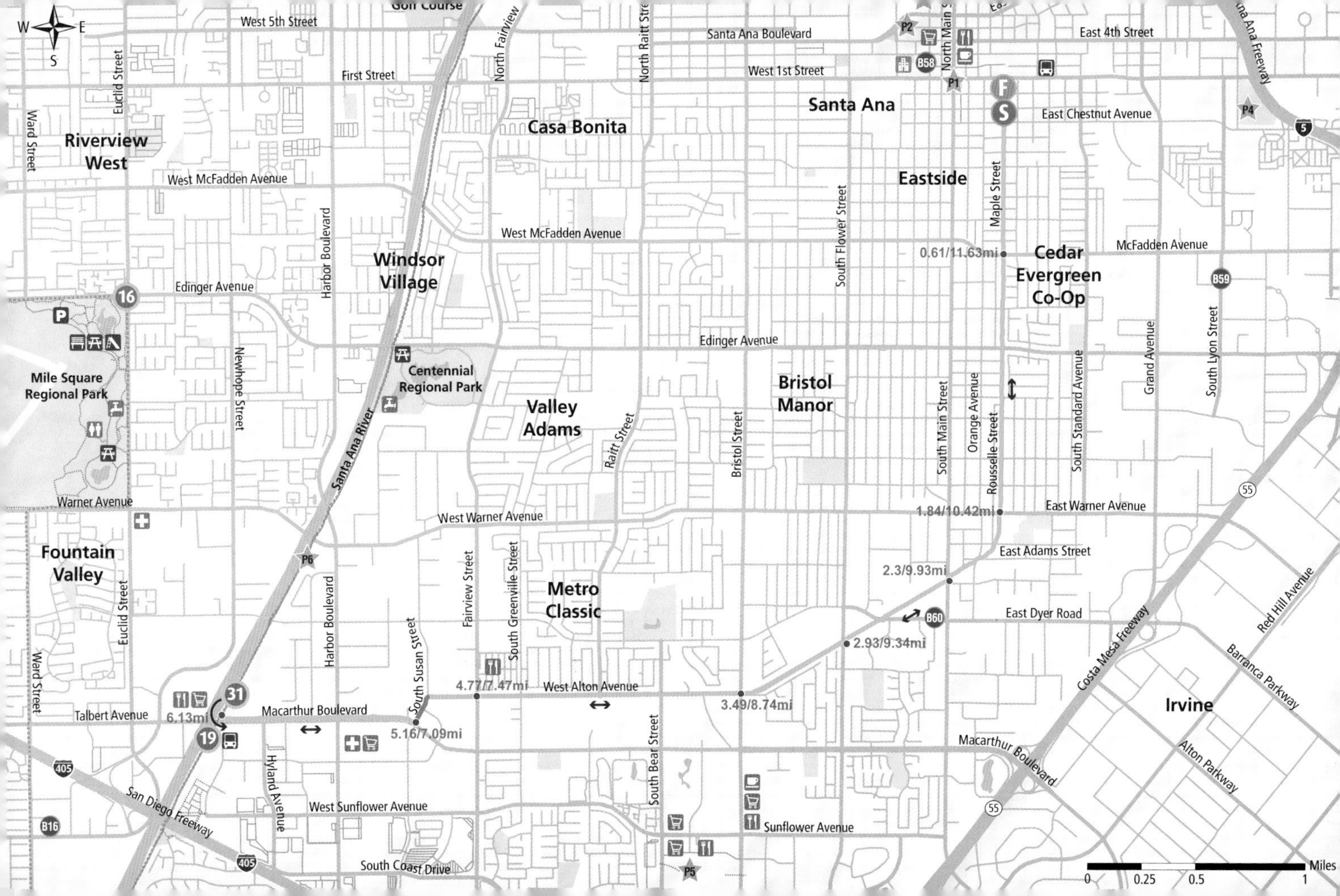

Santa Ana
Eastside
Cedar Evergreen Co-Op
Casa Bonita
Riverview West
Windsor Village
Valley Adams
Bristol Manor
Metro Classic
Fountain Valley
Irvine
Mile Square Regional Park
Centennial Regional Park
Santa Ana River
West 5th Street
First Street
West 1st Street
Santa Ana Boulevard
East 4th Street
East Chestnut Avenue
West McFadden Avenue
McFadden Avenue
Edinger Avenue
Warner Avenue
West Warner Avenue
East Warner Avenue
East Adams Street
East Dyer Road
West Alton Avenue
Talbert Avenue
Macarthur Boulevard
West Sunflower Avenue
Sunflower Avenue
South Coast Drive
Ward Street
Euclid Street
Newhope Street
Harbor Boulevard
Hyland Avenue
North Fairview
Fairview Street
South Susan Street
South Greenville Street
Raitt Street
North Raitt Street
South Bear Street
Bristol Street
South Flower Street
South Main Street
North Main Street
Orange Avenue
Rousselle Street
Maple Street
South Standard Avenue
Grand Avenue
South Lyon Street
Costa Mesa Freeway
San Diego Freeway
Red Hill Avenue
Barranca Parkway
Alton Parkway
0.61/11.63mi
1.84/10.42mi
2.3/9.93mi
2.93/9.34mi
3.49/8.74mi
4.77/7.47mi
5.16/7.09mi
6.13mi
Miles
0
0.25
0.5
1
W
E
S

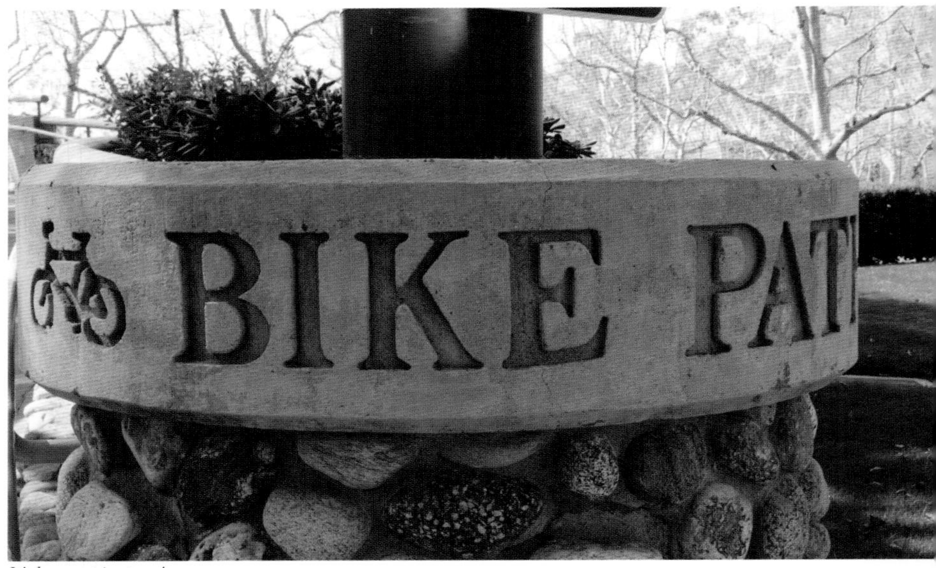

It's been set in stone!

At a Glance

partially

Distance 4.88 miles **Elevation Gain** 50′

Terrain

This ride is almost completely flat and travels along on-road bike paths.

Traffic

Expect light traffic as you pass through this quiet neighborhood.

How to Get There

By bus, OCTA route175 makes a stop at the Windrow Community Park.

By car, take exit 4, University Road, off of Interstate 405 heading north. Travel for 0.6 miles, the road will change its name to Jeffrey Road. Turn left onto Alton Parkway, then right on East Yale Loop. Turn right into Windrow Community Park.

Food and Drink

At the center of the loop, Woodbridge shopping cent is your best bet for food. Options range from Ruby Diner to a bit more upscale Champagne French Ba ery. Another option is El Cholo's, located in Alt Square shopping center.

Side Trip

Yale Loop circles two bodies of water, named Nor and South lakes. Surrounded by a number of parks, is all connected by a maze of bike paths that bisect t loop.

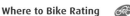

Links to 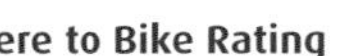 29 34 38

Where to Bike Rating 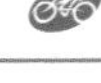

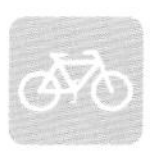    

About...

Beginning and ending at Irvine's Civic Center, this ride travels nearly the entire width of the city. Cutting through the city's heart, this spin is an excellent example of Irvine's commitment to incorporating cycling into its transportation plan. The city boasts 51 miles of off-street bike lanes and a staggering 301 miles of on-road lanes. As a popular commuter and training ride, this route's connectivity serves as the backbone to longer, more challenging rides.

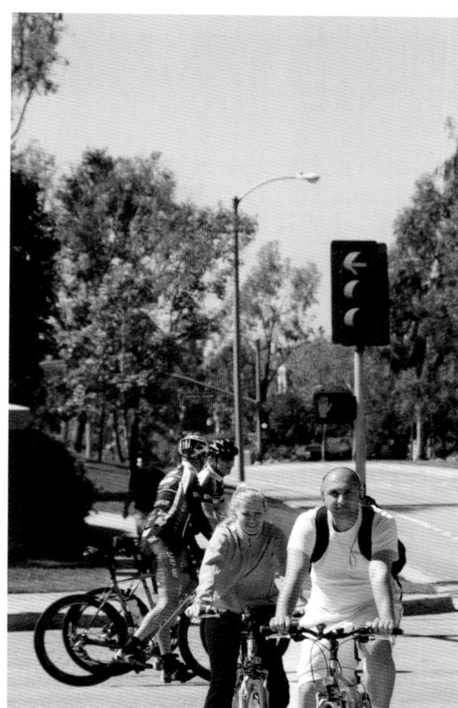

This is a ride for roadies and recreational riders.

his ride launches from Civic Center Park, an attractive public space that is also home to Kids' Ride 23. njoy rose gardens and fountains as you stroll under ellises covered in wisteria and bougainvillea. At the nd of your ride grab your picnic basket, throw out our blanket and enjoy lunch here.

Setting out from the quiet suburbs surrounding the rk, this route moves onto Barranca Parkway with its ergetic ebb and flow of traffic. You will find yourself daling from suburban neighborhoods, through retail nes, then past industrial parks before returning to tractive suburbs. At 6.84 miles this route intersects ith Ride 29 and a left here will allow you to complete grand tour of Irvine past undeveloped Orange County reat Park and from there the more northerly villages Irvine.

This outing travels between North and South lakes, o placid bodies of water surrounded by miles of bike ils.The easiest way to access the bike path is to en- Woodbridge Community Park from Alton Parkway 12.01 miles. The trail into the park will be on your ht and from there meanders around both lakes, all nnected by a large pedestrian bridge over Barranca rkway.

Dining opportunities are plentiful along this route. At the intersection of Alton Parkway and Jeffrey Road are two very large shopping centers with a number of dining options. El Cholo's is famous for its green corn tamales and excellent tacos. They are also well known for their strong margaritas but as you still have a few miles to ride, you may want to pass on the drinks. NY's Upper Crust Pizza is also located here and if pizza is your thing, they do a pretty good job.

At 16.39 miles this ride passes The District at Tustin Legacy. This shopping center is part of the larger plans to develop the land formerly known as the Marine Corp Air Station. The District is comprised of a million square feet of retail space that will tie in to the larger 1,600 acres of parks, homes and commercial uses. Glossy and modern, the shopping center offers plenty of dining and shopping, as well as a bike path cutting through it.

Ride Log

0.0 Begin ride on Harvard Ave where it intersects with Civic Center Plaza. Head north.
0.22 Cross San Juan Rd.
0.39 Turn right on Barranca Pkwy.
0.69 Cross PaseoWestpark.
1.05 Cross Culver Dr.
1.23 Cross West Yale Loop.
1.57 Cross Lake Rd.
1.87 Cross Creek Dr.
2.44 Cross East Yale Loop.
2.64 Cross Jeffery Rd.
3.42 Cross Valley Oak Dr.
3.65 Cross Sand Canyon Ave.
3.97 Cross Laguna Canyon Rd.
4.47 Cross Banting Rd.
4.71 Cross Pacifica Rd.
4.99 Cross Irvine Center Dr.
6.05 Irvine Metrolink station.
6.84 Turn right on Alton Pkwy.
7.33 Cross Ada Rd.
7.46 Cross Technology Way. Be alert here as it is also the beginning of the on ramp to Interstate 5.
8.0 Cross Irvine Center Dr.
8.38 Cross Pacifica Rd.
9.17 Cross Laguna Canyon Rd.
9.63 Cross Sand Canyon Ave.
10.69 Cross Jeffrey Rd.
12.01 Access trail into Woodbridge Community Pa and side trip around the lake, on your right.
12.08 Cross West Yale Loop.
12.27 Cross Culver Dr.
13.19 Cross Harvard Ave.
13.61 Cross Jamboree Rd.
14.12 Cross Von Karman Ave.
14.86 Turn right on Red Hill Ave.
15.11 Cross Deere Ave.
15.34 Turn right on Barranca Pkwy.
16.39 Cross Millikan Ave. The District at Tustin Le acy is located here.
16.57 Cross Jamboree Rd.
17.18 Turn right on Harvard Ave.
17.34 Cross San Juan Rd.
17.57 End.

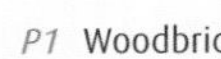

P1 Woodbridge Community Park
P2 San Diego Creek Trail
P3 Great Park Balloon Ride
P4 Irvine Valley College
P5 The District at Tustin legacy
P6 University of California, Irvine
P7 William R Mason Regional Park
P8 Irvine Spectrum Center
P9 Peters Canyon Trail
P10 Jeffrey Open Space Trail

Alton & Barranca Parkway Loop

Altitude ft: 0, 100, 200, 300, 400
Distance miles: 0, 3, 6, 9, 12, 15

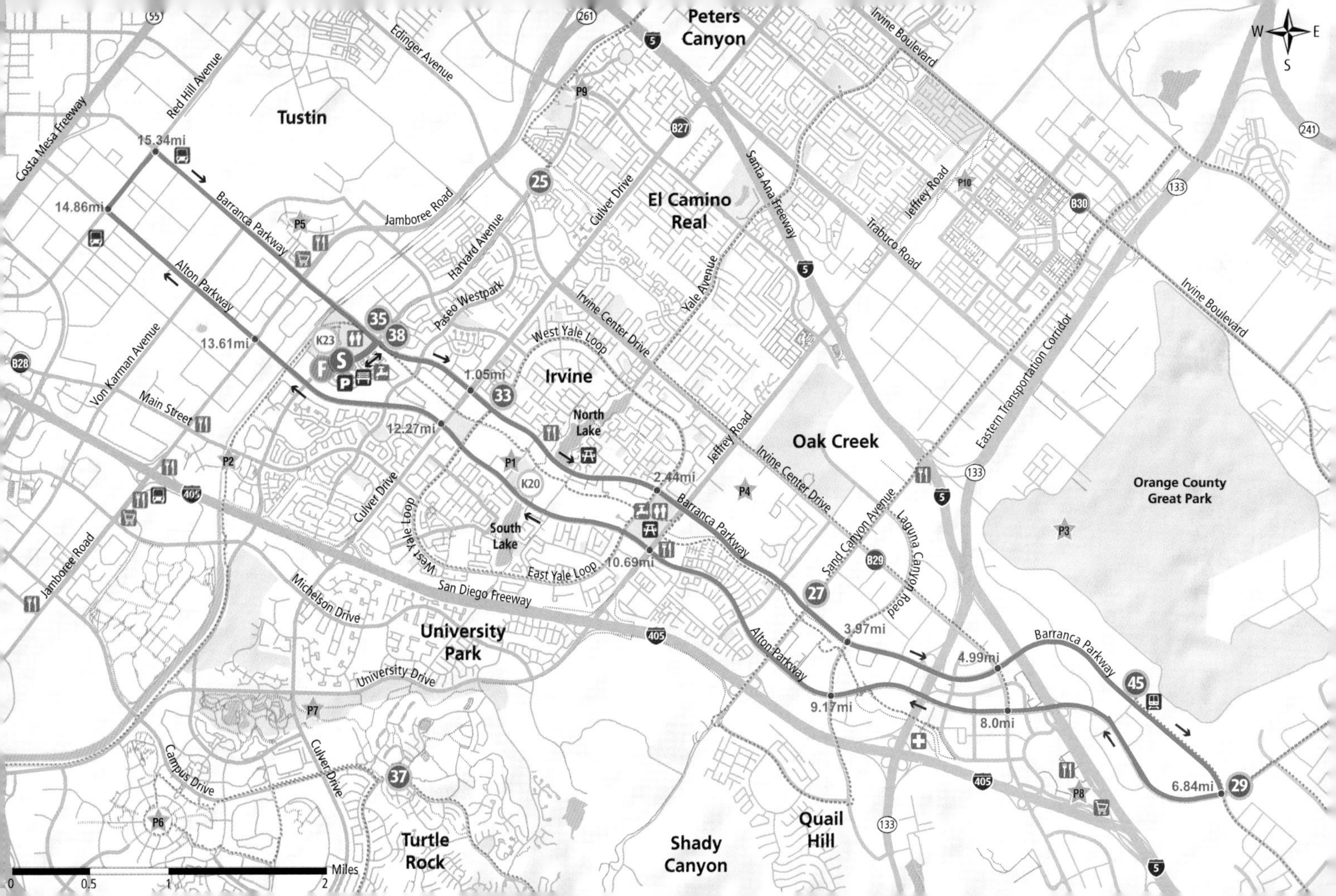

Peters Canyon
Tustin
El Camino Real
Irvine
North Lake
South Lake
Oak Creek
Orange County Great Park
University Park
Turtle Rock
Shady Canyon
Quail Hill
Costa Mesa Freeway
Red Hill Avenue
Edinger Avenue
Jamboree Road
Harvard Avenue
Paseo Westpark
Culver Drive
Irvine Center Drive
Yale Avenue
West Yale Loop
East Yale Loop
Santa Ana Freeway
Jeffrey Road
Trabuco Road
Irvine Boulevard
Eastern Transportation Corridor
Sand Canyon Avenue
Laguna Canyon Road
Barranca Parkway
Alton Parkway
Von Karman Avenue
Main Street
Michelson Drive
San Diego Freeway
University Drive
Campus Drive
15.34mi
14.86mi
13.61mi
12.27mi
1.05mi
2.44mi
3.97mi
4.99mi
6.84mi
8.0mi
9.17mi
10.69mi
Miles
0
0.5
1
2

Walnut Bike Trail/Incredible Edible Park — Ride 35

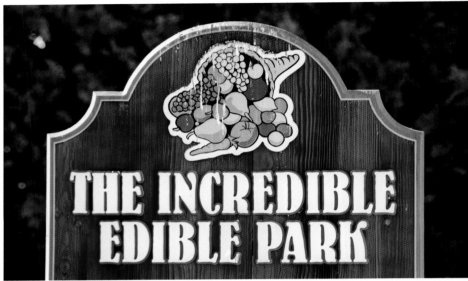

Incredible Edible Park helps to feed thousands of families in need every year.

At a Glance

Distance 8.27 miles **Elevation Gain** 147′

Terrain

This is a flat ride along off-street bike paths.

Traffic

Except for the handful of times the path crosses roads, this ride is free of traffic.

How to Get There

By bus, OCTA bus 473 makes stops along Harvard Avenue, near the ride's start.

By car, take exit 99, Culver Drive, off of Interstate 5 and head south. Turn right onto Deerfield Avenue after 1.2 miles, then right onto Flagstone. Parking is available on the street.

Food and Drink

Although there are no restaurants along the route itself, the District at Tustin Legacy is located about a mile away and offers a number of dining options. Also located nearby in the Culver Plaza at the corner of Cu ver Drive and Irvine Center Drive is Sam Woo servir authentic Cantonese style Chinese food.

Side Trip

This ride is the connector to upper and lower Pete Canyon Trail, also known as the Mountains to the Se Trail. See rides 25 and 38 for more information.

Links to 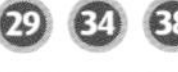

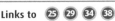

Where to Bike Rating 

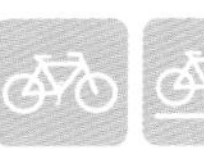 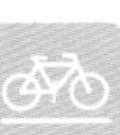   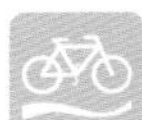

About...

This is one of the finest rides in the book, perfectly suited to novice riders as well as seasoned cyclists looking for a training run. The ride begins where San Diego Creek empties into Newport Back Bay; from there the trail travels beside the creek as it goes through many transformations. First is the channeled, concrete streambed typical of Southern California, followed by a grassy, almost prairie-like streambed until at its upper reaches it travels swiftly through ravines with lush vegetation alongside.

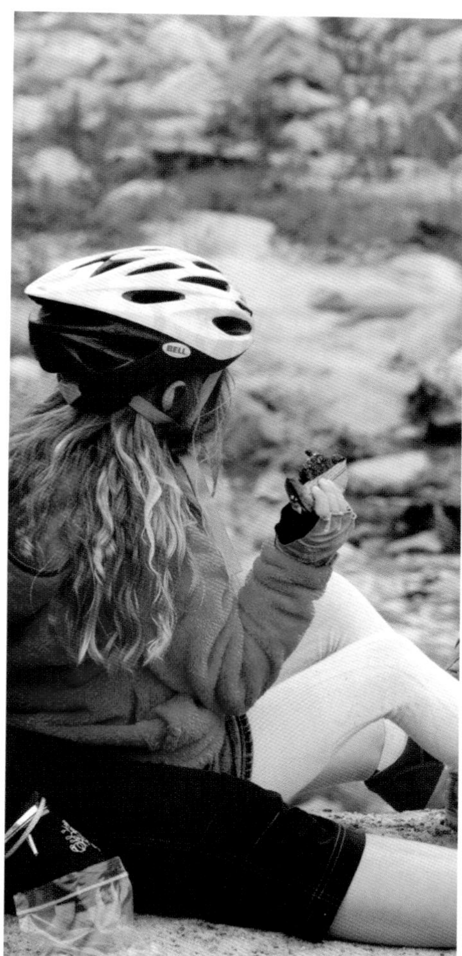
Don't forget to take a break and fuel up.

or the purpose of the ride log, this ride officially starts the corner of Eastbluff Drive and Jamboree Road. ecause parking can be difficult in this area you may nd yourself a considerable distance from this spot, so art your bike's trip odometer at this corner.

To avoid confusion, the San Diego Creek Trail is so known as Lower Peters Canyon Trail and the ountains to the Sea Trail and there are a number of fferent signs along the route indicating such. At 4.77 is ride continues straight, but to follow these other ails you will need to exit onto Harvard Avenue. Rides 4, 25, 35 and 39 cover the various sections of the ountain to the Sea Trail. Altogether these intercon-cted rides comprise nearly 50 miles of bike paths just aiting to be explored.

From this point on, the pedestrian traffic signifi-ntly drops and the creek becomes more attractive d natural looking. As the route passes by way of indrow Community Park, it travels through a tunnel der Jeffrey Road. On the other side of the tunnel you ll need to make a hairpin turn and travel the path ongside Jeffrey Road for about a third of a mile be-re returning to the creek itself. If you reach Barranca rkway, you have missed the turn, as I did on my first ride through here.

Along the upper portion of the trail the creek traverses through a steep ravine and the landscape has the feel of wilderness with large trees and undergrowth crowding the path. This section of the ride is quiet and peaceful until suddenly ending at 9.91 miles. This part of Irvine is under development and even as we turned around for the return trip we could see that the path was under construction and will eventually continue to travel alongside the creek.

Central Coast

Ride Log

0.0 Start ride at the corner of Eastbluff Dr and Jamboree Rd, head downhill.
0.19 Bear left onto San Diego Creek Trail.
0.46 Continue straight.
0.54 Bear left and pass under Campus Dr.
2.73 Bear left and cross pedestrian bridge.
2.86 Bear left and pass under Michelson Dr.
3.18 Continue straight.
3.30 Bear left and pass under Main St.
4.04 Bear left under Alton Pkwy.
4.54 Turn left and cross pedestrian bridge.
4.57 Turn right and return to trail.
4.77 Bear right and pass under Harvard Ave.
5.08 Bear right under PaseoWestpark.
5.41 Bear right and pass under Culver Dr.
6.03 Cross W Yale Loop.
6.15 Continue straight.
6.37 Cross Lake Rd.
6.86 Bear left and pass under E Yale Loop.
7.07 Bear left and pass under Jeffrey Rd.
7.22 Make sharp left turn onto path that runs alongside Jeffrey Rd.
7.40 Turn left back onto San Diego Creek Trail.
8.18 Bear left and pass under Valley Oak Dr.
8.45 Bear left and pass under Sand Canyon Ave.
8.90 Bear left and pass under Laguna Canyon Rd.
9.10 Bear left and pass under Alton Pkwy.
9.29 Bear right.

P
P1 Aldrich Park
P2 John Wayne Airport
P3 Civic Center Park
P4 Peters Canyon Trail
P5 North Lake
P6 South Lake
P7 Irvine Valley College
P8 Irvine Spectrum Center
P9 The District at Tustin Legacy

9.30 Turn right and cross over bridge to other side creek.
9.37 Turn right back onto path.
9.91 Turn around.
10.76 Turn left and cross bridge to other side of cree
10.82 Turn left back onto trail.
10.83 Hairpin left turn back onto trail, watch for o coming pedestrian traffic.
11.29 Bear right and pass under Sand Canyon Ave.
12.44 Turn right and ride path alongside Jeffrey Rd.
12.61 Right hairpin turn back onto trail. Watch f blind corner ahead.
14.23 Bear left and pass under W Yale Loop.
14.91 Bear left and pass under Harvard Ave.
15.25 Turn left and cross pedestrian bridge.
15.66 Bear right and pass under Alton Pkwy.
16.89 Bear right and pass under Michelson Dr.
19.63 After passing under Jamboree Dr, bear rig onto Back Bay Trail.
19.82 End.

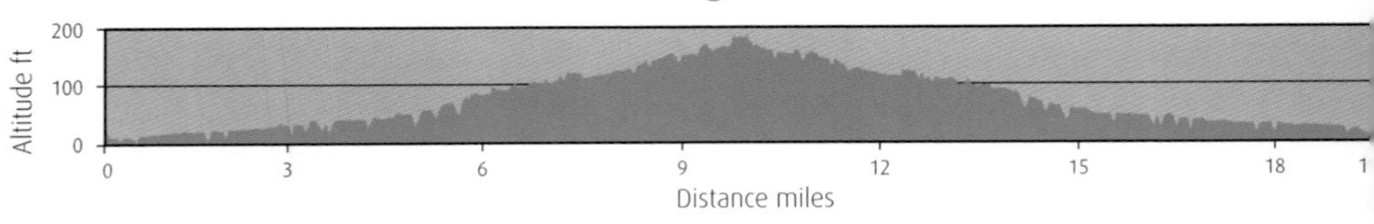

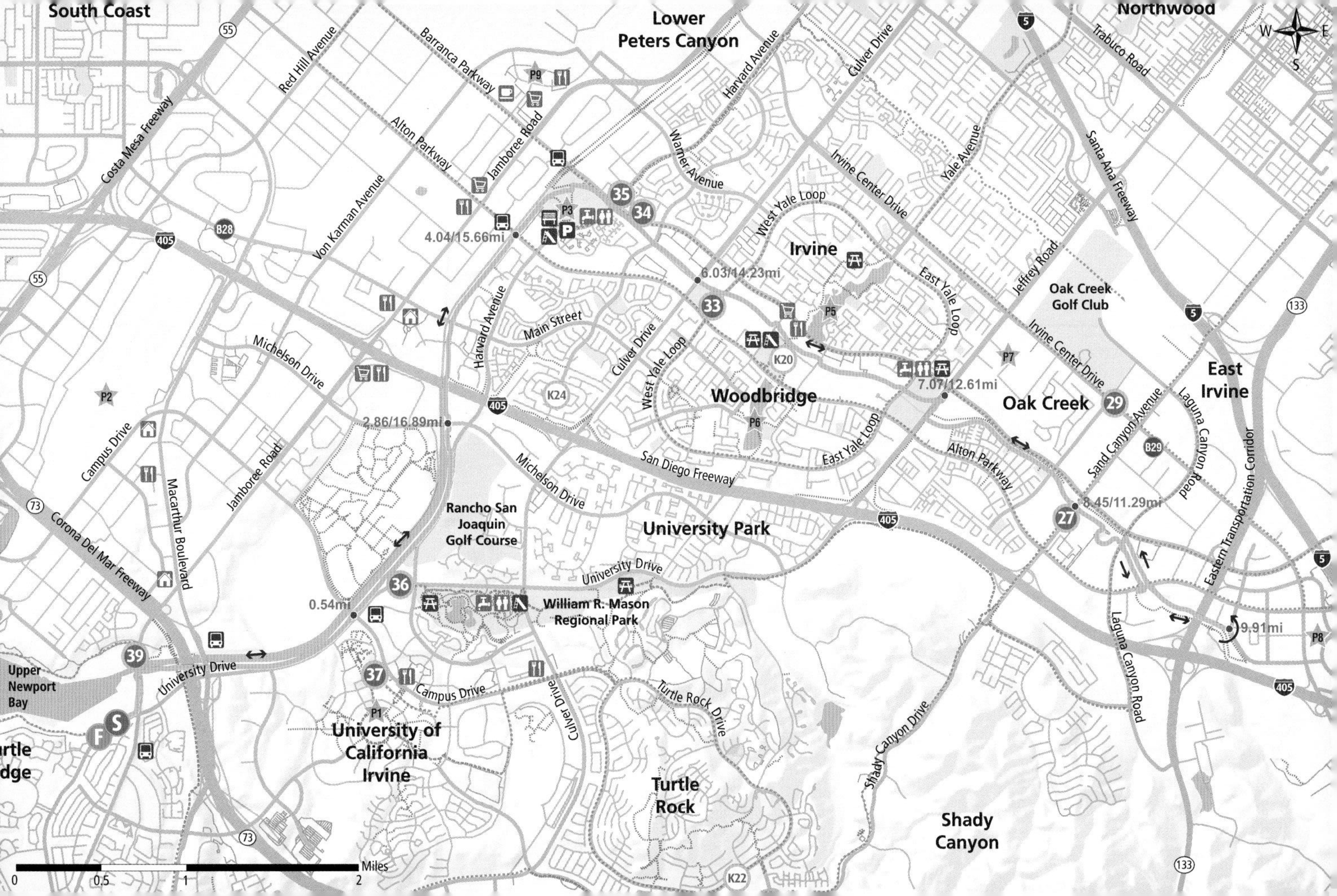
South Coast
Lower Peters Canyon
Northwood
East Irvine
Irvine
Woodbridge
Oak Creek
Oak Creek Golf Club
University Park
Rancho San Joaquin Golf Course
William R. Mason Regional Park
University of California Irvine
Turtle Rock
Shady Canyon
Upper Newport Bay
Costa Mesa Freeway
Red Hill Avenue
Barranca Parkway
Alton Parkway
Jamboree Road
Von Karman Avenue
Harvard Avenue
Culver Drive
Warner Avenue
West Yale Loop
East Yale Loop
Irvine Center Drive
Yale Avenue
Jeffrey Road
Trabuco Road
Santa Ana Freeway
Main Street
Michelson Drive
Campus Drive
Macarthur Boulevard
Corona Del Mar Freeway
San Diego Freeway
University Drive
Turtle Rock Drive
Shady Canyon Drive
Sand Canyon Avenue
Laguna Canyon Road
Eastern Transportation Corridor
4.04/15.66mi
6.03/14.23mi
7.07/12.61mi
8.45/11.29mi
9.91mi
2.86/16.89mi
0.54mi
P1
P2
P3
P5
P6
P7
P8
P9
K20
K22
K24
B28
B29
27
29
33
34
35
36
37
39
F
S
5
55
73
133
405
W
E
S
0
0.5
1
2
Miles

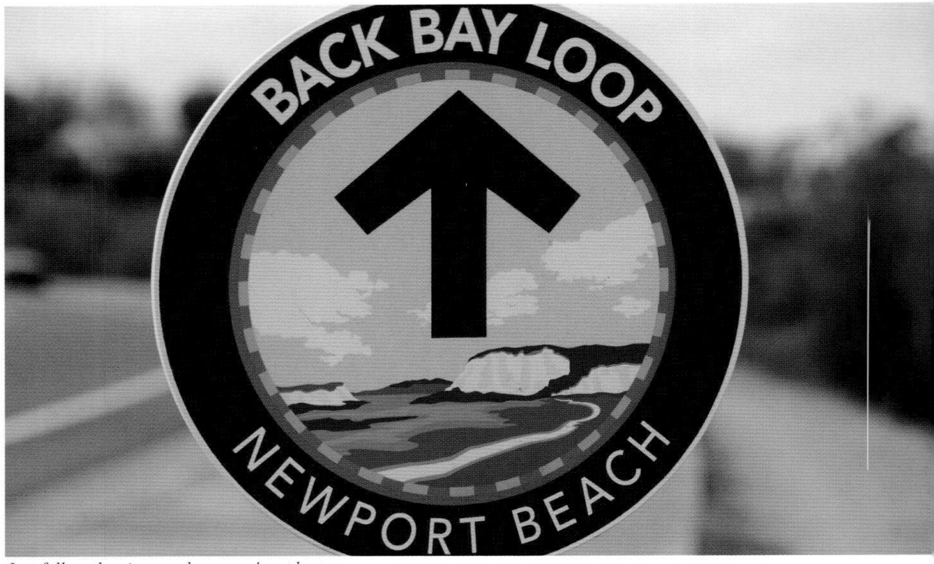

Just follow the signs and you can't get lost.

At a Glance

partially

Distance 10.50 miles **Elevation Gain** 331′

Terrain

This looping ride travels over undulating bike paths and on-street bike lanes.

Traffic

Although most of this ride is car-free with the exception of a one and a half mile section along Dover Street and Irvine Avenue, pedestrian traffic is present all year around, and especially heavy on weekends.

How to Get There

By bus, OCTA bus 55 makes a stop right in front of Castaways Park parking lot.

By car, take CA-55, Costa Mesa Freeway, and turn left onto 16th Street. Travel for 1.2 miles before 16th Street turns into Castaways Lane, parking lot will be on your right.

Food and Drink

There are not a lot of opportunities to eat along t route itself, however along Bayside Drive where crosses Pacific Coast Highway at 9.76 miles there a some fast food places as well as some upscale resta rants.

Side Trip

This route takes you through the Newport Bay Natu Preserve which offers plenty of hiking and bird watc ing opportunities. Visit the interpretive center locat at 3.63 miles or after your ride explore Newport Ha bor.

Links to 36 38

Where to Bike Rating 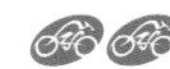

 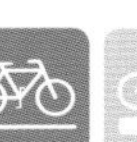 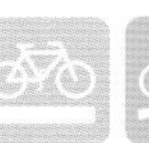  

About...

This ride loops around Newport Beach's Back Bay, a 1,000 acre ecological reserve and certainly one of the most scenic sights in Orange County. As you travel bluffs that rise over the bay, you will be treated to panoramic views while passing through grassland and coastal sage scrub. Over 35,000 species of birds pass through this estuary during winter migrations. And at times it may seem that there are that many people sharing the path with you. Sunrise and sunset are the most peaceful times to visit.

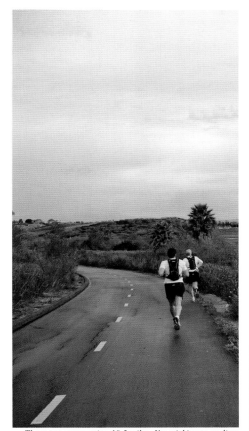

These two are running 10.5 miles. I'm sticking to cycling.

ncorporated in 1906, Newport Beach has long been mecca for beach goers and nature lovers since the acific Electric Railway's Red line ferried passengers rom distant Los Angeles. The harbor is the largest recreational harbor on the west coast and is a favorite to sherman, boaters, kayakers, rowers and paddle boarders, all of which can be rented and enjoyed year round.

This ride is well marked and if in doubt look for Back Bay Loop signs on posts as well as painted on the round indicating direction. Start at Castaways Park vith a jaw dropping view of harbor and bay gloriously aid out before you. Although the path that runs along he bluff is often busy with foot traffic it is well worth he inconvenience to be able to enjoy such a spectacuar view. There are trails that meander through this park s well. Benches are in short supply, but if you can find ne, this is a fine place to have a picnic.

Once leaving the park this route travels for about mile and a half along city streets. The stretch along rvine Avenue is the busiest part of the ride and for bout half a mile the on-street bike lane is a bit narrow vith cars parked in the lane. The possibility of getting oored is very real so riders should stay alert.

To visit the Upper Newport Bay Interpretive Center, turn right into the parking lot at 3.63 on the ride log. This excellent learning center offers year round programs that include guided birding tours with park rangers, restoration projects and wildlife watches.

At 5.11 miles this ride intersects with Ride 38 which runs along San Diego Creek and makes up the lower half of the Mountain to the Seas Trail. Connect Rides 25, 38 and the Back Bay Loop and enjoy a blissful 40 plus miles of cycling, nearly all of it on bike paths.

As you travel along Bayside Drive, at 9.76 miles, continue straight and you will find a coffee shop and healthy minded fast food restaurants on your left. On your right you will see pricier restaurants that include SOL Mexican Cocina which features Baja cuisine.

Ride Log

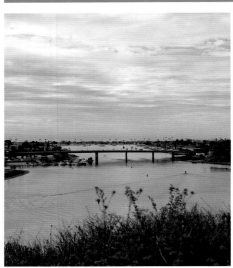
The view of the bay and the harbor.

P1 Upper Newport Bay Interpretive Center
P2 Back Bay View Park
P3 Newport Beach Golf Course
P4 Orange County Fair and Event Center
P5 Fashion Island Shopping Center
P6 Balboa Island Ferry
P7 Orange County Museum of Art

0.0 Begin ride near the parking lot of Castaway Park at the trailhead.
0.06 Turn right.
0.10 Turn left.
0.37 Continue straight.
0.72 Bear left.
1.03 Bike path ends, turn right onto Dover Dr whic has an on-street bike lane.
1.10 Cross Westcliff Dr.
1.53 Cross Mariners Dr.
1.73 Turn right onto Irvine Ave.
1.98 Cross Highland Dr.
2.50 Cross Santiago Dr.
2.54 Bear right onto bike path.
3.63 Passing the Upper Newport Bay Interpreti Center.
3.86 Blind corner, be alert.
4.91 Turn right on path as it travels alongside Jan boree Rd.
5.11 Continue straight.
5.13 Path turns right and runs alongside Eastbluff D
5.58 Turn right onto Back Bay Dr which has an o street bike path.
7.96 Bear right.
8.48 Continue straight.
8.84 Turn right onto trail that runs through Newpo Dunes RV Resort.
9.55 Turn left onto Bayside Dr.
9.76 Turn right onto bike path that runs along Paci Coast Hwy.
10.10 Turn right as path travels alongside Dover Dr.
10.25 Bear right onto path that travels into Castawa Park.
10.39 Turn left.
10.43 Turn left.
10.50 End.

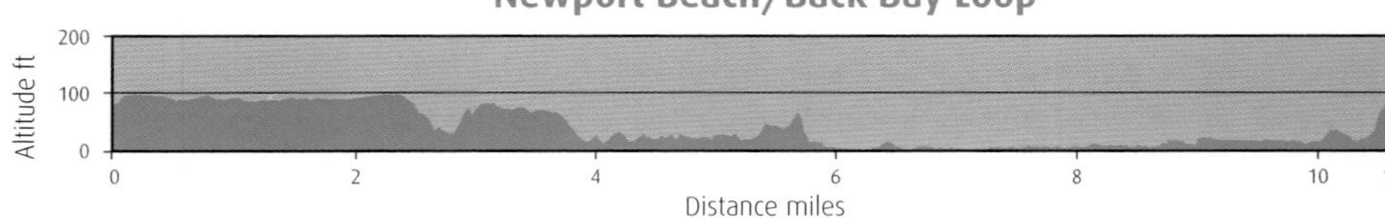

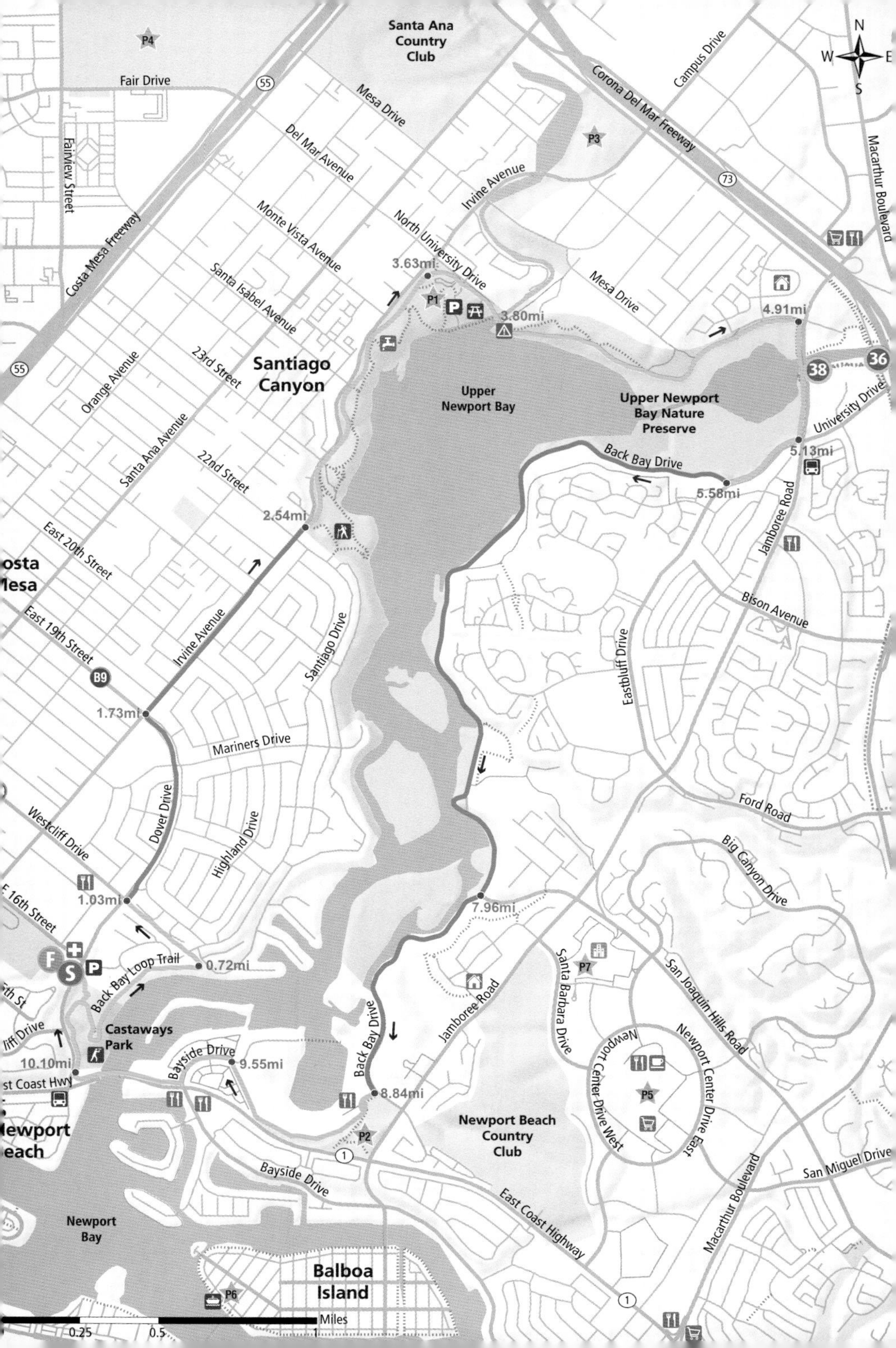
Santa Ana Country Club
Fair Drive
Fairview Street
Costa Mesa Freeway
Mesa Drive
Del Mar Avenue
Monte Vista Avenue
Santa Isabel Avenue
North University Drive
Irvine Avenue
Corona Del Mar Freeway
Campus Drive
Macarthur Boulevard
Mesa Drive
3.63mi
3.80mi
4.91mi
Santiago Canyon
Upper Newport Bay
Upper Newport Bay Nature Preserve
Orange Avenue
23rd Street
Santa Ana Avenue
22nd Street
University Drive
5.13mi
Back Bay Drive
5.58mi
2.54mi
East 20th Street
Costa Mesa
East 19th Street
Irvine Avenue
Santiago Drive
Jamboree Road
Bison Avenue
Eastbluff Drive
1.73mi
Mariners Drive
Dover Drive
Highland Drive
Westcliff Drive
Ford Road
Big Canyon Drive
1.03mi
E 16th Street
7.96mi
Santa Barbara Drive
San Joaquin Hills Road
Back Bay Loop Trail
0.72mi
Jamboree Road
Back Bay Drive
Castaways Park
Bayside Drive
9.55mi
10.10mi
Newport Center Drive West
Newport Center Drive East
East Coast Hwy
8.84mi
Newport Beach
Newport Beach Country Club
Bayside Drive
East Coast Highway
San Miguel Drive
Macarthur Boulevard
Newport Bay
Balboa Island
Miles
0.25
0.5
1

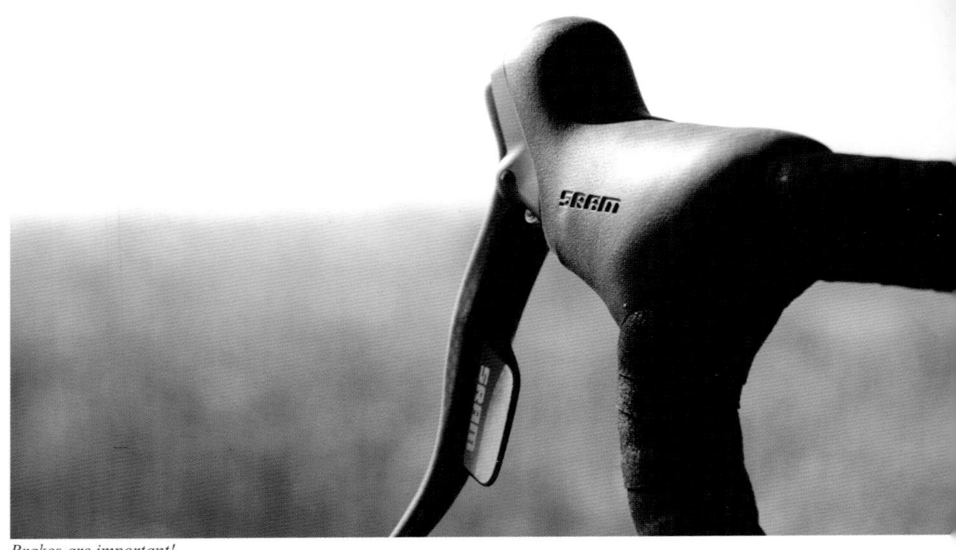

Brakes are important!

At a Glance

partially

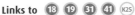

Distance 11.71 miles **Elevation Gain** 367′

Terrain

This is a mostly flat ride over bikes paths and on-street bike lanes.

Traffic

You will encounter modest traffic through most of the ride with a heavier stretch along West Coast Highway.

How to Get There

By bus, OCTA bus routes 1, 43, 47, 71, 78 and 173 all intersect with this ride.

By car, take exit 11, Harbor Boulevard, off of Interstate 405. Travel south on Harbor for 0.5 miles, turn right onto Baker Street, followed by a right onto Mesa Verde Drive. Mesa Verde turns into Placentia Avenue and after 2.2 miles the park will be on your right.

Food and Drink

Along West Coast Highway you find a number of dining options. Spaghetti Bender is a fun, casual neighborhood restaurant that has been around forever and nearby Newport Burger serves quite a bit more than hamburgers.

Side Trip

Besides a picnic on the beach, this ride passes through Talbert Nature Preserve with miles of trails for hiking and cycling. Located near the ride's start is Estancia Park where the Diego Sepulveda Adobe has been restored.

Links to 18 19 31 41 K25

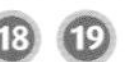

Where to Bike Rating

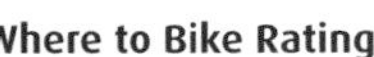
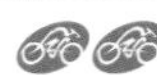

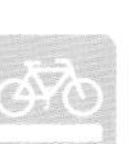
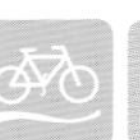

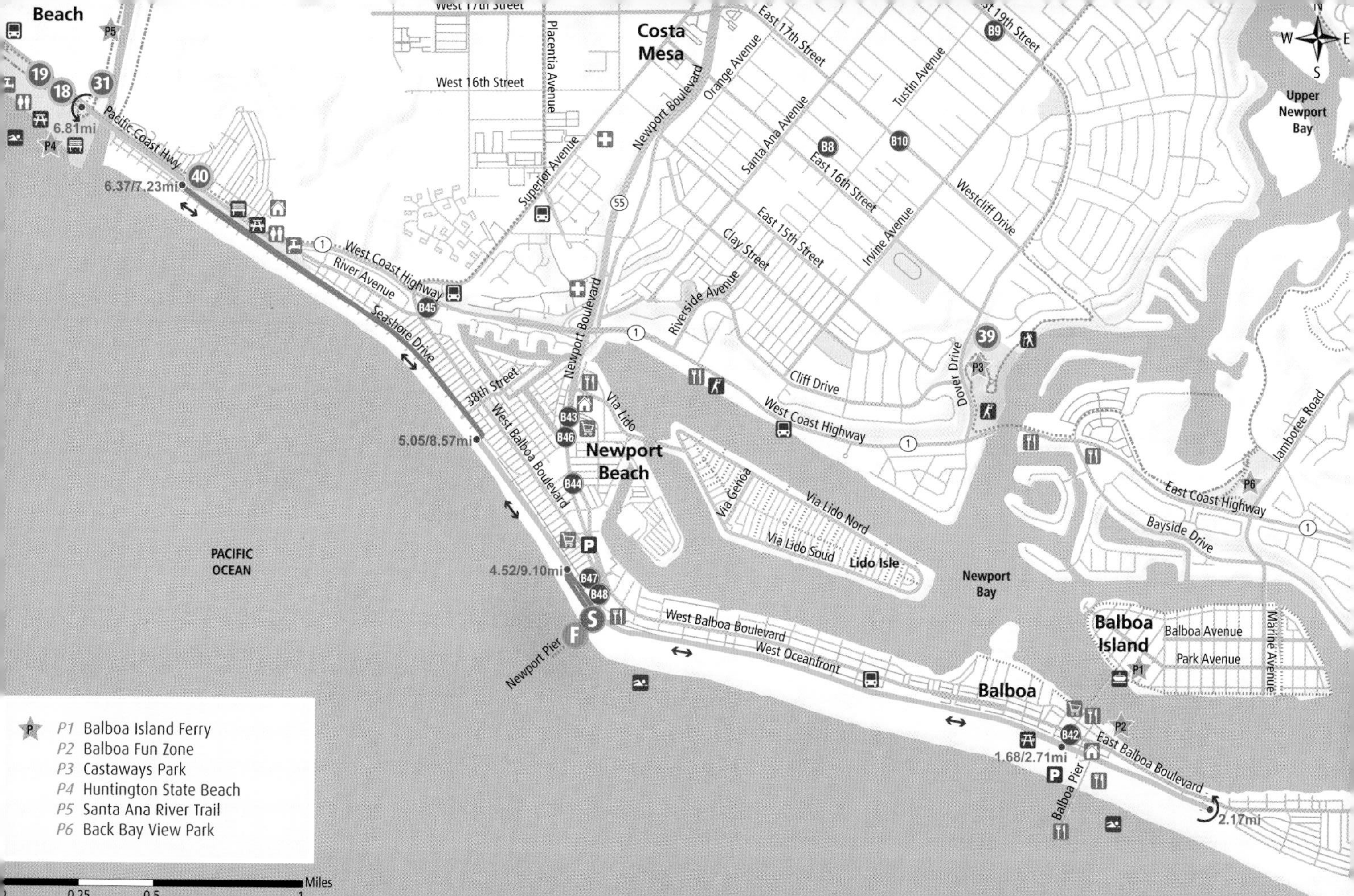

Beach
Costa Mesa
Newport Beach
Balboa
Balboa Island
Lido Isle
Newport Bay
Upper Newport Bay
PACIFIC OCEAN
West 17th Street
West 16th Street
Placentia Avenue
Superior Avenue
Newport Boulevard
Orange Avenue
East 17th Street
Santa Ana Avenue
East 16th Street
Tustin Avenue
19th Street
Westcliff Drive
Irvine Avenue
East 15th Street
Clay Street
Riverside Avenue
Cliff Drive
Dover Drive
Jamboree Road
West Coast Highway
East Coast Highway
Bayside Drive
Marine Avenue
Balboa Avenue
Park Avenue
Pacific Coast Hwy
River Avenue
Seashore Drive
38th Street
West Balboa Boulevard
Via Lido
Via Genoa
Via Lido Nord
Via Lido Soud
West Oceanfront
East Balboa Boulevard
Newport Pier
Balboa Pier
6.81mi
6.37/7.23mi
5.05/8.57mi
4.52/9.10mi
1.68/2.71mi
2.17mi
P1 Balboa Island Ferry
P2 Balboa Fun Zone
P3 Castaways Park
P4 Huntington State Beach
P5 Santa Ana River Trail
P6 Back Bay View Park
0.25
0.5
1
Miles

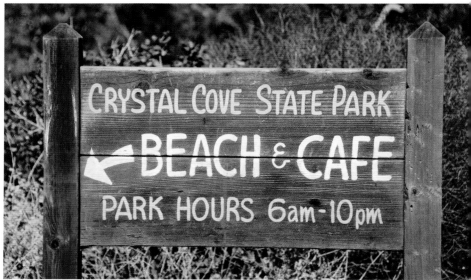

Follow the signs to Crystal Cove's historic district.

At a Glance

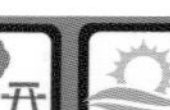

Distance 5.48 miles **Elevation Gain** 295′

Terrain

Mostly flat, smooth bike paths.

Traffic

This ride is completely car-free except the few places where the path crosses roads. Expect quite a bit of pedestrian traffic on weekends.

How to Get There

By bus, OCTA route 1 makes a stop near the Crystal Cove State Park entrance.

By car, take Pacific Coast Highway to where it intersects with Reef Point Drive and turn right into Crystal Cove State Park. After paying, turn left and park in the most southerly lot.

Food and Drink

Two excellent dining opportunities exist on this ride. First is Ruby's Shake Shack with a commanding bluff-top view of the ocean to the distant horizon. Nearb[cut off] is the Beachcomber Café, located right on the beac[cut off] amidst charming cottages built in the 1930s.

Side Trip

Explore the tide pools, hike into the larger hillsid[cut off] section of the park, visit the historic district or simpl[cut off] picnic on the beach. For skin and scuba divers, the of[cut off] shore waters are designated as an underwater park an[cut off] offer spectacular opportunities to do some underwate[cut off] sightseeing.

Where to Bike Rating 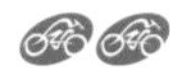

 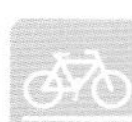   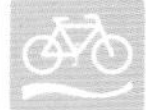

About...

One of this section's premier rides, Aliso Creek Bikeway is the kind of route that will get you excited to hop on your bike. The ride takes off from Sheep Hill Park and meanders northward following Aliso Creek through attractive parks and wetlands with the route often dipping onto the creek bed itself. Car-free and safe, this is a route you are sure to ride many times.

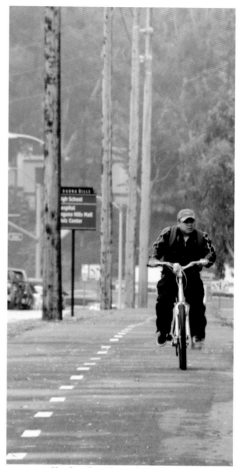

Hey friend, you're on the wrong side of the road!

'he route's start just outside of Sheep Hill Park is lso the start of Ride 46 which heads south, through he park, to follow the lower portion of Aliso Creek ikeway to Aliso and Woods Canyon Regional Park. n addition to that, Sheep Hill Park is the site of Kids' ide 28 making this a cycling epicenter. Not surprising iven the many trails, paths and on-road bike lanes in is part of Orange County.

At the beginning the route runs parallel to city treets before turning away from the road at 1.15 miles nd to travel beside the creek. The first few miles the tream is channelized before it becomes a more natural oking, sandy bottomed creek. At this point vegeta-on increases and a whole range of birds can be found om red tail hawks to sandpipers to snowy egrets. hrough this section the trail dips down to run beside e creek and if you are riding after recent storms you ay find these parts under water or covered in mud. this happens, follow signs that indicate alternative outes that bypass these hazards.

The last couple of miles the path gets steeper as the eek passes between Whiting Ranch Wilderness and 'Neill Regional Park. For mountain bikers and hik-s, there are some excellent trails connected to this de. At 9.37 miles the route connects to Live Oak anyon Trail which if taken will eventually connect to Ride 44 in O'Neill Regional Park, however, this is only an option for mountain bikers. Expect some very steep climbs along this trail.

The turnaround point at 9.43 miles marks the end of the Aliso Creek Bikeway and for those looking for a serious challenge with heart-pounding climbs, you could continue north and take on Ride 22, Santiago Canyon, in reverse. For those already satisfied with the nearly 1,000 feet of climbing they have already done, turn around and enjoy the gentle downhill back to the start.

Ride Log

0.0 Begin ride where path exits from Sheep Hill Park running alongside Laguna Hills Dr.

0.07 Cross Indian Hill Ln.

0.57 Turn left at Paseo De Valencia and pick up trail again catty corner.

0.89 Cross Beckenham St.

1.15 Follow trail as it turns right away from street and travels besides creek.

1.36 Follow the middle path, DO NOT turn left or right here.

1.84 Bear left.

2.32 Bear right and pass under bridge.

2.44 Cross right over creek.

2.46 Bear left.

2.57 Continue straight.

2.68 Bear left and pass under Muirlands Blvd.

3.45 Bear left and pass under bridge.

3.63 Turn left and cross pedestrian bridge.

3.66 Turn right and return to trail.

4.32 Turn right and cross pedestrian bridge.

4.33 Turn left and return to path, then bear left and pass under Trabuco Rd.

5.00 Cross Creekside Rd, this is a blind intersection, be alert.

5.47 Turn left and head under El Toro Rd.

6.28 Bear left and pass under bridge.

6.87 Bear left and pass under Santa Margarita Pkwy.

8.96 Bear left.

9.37 Continue straight. A right here intersects wi Live Oak Canyon Trail.

9.43 Turn around.

13.30 Bear right and pass under bridge.

13.37 Turn right and continue on trail.

13.85 Cross Creekside Rd, beware blind intersectior

14.43 Turn right and cross pedestrian bridge.

15.21 Turn left and cross bridge.

15.33 Bear right, pass under bridge.

16.09 Bear right and pass under Murilands Blvd.

16.40 Bear right and travel along stream.

17.49 Continue straight.

17.69 Trail turns left and follows Paseo De Valencia

18.25 Turn right at Laguna Hills Dr and pick up tra catty corner.

18.86 End.

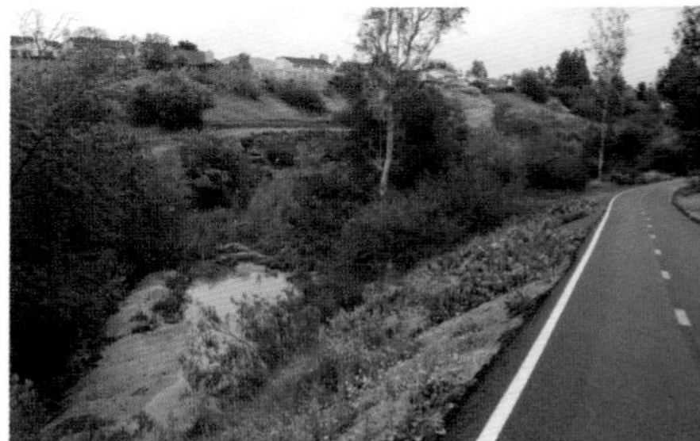

Pause occaisonally to enjoy the lush vegetation along the wa

Aliso Creek Bikeway

Please note: the profile for Ride 43 is depicted in 250ft vertical increments due to unusually high elevation.

About...

This route connects central Orange County to its southern portions by way of Muirlands Boulevard, cutting through the cities of Irvine, Lake Forest and Mission Viejo. This is an ideal commuter ride. Setting out from Irvine Transportation Center, on-street bike lanes travel wide roads over rolling hills. For those looking for a training opportunity, the ascent up La Paz Road will challenge even the most experienced riders. The ride then loops back to its start with lots of downhill sections.

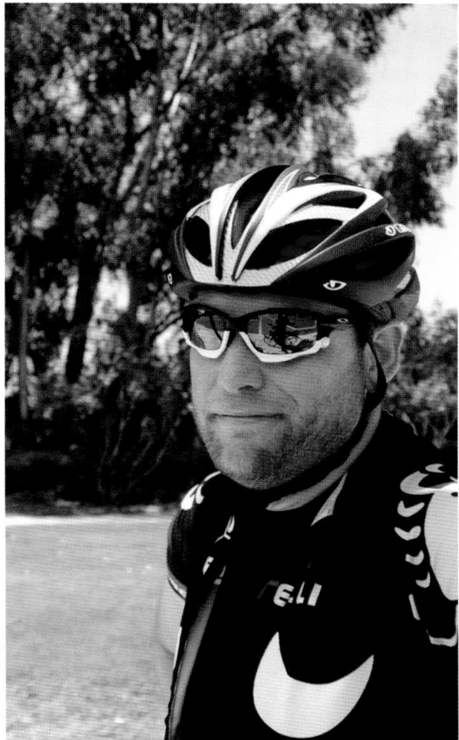

Jim looks fresh for a guy who just rode 70 miles.

Near the ride's start are two attractive side trips. Orange County Great Park, once known as El Toro Marine Corp Air Base, is an ambitious project that intends to remake 1,347 acres into a premier public park. The designs are grand and costly and while it is still in development, you can get a taste of things to come by visiting the Great Park Balloon. This free attraction floats 500 feet into the air and offers spectacular panoramic views of central Orange County. Located amidst the attractive landscaping are a carousel, Kid Rock playground and on Sundays, a farmers' market.

Also nearby is the Irvine Spectrum Center with over 130 retail and dining outlets catering to a well-heeled crowd. Located within this complex is the Giant Wheel, a 108 foot tall Ferris wheel.

At 6.49 miles La Paz Road crosses Marguerite Parkway. For those looking to avoid a long and steep climb, turn left here and follow Marguerite until it intersects with Jeronimo Road approximately 0.7 miles away. This alternate route is also hilly, but tame compared to what lies ahead. From this point La Paz starts climbing. And it climbs. And climbs. Over a two mile stretch this hill ascends 400 feet! La Paz ends at Olympiad Road and following the Ride Log, turn left. Pavion Park is located nearby at the corner of Olympiad and Jeronimo roads and is a pleasant, shaded place to take a break.

A left onto Jeronimo Road means the ride is returning to Irvine. From here generally expect downhill riding with a few rolling sections. At the El Tore Road intersection, to your left is a nondescript shopping center where you will find Chili Chutney Restaurant, featuring Afghan cuisine. This modest looking restaurant is the most interesting dining option located along the route. Kebabs, flatbreads and leek dumplings called ashak await you along with a range of flavorful chutneys.

The last four miles from here are flat. At 16.23 miles the ride returns to Barranca Parkway, a keystone intersection with Rides 29 and 34. If those legs still have some energy left, connect with either route and take a tour through the heart of Irvine.

Ride Log

P1 Great Park Balloon Ride
P2 Aliso Creek Bikeway
P3 Irvine Spectrum Center
P4 Florence Joyner Olympiad Park
P5 Heroes Park
P6 Serrano Creek Park

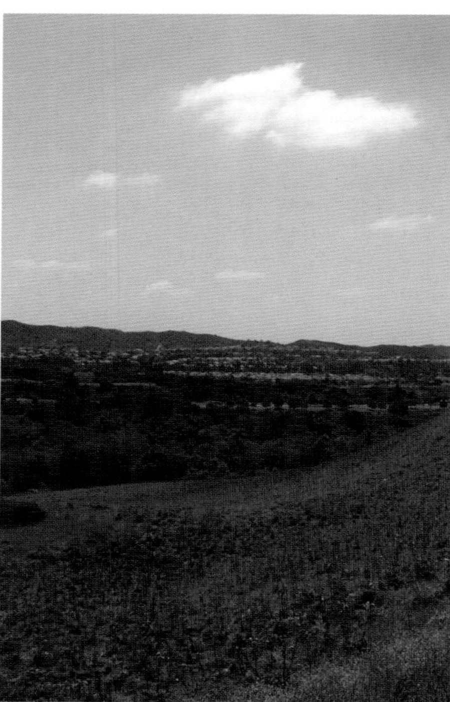
The panoramic view from the top of La Paz Road.

0.0 Begin ride where Ada ends in front of Irvine Metrolink station.

0.04 Turn left onto Barranca Pkwy.

0.87 Cross Alton Pkwy. This is where Barranca Pkwy turns into Muirlands Blvd.

1.66 Cross Bake Pkwy.

2.20 Cross Lake Forest Dr.

2.70 Cross Ridge Route Dr.

3.27 Cross El Toro Rd.

3.79 Cross Los Alisos Blvd.

4.40 Cross Alicia Pkwy.

5.41 Left on La Paz Rd.

5.63 Cross Cristanta Dr.

6.49 Cross Marguerite Pkwy. Alternate route up to Jeronimo Rd here.

8.02 Turn left on Olympiad Rd.

8.98 Turn left on Jeronimo Rd.

9.02 Pavion Park on your left, good place to break.

10.62 Cross Marguerite Pkwy.

12.23 Cross Alicia Pkwy.

12.96 Cross Los Alisos Blvd.

13.46 Cross El Toro Rd.

13.97 Cross Ridge Route Rd.

14.61 Cross Lake Forest Dr.

15.01 Cross Bake Pkwy.

15.84 Turn left on Alton Pkwy.

16.23 Turn right onto Barranca Pkwy.

17.02 Turn right onto Ada.

17.09 End.

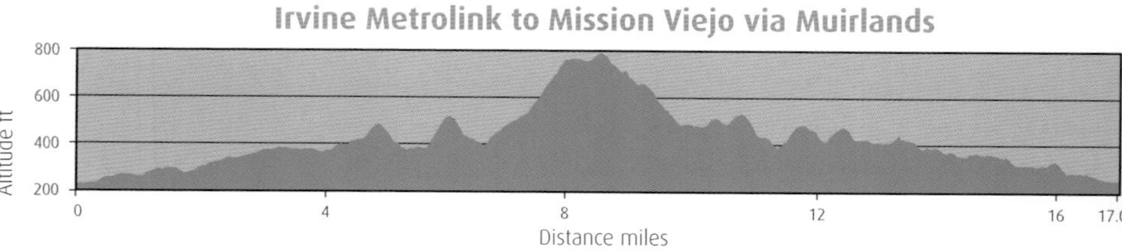

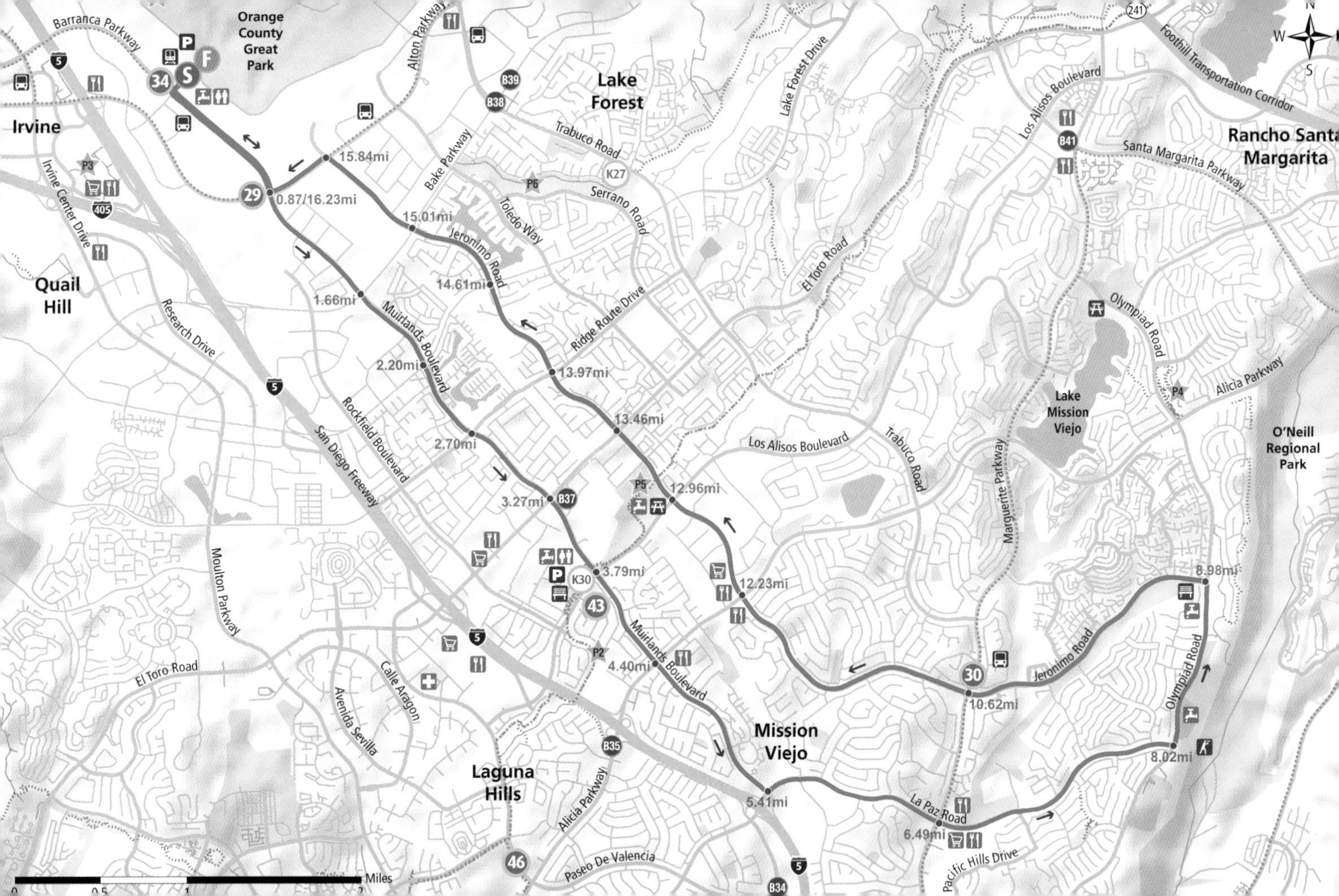
Orange County Great Park
Lake Forest
Rancho Santa Margarita
Irvine
Quail Hill
Lake Mission Viejo
O'Neill Regional Park
Mission Viejo
Laguna Hills
Barranca Parkway
Alton Parkway
Trabuco Road
Lake Forest Drive
Los Alisos Boulevard
Santa Margarita Parkway
Foothill Transportation Corridor
Irvine Center Drive
Bake Parkway
Toledo Way
Serrano Road
El Toro Road
Jeronimo Road
Ridge Route Drive
Olympiad Road
Alicia Parkway
Research Drive
Muirlands Boulevard
Rockfield Boulevard
San Diego Freeway
Marguerite Parkway
Moulton Parkway
Calle Aragon
Avenida Sevilla
La Paz Road
Pacific Hills Drive
Paseo De Valencia
0.87/16.23mi
15.84mi
15.01mi
14.61mi
13.97mi
13.46mi
12.96mi
12.23mi
10.62mi
8.98mi
8.02mi
6.49mi
5.41mi
4.40mi
3.79mi
3.27mi
2.70mi
2.20mi
1.66mi
34
29
30
43
46
B34
B35
B37
B38
B39
B41
K27
K30
P2
P3
P4
P5
P6
241
405
5
N
W
S
Miles
0
0.5
1
2

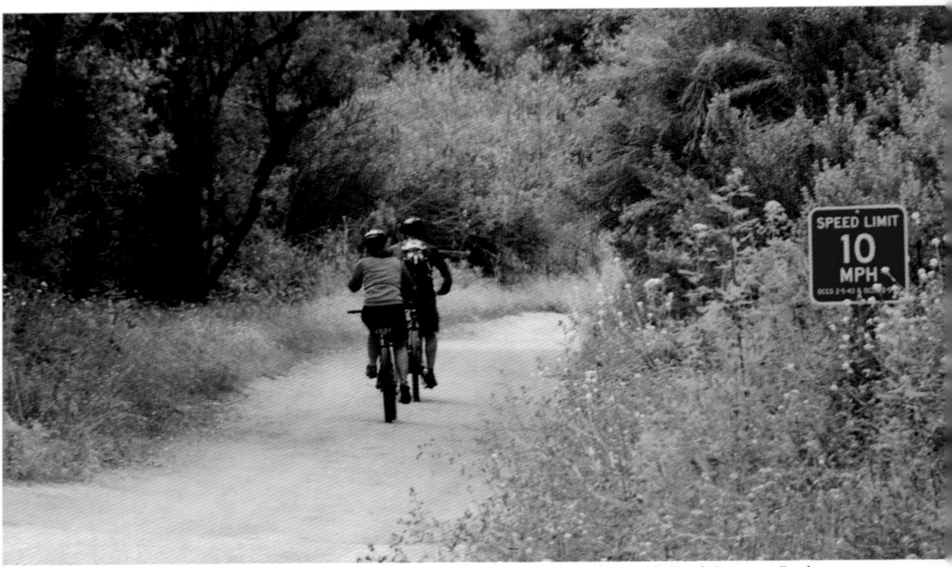

For those with fat tires, turn right at the turnaround point and start exploring Aliso and Wood Canyons Park.

At a Glance

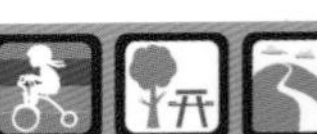

Distance 11.31 miles **Elevation Gain** 329′

Terrain

Traveling along off-street bike lanes almost entirely, this ride flows gently downhill until the turnaround point.

Traffic

This ride is car-free except for the few intersection where the path crosses roads.

How to Get There

By bus, OCTA route 188 makes a stop near Sheep Hill Park.

By car, take exit 90, Alicia Parkway, off of Interstate 5, and head south for 1.7 miles. Turn right onto Moulton Parkway and after 0.6 miles turn right on Laguna Hills Drive. Park on street next to Sheep Hill Park.

Food and Drink

Although there are not many dining opportunities along this route, Aliso and Wood Canyons offers an incredible backdrop to the perfect picnic location. For dining, head over to Laguna Hills Mall where there are plenty of options. For a truly unique experience, visit Break of Dawn with its ever-changing, Vietnamese influenced menu.

Side Trip

Aliso and Wood Canyons Park is massive and crisscrossed by hiking and mountain biking trails. At the Laguna Hills Community Center and Sports Complex check out the skate park or for youngsters visit the epic Prehistoric Playground.

Links to  

Where to Bike Rating  

   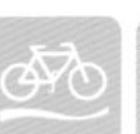 

About...

Flat and short enough for families and inexperienced riders, this ride is still interesting enough for advanced riders looking to add some miles. The route takes off from Sheep Hill Park, site of Kids' Ride 28 as well as starting point of Ride 43, and follows the lower portion of Aliso Creek Trail until it disappears into Aliso and Wood Canyons Park.

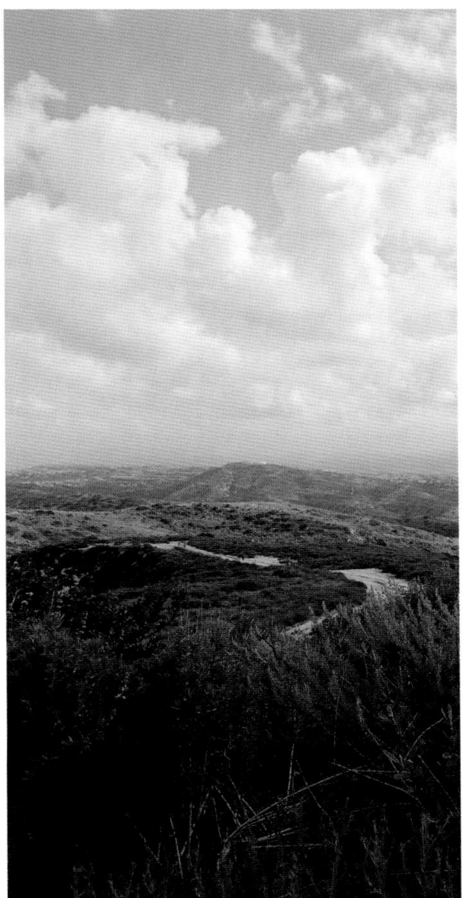

The view from the top of the world!

'or families interested in safe rides that build stamina nis is an excellent choice. Start by doing a few laps round Sheep Hill Park then pass under the bridge and ycle this trail as it follows meandering Aliso Creek. \t 3.34 miles the trail officially ends at Awma Road nd for the most inexperienced riders this is probably good turnaround point. For those venturing on, pass hrough the unpaved parking lot and pick up the paved rail that heads into the park.

Aliso and Wood Canyons Park is a spectacular wildife refuge comprised of over 3,900 acres. The trail continues gently downhill as chaparral-covered peaks ower above on either side. Once the tribal home to a umber of Native American tribes, the park is now part f the 38,000 acre Nature Reserve of Orange County vhose aim it is to preserve plants, animals and the naive environment for future generations. With over 30 niles of trails this is a paradise for hikers and mountain bikers. Pick up a map at the park entrance and hike/ bike to the aptly named Top of the World peak. At the urnaround the road continues on, however this moves onto private property and is clearly marked as trespassng.

At 9.23 miles the trail forks and a left here will reurn you to the start in the shortest possible time. For a slightly longer ride follow the Ride Log and bear right heading up the trail. This section of the route runs alongside Alicia Parkway and does cross a number of roads along the way so stay alert.

At 10.36 miles the path passes by Laguna Hills Community Center and Sports Complex and traffic in and out of here can be heavy, especially on weekends. The sports complex is vast with soccer fields, baseball diamonds and basketball courts. In one corner you will find the large skate park and nearby is the Prehistoric Playground where kids can climb through 'fossils' and over large stone turtles. Bring a picnic and let the kids explore.

Ride Log

P1 Laguna Hills Community Park and Sports Center
P2 Laguna Niguel Lake
P3 Chet Holifield Federal Building

0.0 Begin ride where Aliso Creek Trail enters Sheep Hill Park, heading into park.
0.03 Bear left into park.
0.16 Bear right and pass under Moulton Pkwy.
0.29 Continue straight. Hiking trailhead here.
0.64 Turn right and cross pedestrian bridge.
0.77 Continue straight.
3.34 Turn right onto Awma Rd.
3.41 Bear left into Aliso and Wood Canyons Park, off-street bike path resumes here.
4.22 Bear left.
4.93 Trail ends here, even though road you are traveling continues. This is private property. Mountain bikers and hikers can turn right here and explore the park.
5.64 Bear right.
6.43 Exit park.
6.45 Bear left onto Awma Rd.
6.50 Turn left back onto Aliso Creek Trail.
9.10 Continue straight.
9.19 Cross pedestrian bridge.
9.23 Bear right. A left here will take you the shortest route back to Sheep Hill Park.
9.57 Cross Laguna Ct, be alert, blind corner.

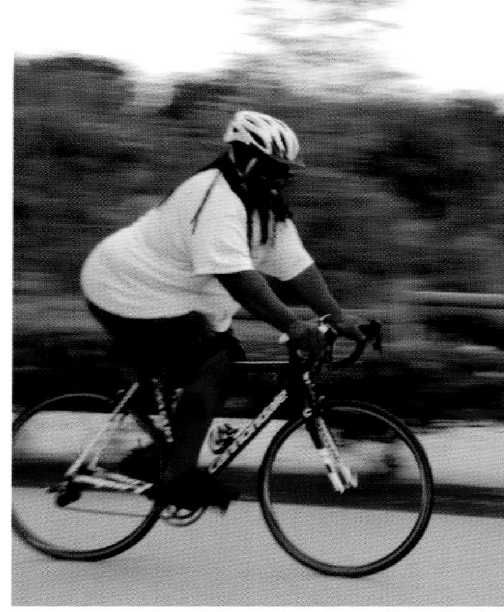

He's a blur passing through Sheep Hill Par

9.62 Bear right and pass under Moulton Pkwy.
10.08 Bear right and pass under Via Lomas.
10.36 Cross Community Center Dr.
10.44 Bear left as trail turns to parallel Paseo de Va-lencia.
10.64 Cross Hawk High Way, Laguna Hills Hig School to your left.
11.21 Cross Indian Hill Ln.
11.31 End.

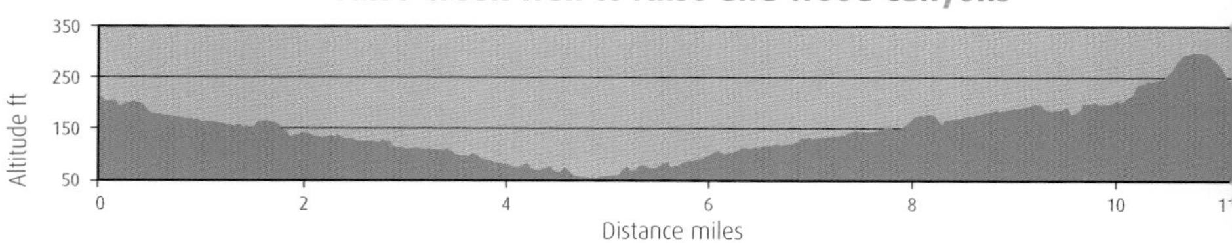

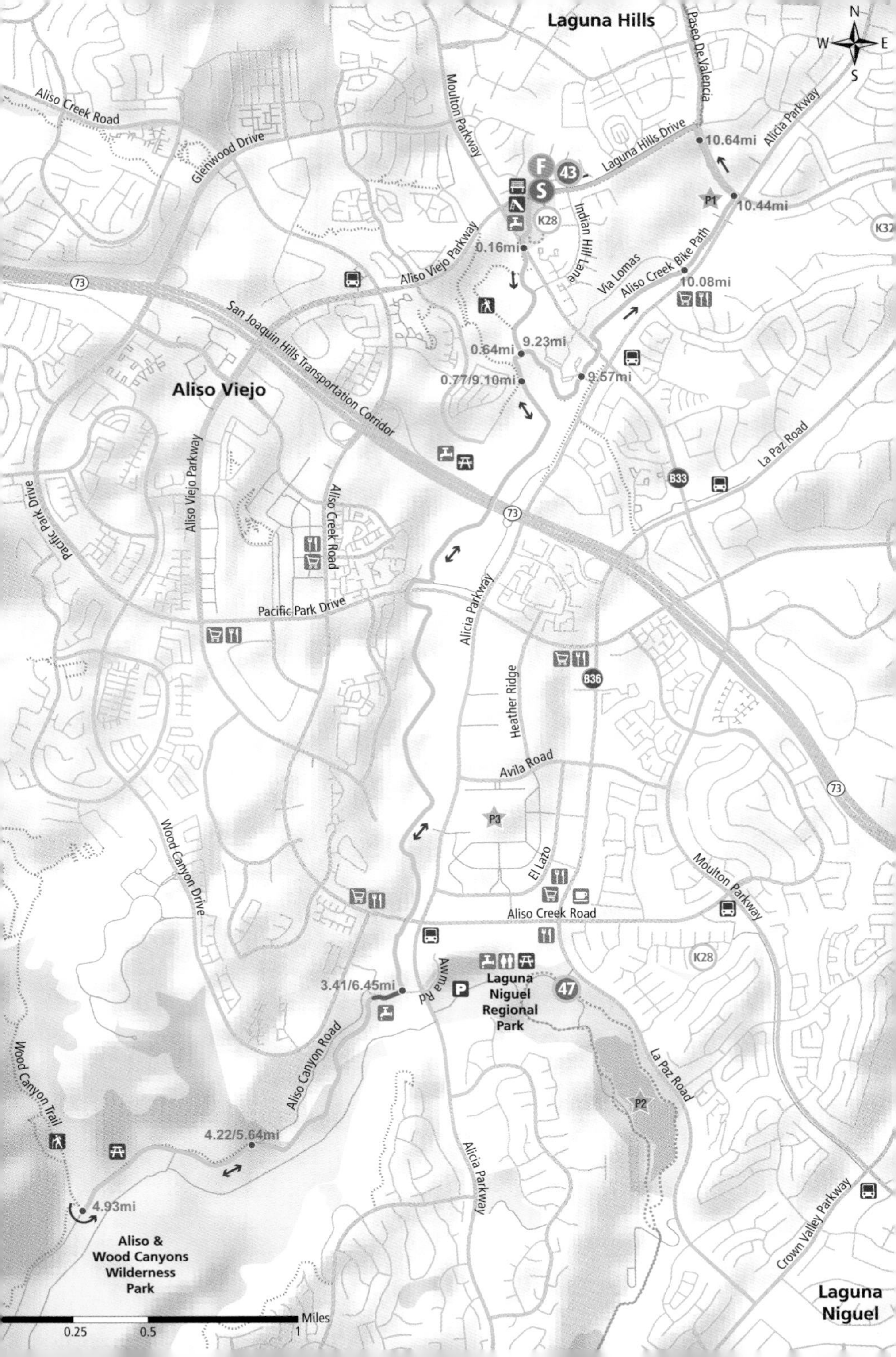
Laguna Hills
N
W
E
S
Paseo De Valencia
Aliso Creek Road
Glenwood Drive
Moulton Parkway
Laguna Hills Drive
Alicia Parkway
10.64mi
10.44mi
P1
F
S
43
K28
K32
Indian Hill Lane
Aliso Viejo Parkway
0.16mi
73
Vía Lomas
Aliso Creek Bike Path
10.08mi
San Joaquin Hills Transportation Corridor
0.64mi
9.23mi
0.77/9.10mi
9.57mi
Aliso Viejo
La Paz Road
B33
Pacific Park Drive
Aliso Viejo Parkway
Aliso Creek Road
Alicia Parkway
Pacific Park Drive
Heather Ridge
B36
Avila Road
P3
El Lazo
Wood Canyon Drive
Moulton Parkway
Aliso Creek Road
K28
Awma Rd
Laguna Niguel Regional Park
47
3.41/6.45mi
Aliso Canyon Road
La Paz Road
P2
Wood Canyon Trail
4.22/5.64mi
Alicia Parkway
4.93mi
Crown Valley Parkway
Aliso & Wood Canyons Wilderness Park
Laguna Niguel
Miles
0.25
0.5
1

This is definitely more fun than playing bridge.

At a Glance

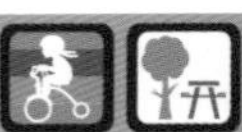
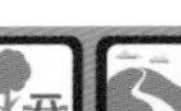 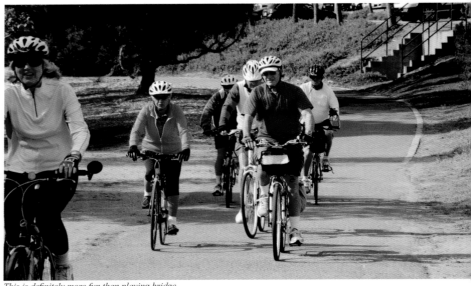

Distance 4.44 miles **Elevation Gain** 194′

Terrain

This flat ride travels off and on-street bike paths, with a short section that passes over hard-packed gravel roads.

Traffic

Expect very light, slow traffic along park roads.

How to Get There

By bus, OCTA route 187 makes a stop along La Paz Road near the entrance to Laguna Niguel Regional Park.

By car, take exit 3, La Paz Road, off of CA 73 and head southbound. Travel for 1.4 miles, the park will be on your right. Park in the lots to the immediate right upon entering.

Food and Drink

The Laguna Lake concession stand is located at 0.73 miles and carries drinks and pre-packaged foods. A the nearby intersection of La Paz Road and Aliso Cree Road is the Laguna Niguel Promenade where you wi find Avila's El Ranchito Restaurant among many othe dining choices.

Side Trip

Explore Laguna Niguel Lake. The concession stand of fers boat rentals as well as everything needed to fish Taking the first right along the park access road wi allow you to connect to Ride 46 and Aliso and Woo Canyons Park.

Links to  

Where to Bike Rating 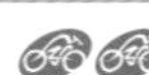

About...

This outing starts and finishes in Dana Point but not before looping through the City of Laguna Niguel. Setting out from Salt Creek Beach, one of the most beautiful settings in Orange County, the ride steadily climbs through Salt Creek Corridor before returning along wide thoroughfares. Expect panoramic ocean views, mansions perched above the ocean, stunning natural habitat and posh resorts.

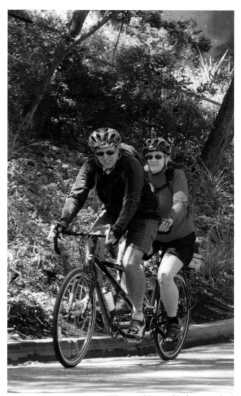

What could possibly be more fun?

rom the parking lot of Salt Creek Beach Park, head rough the mural-painted tunnel towards the beach, 'atching your downhill speed. Before the traffic turnaound, turn right on the path that cuts through the green wns. This is the beginning of Salt Creek Trail and it a beloved path used by pedestrians, joggers, surfers nd cyclists. For the first mile expect a great deal of edestrian traffic. The views through here are distracting, stay alert.

Straddling the trail are Monarch Beach and Ritz arlton resorts with golf links, spas and glitzy reputaons as a playground for the wealthy and famous. The esorts may be expensive, but parking is cheap here nd the beach is free; throw out a blanket, bring a pic-ic and enjoy the surf. Niguel Marine Life Refuge is st to the south, turn left instead of right at the bottom f the hill and you will reach it in minutes. For history uffs, Monarch Beach was the location of the Nixon terviews in 1977.

Leaving the beach the route soon passes over unlating hills. Expect short but steep climbs through alt Creek Corridor Regional Park. Hiking trails pass rough the creek and birders will find hawks soaring bove while California thrashers and roadrunners hunt own the ridiculous number of lizards that prefer to in themselves along the bike path.

At the top of Salt Creek Corridor the route heads through a tunnel under Niguel Road. Before entering the tunnel, bearing left up to the road will take you to Clubhouse Plaza where you will find Fratello's Italian Restaurant and Amber's Cantina, both with more modestly priced menus than you are likely to find at the Ritz.

Near the top of your ascent is Marina Hills Park, a long, welcoming green space. Pause for water and restrooms, take in a game of bocce. From here, one last climb and the route reaches Golden Lantern and then it is downhill to the sea. As you travel along Golden Lantern stay alert as the right turn onto the bike path at 6.43 miles, shortly after Sardina Lane, arrives just as you are hitting top speeds and there are no signs to warn you.

Ride Log

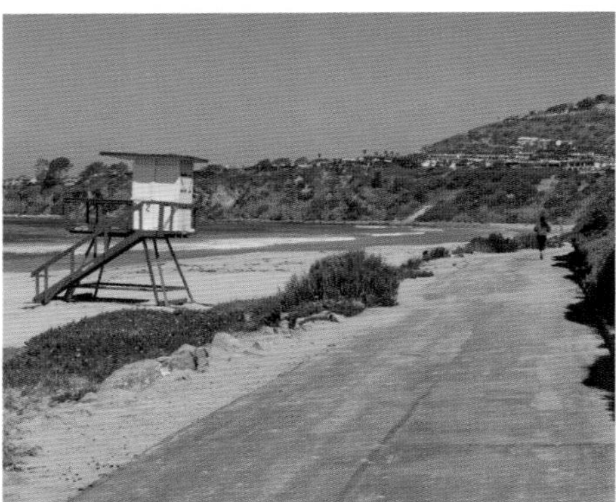

This beach path will take you to Niguel Marine Life Refuge.

- *P1* Niguel Marine Life Refuge
- *P2* Salt Creek Beach
- *P3* Ritz-Carlton Resort
- *P4* Monarch Beach Golf Links
- *P5* Laguna Niguel City Hall
- *P6* Niguel Botanical Preserve
- *P7* San Juan Creek

0.0 Begin ride at the Salt Creek Beach Park parking lot, on the path heading under the bridge towards the beach.

0.14 Turn right.

0.58 Bear left. Be alert, path is also used by electric vehicles here.

0.65 Continue straight.

1.61 Turn left after passing under bridge.

1.71 Turn right.

1.81 Bear right.

2.82 Turn right. To reach Frutello's Italian Restauran and Amber's Cantina, bear left up to Niguel Rd.

2.86 Continue straight through the tunnel.

2.93 Turn left, this is a blind corner, be careful.

3.12 Path comes to a 'T', turn left.

3.91 Turn right and follow path as it travels along Ma rina Hills Dr.

4.12 Cross Parc Vista.

4.37 Marina Hills Park on your right, water and re strooms available here.

5.09 Turn right on Golden Lantern and onto on-roa bike lane.

5.25 Cross Sweet Meadow Ln.

5.75 Cross St. Christopher.

6.32 Cross Sardina Ln.

6.43 Turn right onto bike path. Stay alert as it is eas to fly right past this turn.

7.24 Turn left onto Chapparosa Park Ln.

7.50 Chapparosa ends, move onto off-road bike path

8.32 Turn left.

8.53 Turn right.

8.70 Turn left onto path that runs alongside Niguel Rc

9.34 Cross Ridgeway Ave.

9.85 Cross Camino Del Avion.

10.62 Cross Stonehill Dr, path ends, move to on-roa bike lane.

10.80 Cross Mariner Dr.

10.91 Turn right at Pacific Coast Hwy, moving on sidewalk.

11.12 Turn hard right into Sea Terrace Park.

11.22 Turn right and pass through tunnel.

11.30 End.

Salt Creek Trail

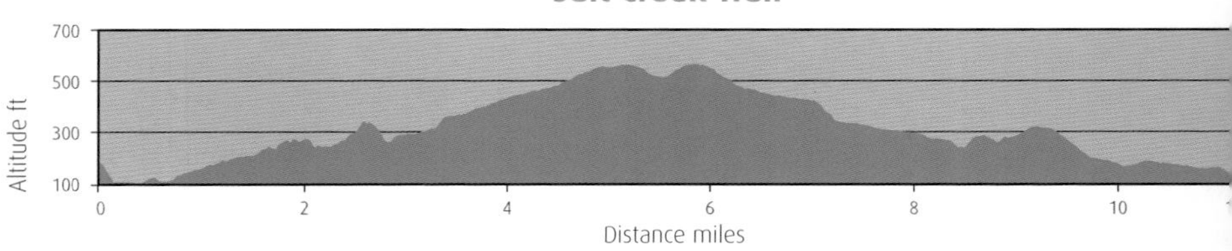

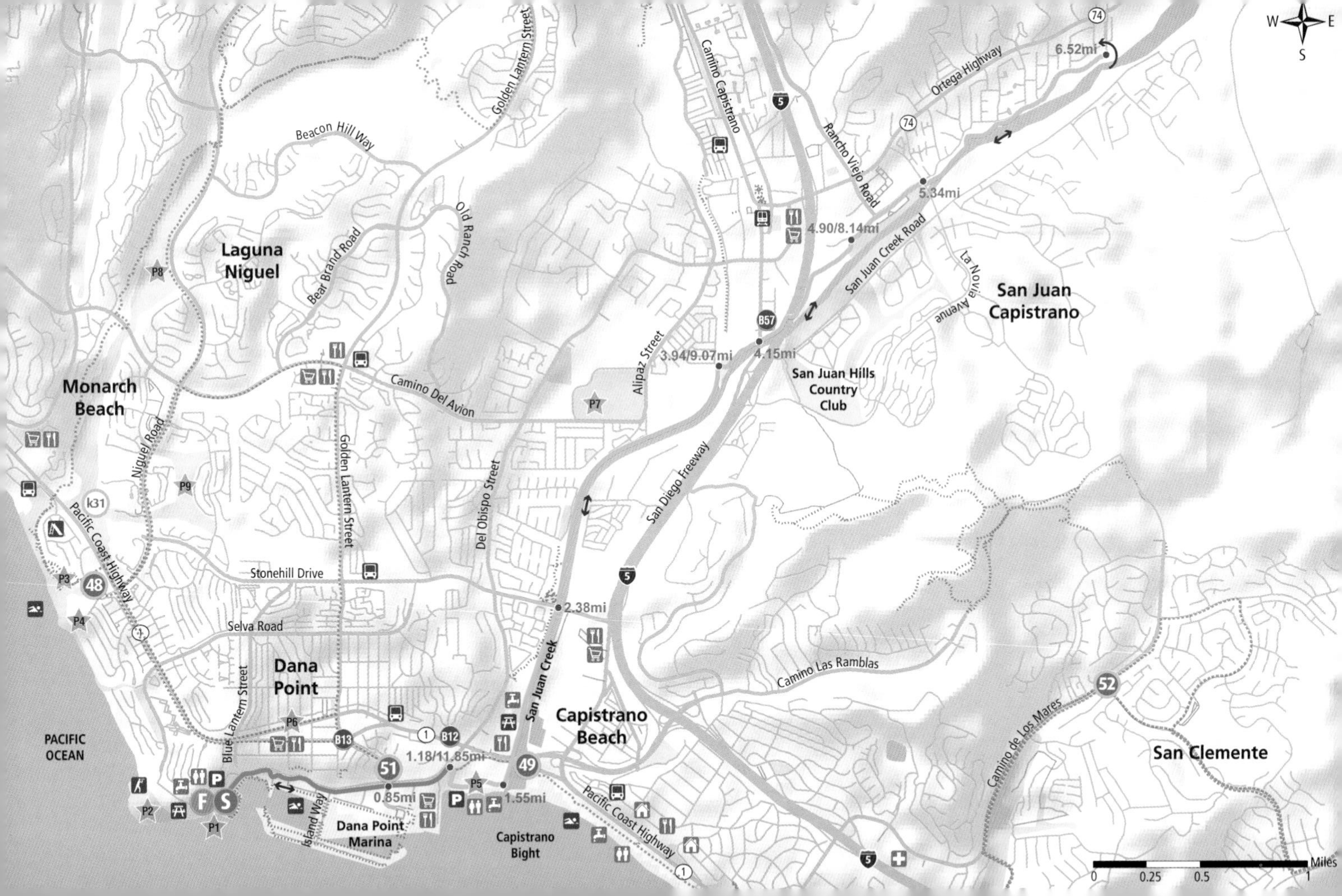

Laguna Niguel
Monarch Beach
Dana Point
Capistrano Beach
San Juan Capistrano
San Clemente
San Juan Hills Country Club
Dana Point Marina
Capistrano Bight
PACIFIC OCEAN
Golden Lantern Street
Beacon Hill Way
Old Ranch Road
Bear Brand Road
Camino Del Avion
Niguel Road
Del Obispo Street
Alipaz Street
Camino Capistrano
Rancho Viejo Road
Ortega Highway
San Juan Creek Road
La Novia Avenue
San Diego Freeway
San Juan Creek
Camino Las Ramblas
Camino de Los Mares
Stonehill Drive
Selva Road
Blue Lantern Street
Island Way
Pacific Coast Highway
6.52mi
5.34mi
4.90/8.14mi
4.15mi
3.94/9.07mi
2.38mi
1.18/11.85mi
0.85mi
1.55mi
48
49
51
52
B12
B13
B57
k31
P1
P2
P3
P4
P5
P6
P7
P8
P9
F
S
W
E
S
Miles
0
0.25
0.5
1

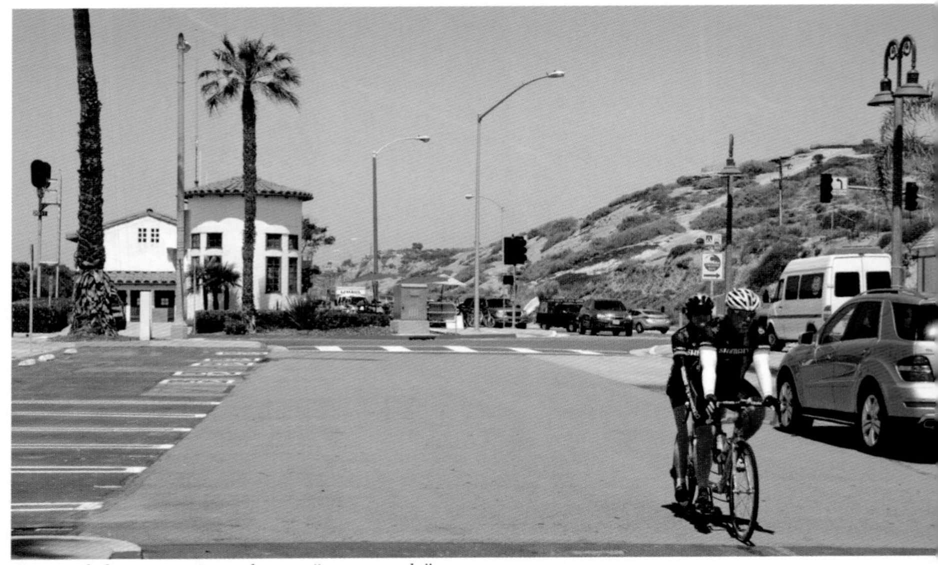

Gives a whole new meaning to the term "power couple".

At a Glance

partially

Distance 12.79 miles **Elevation Gain** 345′

Terrain

This predominantly flat route travels over a combination of on and off-street bike paths. There are two steep sections passing through Dana Point.

Traffic

The stretches at the beginning and end of the ride have heavy traffic.

How to Get There

By bus, OCTA routes 1 and 85 make stops at the intersection of Pacific Coast Highway and Laguna Niguel, near the ride's start.

By train, the ride turns around at the San Clemente Metrolink station.

By car, take exit 79, Pacific Coast Highway, off of Interstate 5 and head northbound. After 3.5 miles turn left onto Ritz Carlton Drive then take the first right into the parking lot.

Food and Drink

This ride passes through historic Dana Point with dc ens of dining opportunities. At the turnaround poi Kaylani Coffee offers a limited menu and a spectacul view.

Side Trip

At the ride's start visit Salt Creek Beach or on the w back pause to visit Dana Point wharf or historic La tern Village. Looking for more miles? Ride 53 starts the turnaround.

Links to 

Where to Bike Rating

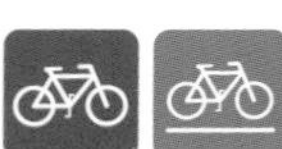

About...

This ride launches from Salt Creek Beach parking lot which is also the start of Ride 48. Where the Salt Creek Trail ride travels inland with plenty of hills to scale, this flat ride heads south to San Clemente, traveling most of its length within sight of the ocean. Palm trees, sand and waves; this is a ride through paradise.

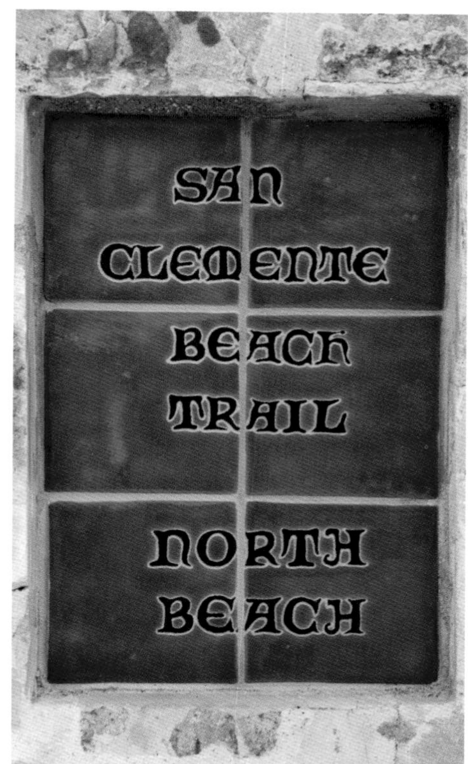

Hike the beach trail to the San Clemente Pier.

The first length of this route travels along Pacific Coast Highway and while traffic can be heavy through here, he bike lanes are nearly as wide as the car lanes. It does, however, narrow and get much busier as the route enters historic Dana Point. On-street parking and numerous exits/entrances to shopping centers make his section frenetic. Stay alert.

At 1.66 miles the Ride Log indicates a right on Golden Lantern. The road here does continue straight and you will find many cyclists continue on here. This s not recommended as the road changes to three lanes, he on-street bike lanes disappear and traffic is extraordinarily heavy. Instead, follow the recommended path and travel through safer and more pleasant Doheny State Park before rejoining Coast Highway beyond.

At 3.74 miles the route returns to Coast Highway along a protected on-street bike lane. To get in the lane you must cross train tracks and an access road. This rea can be confusing so it is especially important to follow all signs and signals and stay alert.

The turnaround is at San Clemente Metrolink station. Enjoy the outdoor seating at Kaylani Coffee as you sip lattes and look out over the tracks, expensive beach homes and the Pacific Ocean. At the end of the parking lot is the beach entrance and the San Clemente Pedestrian Beach Trail, a hard packed gravel path that ravels to the pier 1.1 miles away or to San Clemente State Beach, 2.6 miles away. Although bicycling is permitted, this gravel path is usually so crowded that it is best reserved for pedestrians.

The Metrolink station is also the beginning of Ride 53 and continues south through San Onofre State Beach all the way to Camp Pendleton Marine Corp Base. For those heading south, much like in Dana Point, cyclists do ride Coast Highway which turns into El Camino Real. However, the road is so narrow and impacted with traffic, it is not considered safe for the recreational rider. Instead follow the official bike route as indicated by signs.

On the way back make a food stop at the base of Golden Lantern and visit RJ's café for breakfast or lunch. In historic Dana Point enjoy a hearty breakfast at the Harbor House Café.

Ride Log

0.0 Begin ride at the Salt Creek Beach where Ritz Carlton Dr intersects with the public parking lot exit. Head south.
0.16 Turn right onto Pacific Coast Hwy.
0.55 Cross Selva Rd.
1.13 Cross Blue Lantern St.
1.50 Cross Amber Lantern St.
1.66 Right on Golden Lantern St.
2.01 Left on Dana Point Harbor Dr.
2.30 Right on Park Lantern Rd.
2.63 Narrow bridge, watch for cars and pedestrian traffic.
2.74 Bear right.
2.85 Continue straight.
3.00 Pass through parking lots.
3.61 Off-street path.
3.72 Turn left where path ends and cross train tracks.
3.74 Cross over Beach Rd and resume riding protected on-street path.
5.38 Protected on-street path ends at Camino Capistrano. Continue straight along on-street bike path.
6.29 Turn right onto Avenida Estacion. Bicycles San Clemente is located here as is Kaylani Coffee.
6.35 Turn around.
6.40 Cross Pacific Coast Hwy and turn left.
7.16 Cross Camino San Clemente.
7.32 At Camino Capistrano cross over Pacific Coast Hwy and return to protected on-street bike path.
8.95 Turn left at Beach Rd.

P1 Salt Creek Beach
P2 Ocean Institute
P3 Historic Dana Point
P4 San Juan Creek Trail
P5 Dana Point Marine Life Refuge
P6 San Clemente Pedestrian Beach Trail

8.99 Turn right onto trail.
9.86 Continue straight.
9.96 Turn left onto Park Lantern St.
10.41 Turn left onto Dana Point Harbor Dr.
10.71 Turn right onto Golden Lantern.
10.92 Cross Del Prado Ave.
11.15 Left on Pacific Coast Hwy.
11.65 Cross Blue Lantern St.
12.22 Cross Selva Rd.
12.63 Turn left onto Ritz Carlton Dr.
12.79 End.

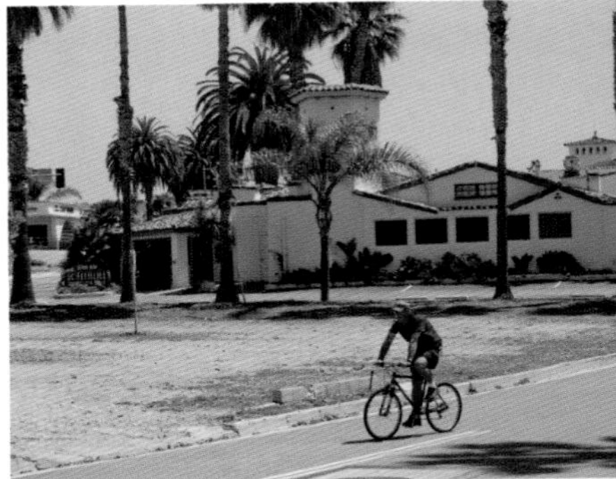

White stucco exteriors and red terra cotta tiles give Sa Clemente a Spanish village fee

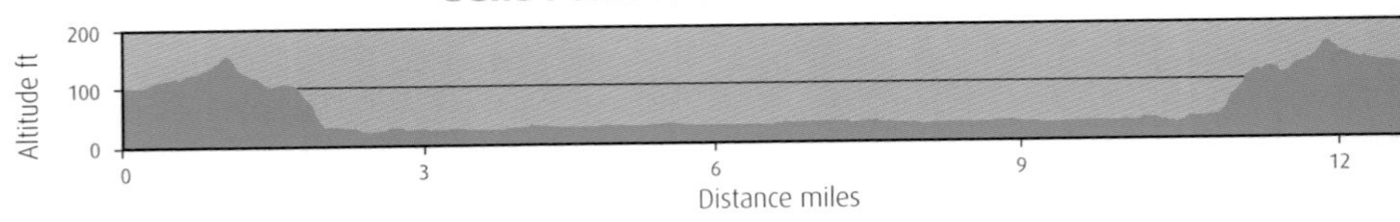

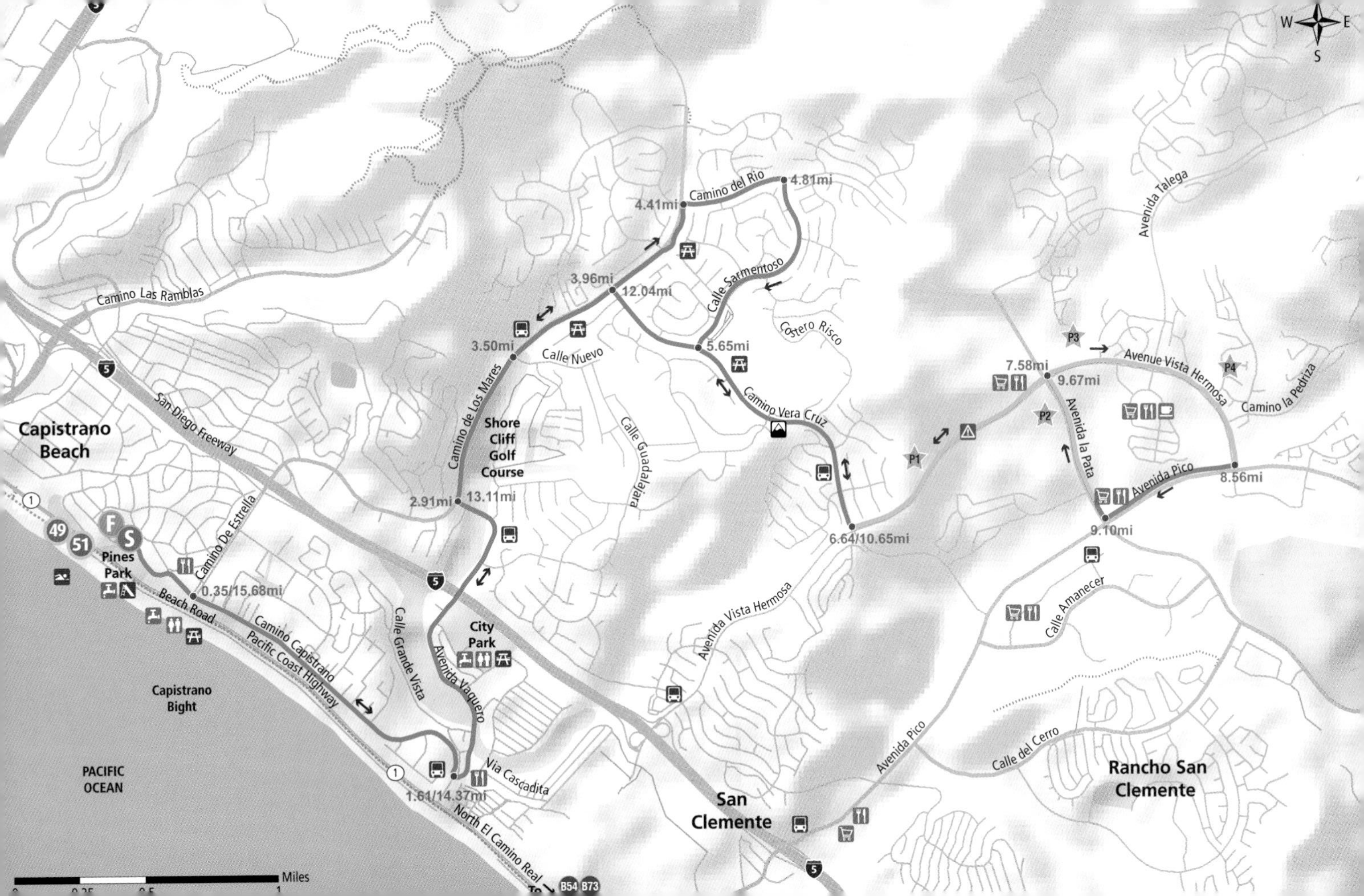

W
E
S
Capistrano Beach
San Clemente
Rancho San Clemente
Shore Cliff Golf Course
City Park
Pines Park
Capistrano Bight
PACIFIC OCEAN
Camino Las Ramblas
San Diego Freeway
Camino De Estrella
Beach Road
Camino Capistrano
Pacific Coast Highway
North El Camino Real
Via Cascadita
Avenida Vaquero
Calle Grande Vista
Camino de Los Mares
Calle Nuevo
Calle Guadalajara
Camino del Rio
Calle Sarmentoso
Costero Risco
Camino Vera Cruz
Avenida Vista Hermosa
Avenue Vista Hermosa
Avenida Talega
Camino la Pedriza
Avenida la Pata
Avenida Pico
Calle Amanecer
Calle del Cerro
0.35/15.68mi
1.61/14.37mi
2.91mi
13.11mi
3.50mi
3.96mi
12.04mi
4.41mi
4.81mi
5.65mi
6.64/10.65mi
7.58mi
9.67mi
8.56mi
9.10mi
P1
P2
P3
P4
F
S
49
51
1
5
To B54 B73
Miles
0
0.25
0.5
1

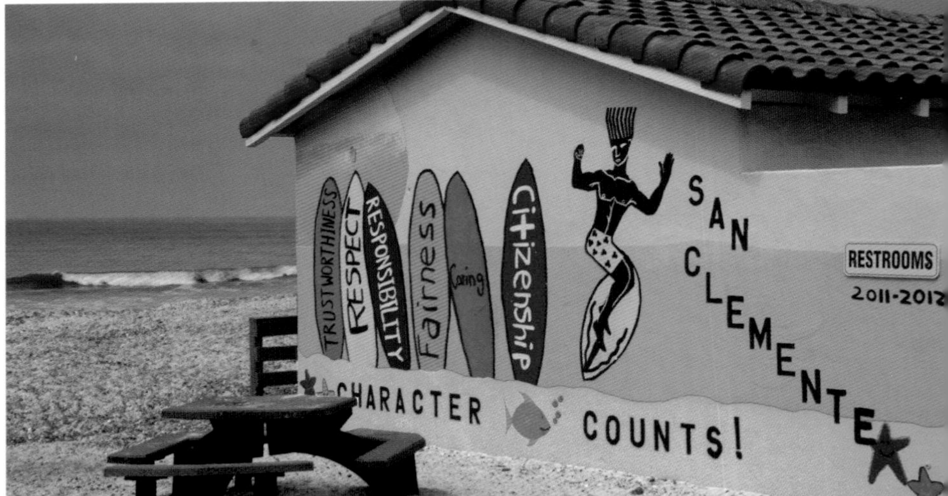

Character counts, that's why we ride our bikes!

At a Glance

Distance 29.01 miles **Elevation Gain** 1034′

Terrain

This route makes use of on and off-street bike lanes. Although there is over 1,000 feet of climbing, most of it is of the long, low-grade variety.

Traffic

Traffic on this route is light.

How to Get There

By bus, OCTA routes 1, 91, 191 and 191 all make stops near ride's start.

By train, Metrolink stops at the San Clemente station located at ride's start.

By car, take exit 76, Avenida Pico, off of Interstate 5 and head southbound. After 0.7 miles, turn right onto Calle Deshecha. Turn left at bottom of hill into parking lot.

Food and Drink

Near the ride's start, Kaylani Coffee offers a limited menu and an excellent view. For more hearty opportunities, visit Avenida Del Mar where you will find the colorful and energetic town center with a number of dining options.

Side Trip

Visit San Clemente pier and spend some time strolling white sand beaches and playing in blue surf. Stroll historic downtown San Clemente or visit world famous surf spots, Trestles and San Onofre.

Links to 51

Where to Bike Rating 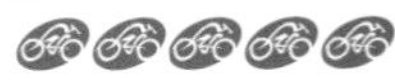

About...

As the most southerly route in this book, this ride actually leaves the cozy confines of Orange County and travels into adjacent San Diego County. Setting out from the Metrolink station, this route wanders through residential San Clemente before passing through massive San Onofre State Beach and from there through the northern portion of Camp Pendleton. With rolling hills, off-street bike lanes, bluff top views of the ocean and coastal wilderness, this is one of the finest rides of the book.

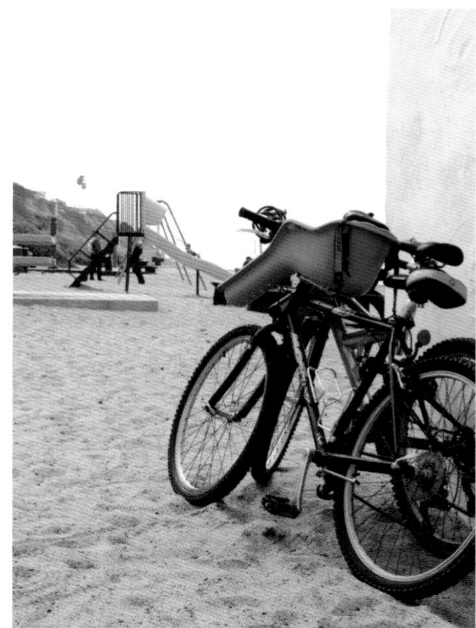

Sand, playground, ocean and bikes: a perfect family outing.

n the 1920s city founder Ole Hanson envisioned a panish-style resort town, a place where Californians ould get away from the big city. A "Spanish Village y the sea," he proclaimed. With its white stucco uildings and red tiled roofs, rocky coast line and mild limate, San Clemente definitely has a Mediterranean uality about it.

The first leg of the ride travels over the safe and leasant residential streets of San Clemente. This section of the route was laid out with the idea that it would rovide riders with an alternative to narrow, congested, angerous El Camino Real, which it parallels. Although many cyclists do ride El Camino Real, it is not ecommended.

At 4.2 miles the ride travels along an off-street path assing through Trestles Wetlands Natural Preserve, art of San Onofre State Beach. Famous as a surf spot, his 160 acre preserve features a fresh water lagoon, a ristine creek and a number of distinct plant communities. Oh, and beautiful beaches. This is also the county ne, from here on you are riding in San Diego County.

At 5.28 miles the trail ends and the ride travels along ld Highway 101 past San Onofre Nuclear Power lant before re-entering San Onofre State Beach. The next three miles pass through empty parking lots with Interstate 5 buzzing on the left and scrub covered cliffs on the right. Camping and day use is available through here as well as six trails that lead steeply to the beaches below.

At 11.16 miles the path leaves San Onofre and enters Camp Pendleton Marine Corp Base, definitely the prettiest part of the ride. Rugged and stark, the trail is a single strip of asphalt and concrete passing through coastal wilderness. There are no amenities along this section and with the exception of cyclists, no traffic at all.

The turnaround point comes at 14.5 miles when the trail ends at Las Pulgas Road. For those looking to ride further into San Diego County, turn left here and head towards the sentry post a quarter of a mile up the hill. Cyclists are permitted to travel through Camp Pendleton but absolutely must stay on designated roads. Also, valid United States Identification is required to enter the base and a Marine will check before you are allowed to pass.

Ride Log

0.0 Begin ride in front of San Clemente Metrolink station, at the convergence of Avenida Estacion and Calle Deshecha. Start by riding up Deshecha.
0.09 Turn right at Avenida Pico.
0.15 Turn left on Boca de la Playa.
0.27 Turn right on Calle Las Bolas.
0.30 Bear right onto Calle Sacremento.
0.44 Bear right onto Calle Florencia.
0.56 Turn left onto Avenida Pelayo.
0.73 Turn right on Calle Puente.
0.78 Continue straight across Avenida Aragon.
1.05 Continue straight across Mariposa.
1.21 Turn right on Avenida Palizada.
1.23 Turn left on Calle Seville.
1.56 Continue straight.
1.66 Turn right onto Ola Vista.
2.27 Continue straight on Ola Vista.
2.44 Bear left, still on Ola Vista.
3.06 Turn left on Avenida Califia.
3.13 Turn right on Avenida Del Presidente.
4.18 Turn left onto Cristianitos Rd.
4.20 Turn right onto off-street bike path running parallel to Interstate 5.
4.48 Entrance to Trestles Wetlands Natural Preserve, trail to the beach.
5.21 Bear left to continue ride, do not go right.
5.28 Leave bike trail and ride onto Old Hwy 101 along the on-street bike path.
7.97 Enter San Onofre State Park.
11.16 Leave park, ride onto off-street bike path, into Camp Pendelton.
12.92 Path turns left and passes through tunnel.

P1 San Clemente Pier
P2 Downtown San Clemente
P3 San Onofre Nuclear Generating Station
P4 San Onofre Mountain

13.02 Bear right.
14.50 Turn around at Las Pulgas Rd.
16.07 Bear right.
17.82 Return to San Onofre State Park.
23.72 Cross to other side of Old Hwy 101 to return t the off-road bike path.
24.79 Path ends, cross road and turn left onto Crist anitos Rd.
24.81 Turn right onto Avenida Del President.
25.57 Cross San Luis Rey. San Clemente Cyclery lo cated across bridge.
25.86 Turn left onto Avenida Califia.
25.90 Turn right on Ola Vista.
26.71 Continue straight on Ola Vista.
27.32 Turn left onto Avenida Santa Barbara.
27.56 Cross Avenida Del Mar, community center o your right.
27.66 Turn right on Avenida Palizada.
27.78 Turn left Calle Puente.
28.26 Turn left Avenida Pelayo.
28.43 Turn right onto Avenida Florencia.
28.55 Left on Calle Sacramento.
28.74 Bear left onto Calle Bolas
28.79 Travel through the traffic circle onto Boca D La Playa.
28.84 Turn right onto Avenida Pico.
28.90 Turn left onto Calle Deshecha.
29.01 End.

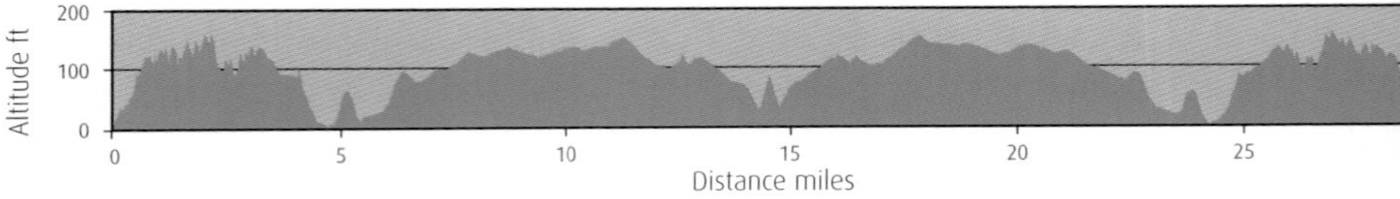

Ride K2 - Clark Park, Fullerton

Distance 0.65 miles

Terrain

Flat, smooth cement path completely car-free.

How to Get There

By car, from Interstate 5 exit onto Beach Boulevard north and travel for two miles. Turn right onto Rosecrans Avenue and then turn right into Clark Regional Park after a half mile. Street parking is free; to park inside is $3-$7.

Amenities and Things to Do

This park is loaded with things to do: barbecue pits, baseball fields, picnic areas, playgrounds, hiking trails, amphitheater, lake fishing, horseshoe pits and an interpretive center.

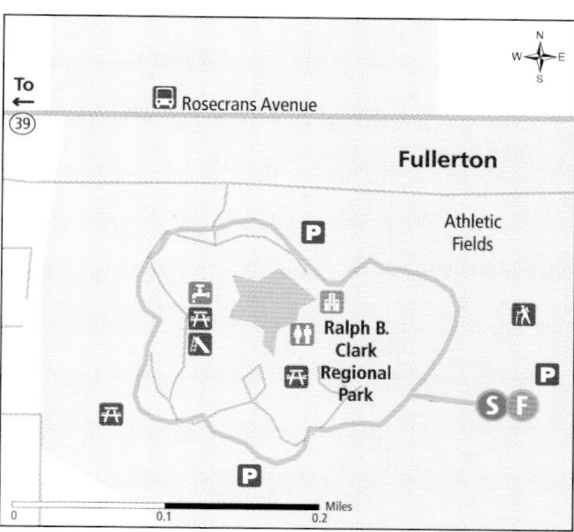

About

With 105 acres of serene, landscaped lawns between rolling hills covered in indigenous chaparral, this park is a delightful place to ride your bikes and spend a day. Amazingly, this patch of earth has yielded a large selection of fossils dating from around 10,000 years ago, back when this area was comprised of marshes and grassy woodlands. The Interpretive Center houses fossils of camels, sloths, whales, bison and wooly mammoths.

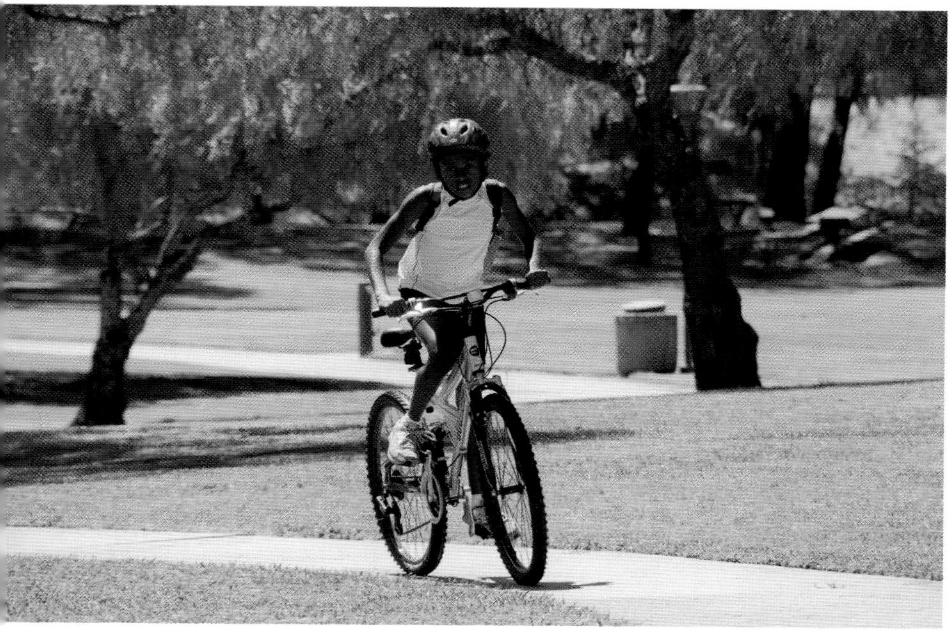

He's focused and moving fast.

Ride K3 - Gardner Park, Fullerton

Distance 0.84 miles

Terrain

A looping trail with a gentle incline in one direction, a gentle decline in the other.

How to Get There

By car, take the 91 Freeway to exit 26, Brookhurst Street, north bound. Drive 1.2 miles before turning lef onto Commonwealth Avenue. After half a mile turr right onto North Gilbert Street, then right onto Pionee Avenue after 1.3 miles. At 1.6 miles turn right ontc Benchley Street and park on your right.

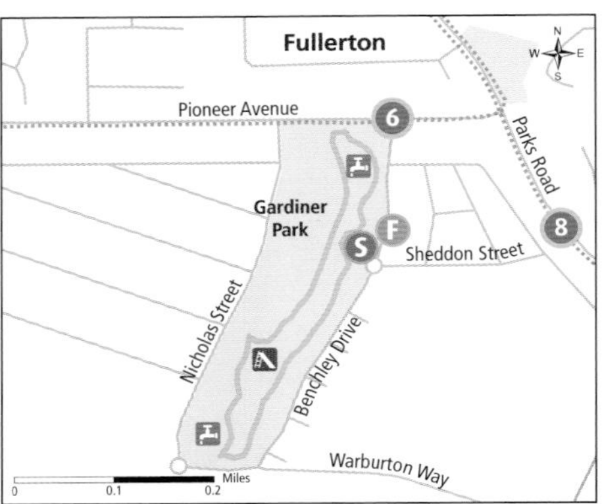

Amenities and Things to Do

This park has a wonderful playground and a joggin path alongside the bike path.

About

Long and narrow this tranquil green space is reminis cent of a Japanese garden. Through the middle of th park a ravine runs, filled with large boulders stylisti cally placed to visually imply rapids. The green gras around each rock appears to ripple away. Gracefu sycamores and pines lean over from each side of th ravine and you expect a stream to appear at any mo ment. This park is a favorite with locals as they do lap along the path. Bring your running shoes and take a jo on the gravel path as your kids pace you on their bikes

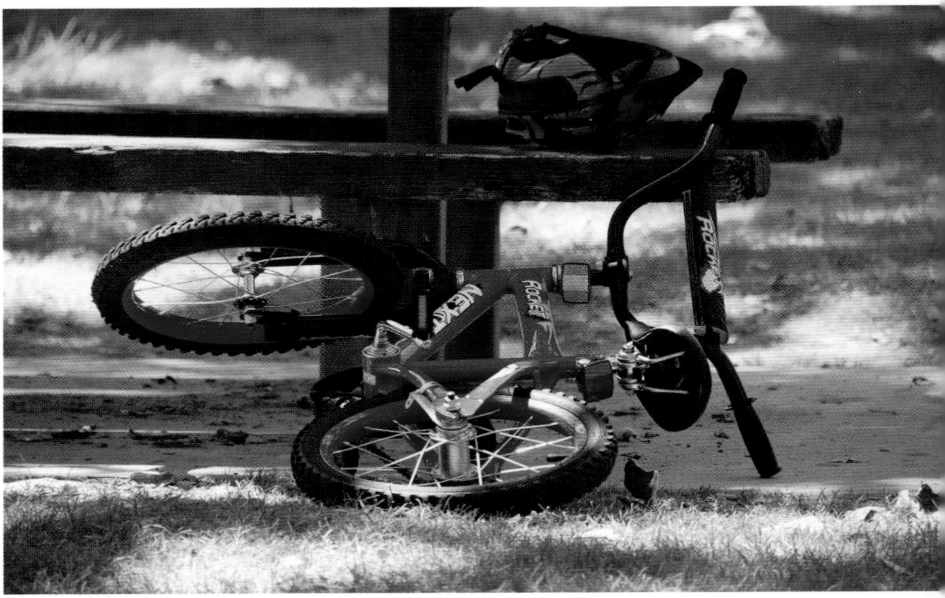

Oh to be a kid again...

Ride K4 - Acacia Park, Fullerton

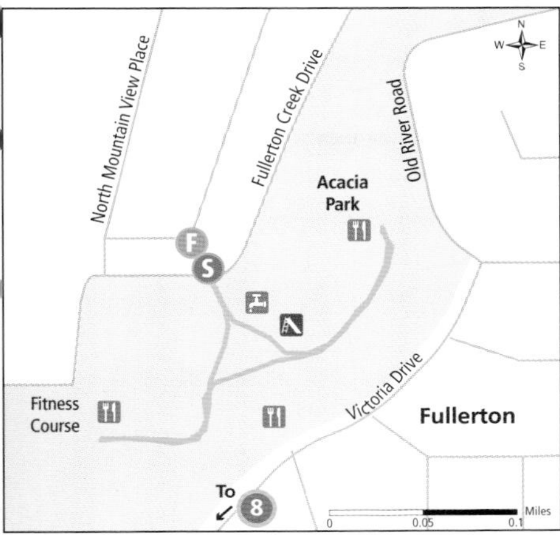

Distance 0.55 miles

Terrain

Flat, smooth cement bike paths.

How to Get There

By car, take Highway 57 to Yorba Linda Boulevard and head west. Yorba Linda ends just past State College Boulevard. Turn left onto Fullerton Creek Road, Acacia Park will be on your left.

Amenities and Things to Do

Along with a fort-like playground and a fitness course, this park has a longer family friendly ride along Fullerton Creek. Amenities include picnic tables, barbecues, and soccer fields.

About

Quiet, shady and peaceful this park is a beautiful green space complete with a creek running the park's length. Keep your eyes open and you are sure to spot ducks, cat tails, wildflowers and in the evening you will hear croaking frogs. The route follows the path running through the park's center. At its northern end, the bike path continues beyond the park and this would make for a pleasant family ride.

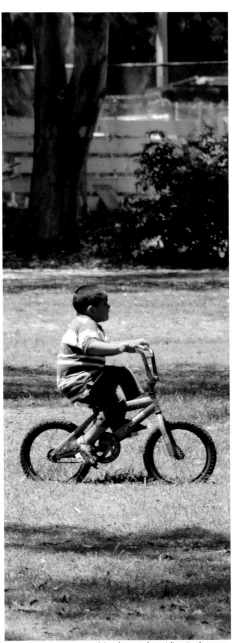

It's a lot tougher riding in the grass.

Ride K5 - Craig Regional Park, Fullerton

Distance 1.11 miles

Terrain

Mostly flat and smooth with a single, moderate hill to climb.

How to Get There

By bus, OCTA bus number 57 stops at this park.

By car, take 57 Freeway to exit 8, Yorba Linda Boulevard, eastbound. Turn right on State College Boulevard and drive 1.6 miles. The park will be on your right. Follow sports complex signs downhill to find the start.

Amenities and Things to Do

Besides being crisscrossed by bike paths, this park has barbecues, picnic tables, baseball fields, lakes, a rose garden, equestrian trails and an interpretive center.

About

As you ride through the valleys and hills of this verdant park it is almost impossible to imagine a time when oil towers, tanks and scrub covered this land. But in the early 1900s the oil boom was on and this was oil coun try. In the 1930s a series of devastating floods led t the building of the Fullerton Dam and this flood basi eventually became a regional park in 1971. For olde kids, ride the moderately steep trail up to the top of th dam for a scenic view of the valley and hills.

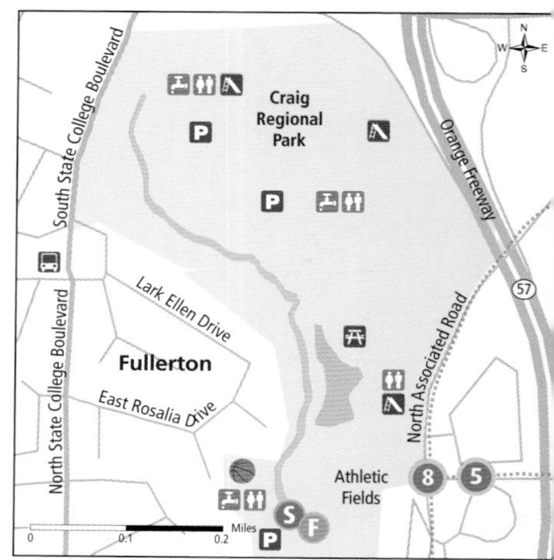

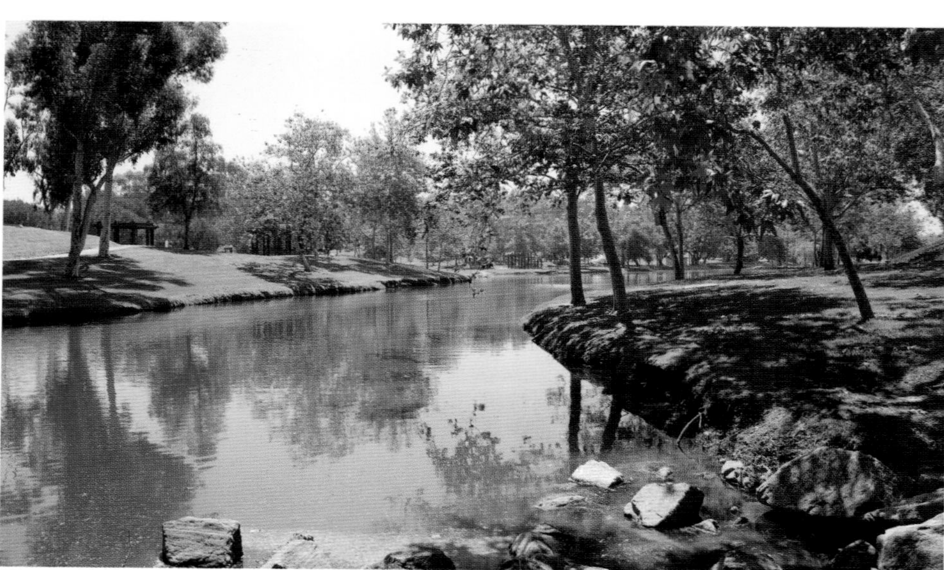

Where are the fish?

Ride K6 - Pearson Park, Anaheim

Distance 0.36 miles

Terrain

This ride is on a flat, smooth cement path.

How to Get There

By bus, OCTA bus number 43 passes Pearson Park along Harbor Boulevard.

By car, take the 91 Freeway to exit 28, Harbor Boulevard, and head south for one mile. The park will be on your left.

Amenities and Things to Do

Located within these 19 acres, Pearson Park has playgrounds, tennis courts, a baseball field, cactus gardens and a lagoon. But the highlight is the beautiful Pearson Amphitheatre built in 1927.

About

This urban park, the first built in the city of Anaheim, is an easy, flat ride that features a remarkable cactus and lagoon garden designed and installed in 1921 by horticulturist Rudy Boysen, father of the Boysenberry. Also located in the park, is Pearson Amphitheatre. This Spanish style building with red terracotta tiles and arbors of mature Bougainvillea and wisteria vines is an excellent place to take in a show. The season generally runs from May through October and is family oriented. Check their website for a calendar.

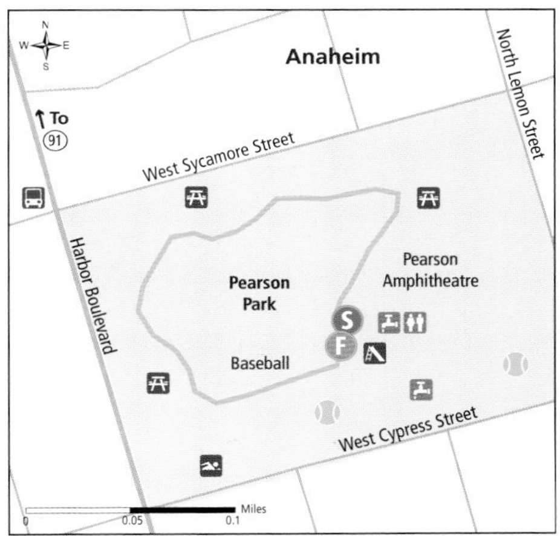

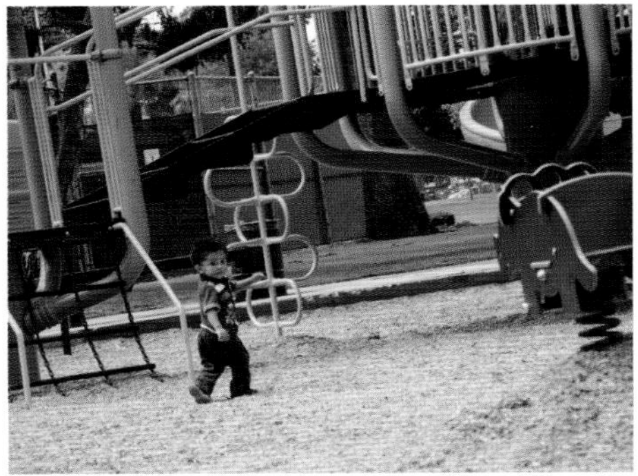

Whoa! It's a topsy-turvy world.

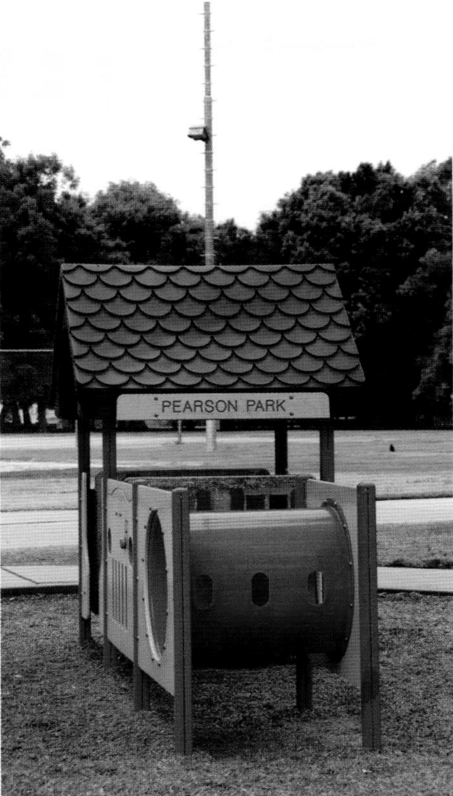

Is this the amphitheatre?

Ride K7 - Yorba Regional Park, Yorba Linda

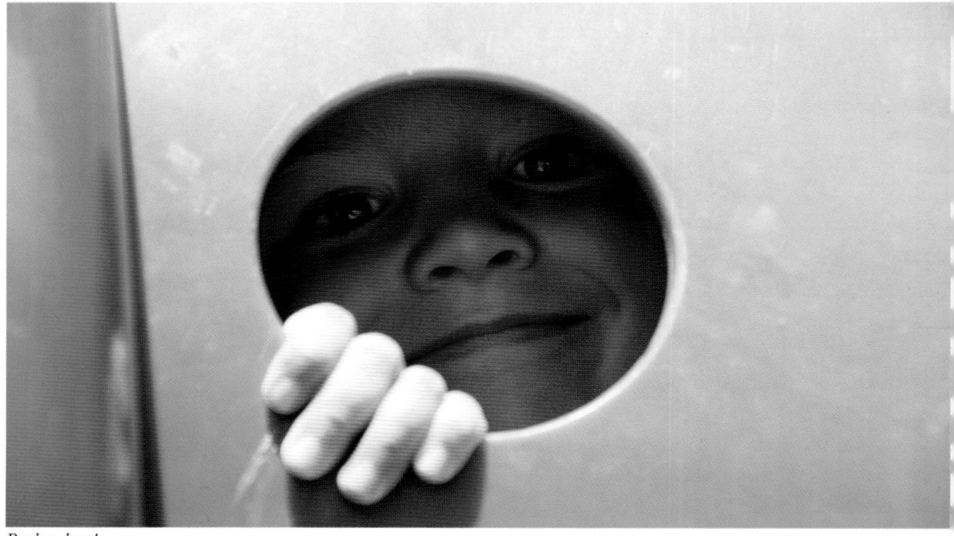

Peek-a-boo!

Distance 0.54 miles

Terrain

Flat loop that travels on well-maintained paths.

How to Get There

By bus, OCTA 38 stops near the park entrance.

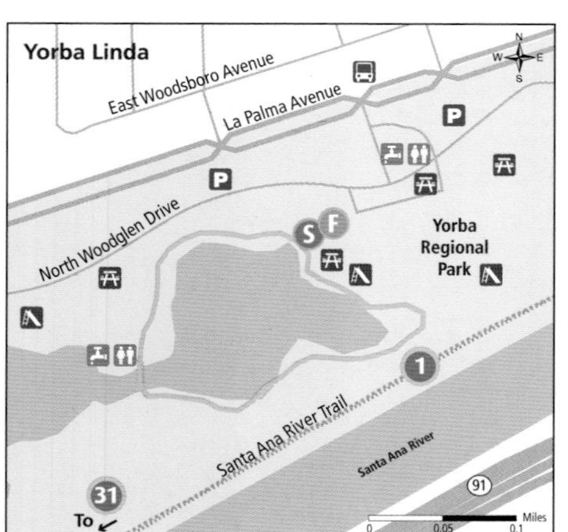

By car, take Highway 91 to exit 31, Imperial Highway. After 0.5 miles, turn right on East La Palma Avenue and travel for 2.2 miles. Park entrance is at North Woodglen Avenue on your right.

Amenities and Things to Do

Over 400 picnic tables, plus lakes, streams, playgrounds, baseball diamonds, volleyball courts, bike rentals and barbecues fill this enormous park.

About

Originally part of a cattle ranch, this 166 acre park at the mouth of Sana Ana Canyon is a cyclist's paradise. For the kid's ride the route loops around the smaller lake, but as a family outing you could ride miles and miles and never leave the park. The larger, outer route is over 3.1 miles but does cross over park roads a couple of times.

The Santa Ana River flows past the park and is quite a sight to pause beside, especially after a rainfall. Interpretive signs explain the history of the people and the river and how its use has changed over the years.

Ride K8 - Central Park and El Rancho Verde, La Palma

Distance 0.71 miles

Terrain

Smooth, flat cement bike path.

How to Get There

By car, take the 91 Freeway to the Orangethorpe exit, westbound, then turn left on Walker Street. Drive half a mile and then turn into Central Park parking lot.

Amenities and Things to Do

The La Palma Community Center is connected to Central Park. Facilities include tennis courts, baseball fields, soccer fields, basketball courts, two playgrounds and bike paths that connect the park to a long greenbelt. Under gazebos you will find plenty of picnic tables as well as fixed barbecue pits.

About

This peaceful park is a pleasant environment to enjoy with the family. Well maintained and clean, the park is part of the City of La Palma's civic center with a community center, police station and hospital nearby. It also is connected to El Rancho Verde, a greenbelt with a meandering bike path that makes up part of this ride. The greenbelt, however, carries on even further than this route and makes for an excellent family ride. During summer months free concerts in the park are held here at Central Park Amphitheater and spectators are encouraged to bring a picnic and enjoy a show. Central Park also hosts a number of other community events including a fun run, a Halloween parade and a Christmas tree lighting ceremony. Check with the city website to find dates and times.

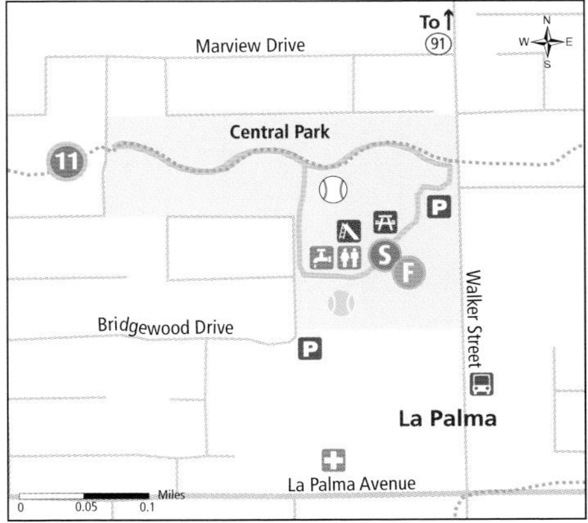

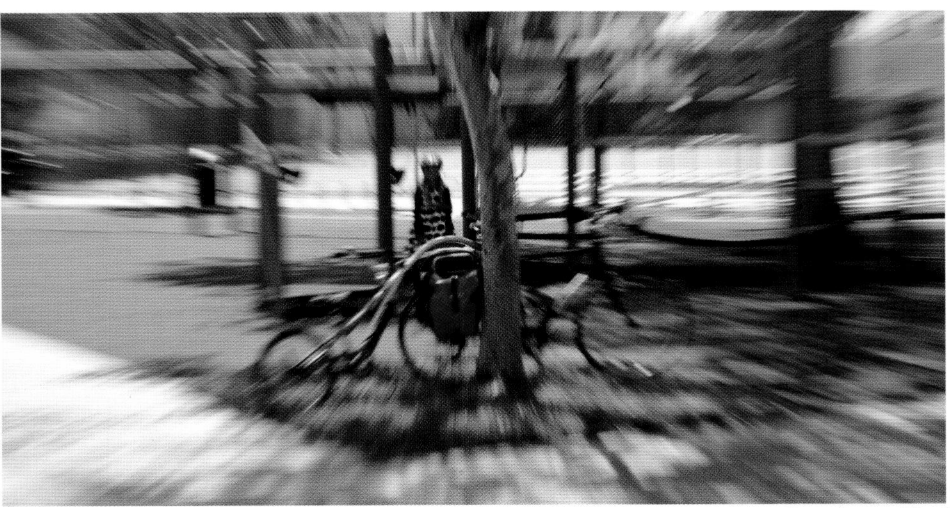

A zooming good time!

Ride K9 - El Dorado Loop, Long Beach

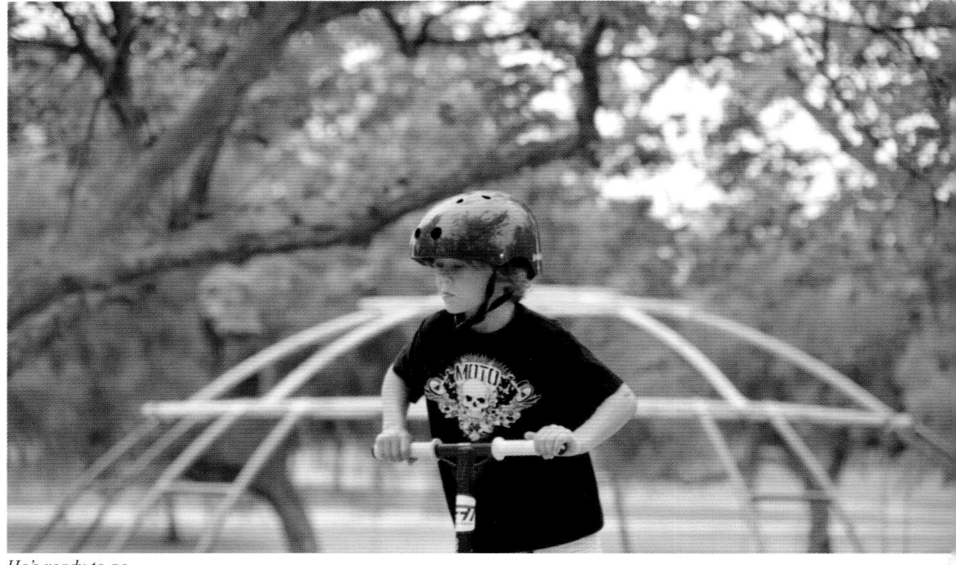
He's ready to go.

Distance 0.5 miles

Terrain

A short loop on a smooth cemented bike path.

How to Get There

By car, take the Interstate 605, exit west on Spring Street. Park entrance is on the right and costs $5 on weekdays, $8 on the weekends and holidays. When you enter you will be in Area 2, follow signs to Area 3. When you reach Area 3, the Golden Groves parking lot that is adjacent to the ride start is on your immediate left after passing under the bridge.

Things to Do

The El Dorado Express, a steam engine train, runs nearby on Saturdays and Sundays. Ride 12 overlaps part of this route and makes for an excellent family ride. The Nature Center in Area 1 of the park is a wonderful way to spend a couple of hours learning about local flora and fauna.

About

This ride loops around three interconnected playgrounds and makes for a perfect place for a family picnic. Sit atop the small knoll and watch your kids play on the swings or time them as they do loops around the playgrounds.

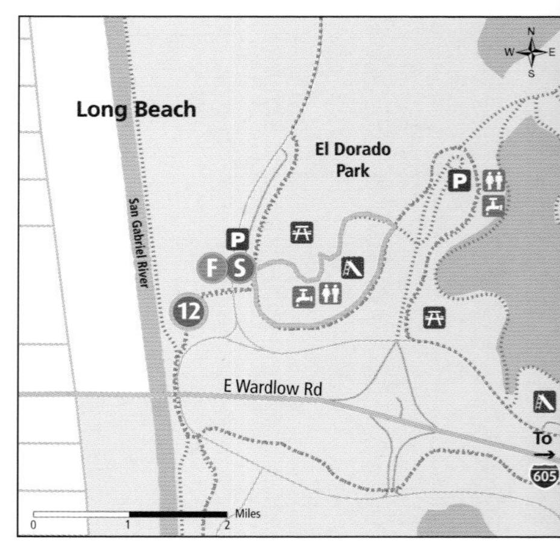

Ride K10 - Garden Grove Park and Atlantis Play Center

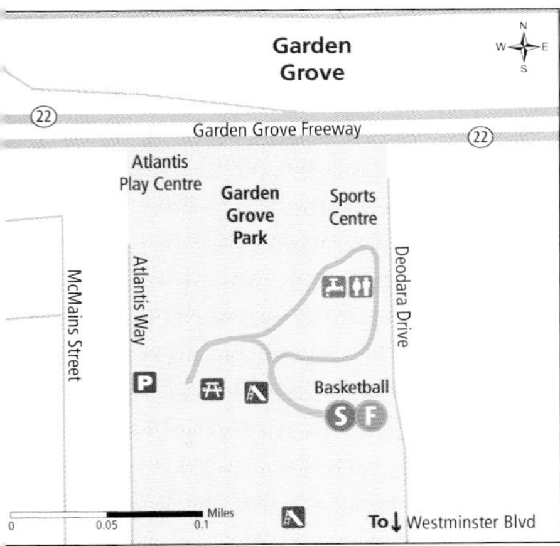

istance 0.43 miles

errain

'lat, cemented paths through a grassy park.

low to Get There

y bus, OCTA bus 60 travels along Westminster Boulvard and stops at Garden Grove Park.

By car, take the 91 Freeway to Magnolia Street, south. Take first left onto Westminster Boulevard then turn left onto Deadara Drive. Parking is plentiful between Deadara and Atlantis Way.

Amenities and Things to Do

Besides the many playgrounds scattered throughout Garden Grove Park, there are baseball fields, basketball courts, a dog park, a recreation center and a skate park. Under the pavilion at the ride's start are picnic tables and fixed barbecue stands. The highlight of the park however, is Atlantis Play Center located off of Atlantis Way in the northwest corner of the park.

About

This park is an excellent place to spend an afternoon. There is not much in the way of food nearby so bring a picnic lunch, or barbecue. After the kids have done the short bike loop and finished playing on the playground equipment, take them over to the Atlantis Play Center where a giant sea serpent slide awaits them along with six lost world themed playgrounds. Atlantis is a well shaded park with plenty of comfortable places to relax while the kids climb, swing and slide to their heart's content. Bikes are not permitted inside Atlantis.

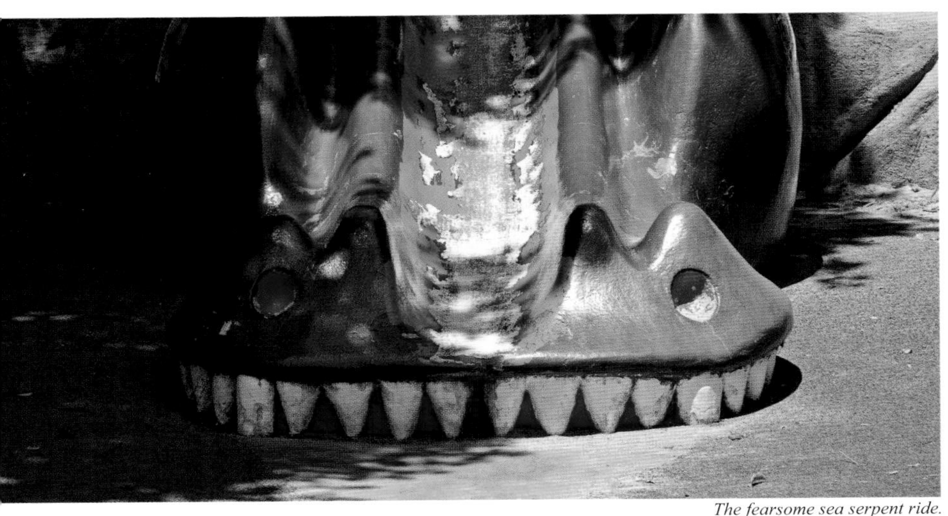

The fearsome sea serpent ride.

Ride K11 - Mile Square Park, Fountain Valley

Distance 0.86 miles

Terrain

Flat, smooth cement sidewalks.

How to Get There

By bus, OCTA bus route 70 stops on Edinger Avenue which runs along the northern boundary of Mile Square Park.

By car, take Interstate 405 and exit onto Brookhurst Street, northbound. Turn right on Edinger.

Amenities and Things to Do

This park screams out for all day picnics and bicycling. There are barbecue pits, playgrounds, a stocked lake for fishing, nature center, bike rentals, fitness course, golf course and archery range. There is no way the kids can get bored here.

About

During World War II the United States Navy Department used this patch of land for military airfields. In 1970 it began its transformation into 640 acres of green-

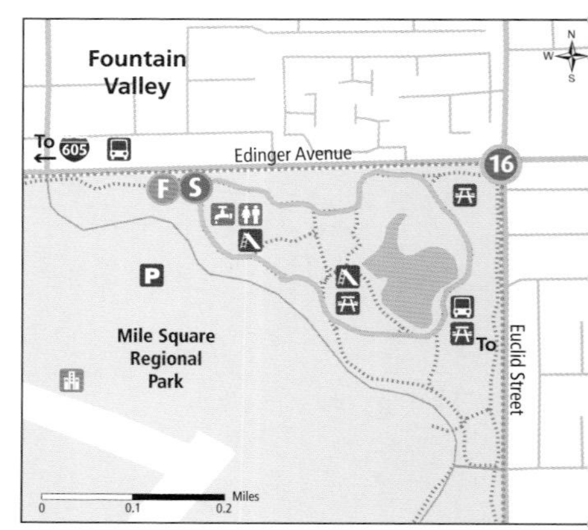

ery, lakes, playgrounds, bike paths and a golf course.

The route described in the log is essentially a bi loop around the lake located in the northern section o the park. However, bike paths abound in this park an there could be any number of routes to ride. There i also a path that circumnavigates the entire park whic makes for a terrific family ride, but not one kids shoul travel unattended. Bikes are available for rent at Whee Fun Rentals, as are paddle boats for the lake.

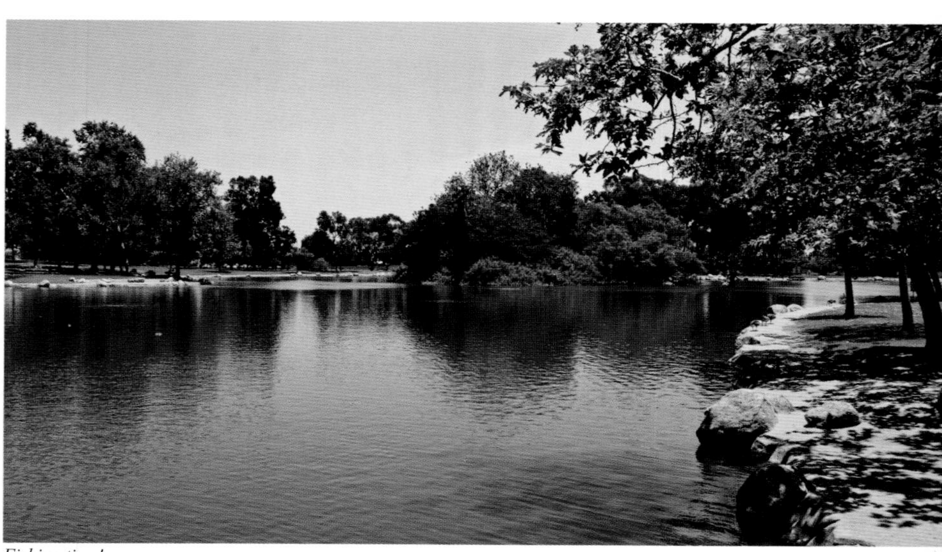

Fishing time!

Ride K12 - Lagenbeck Park, Huntington Beach

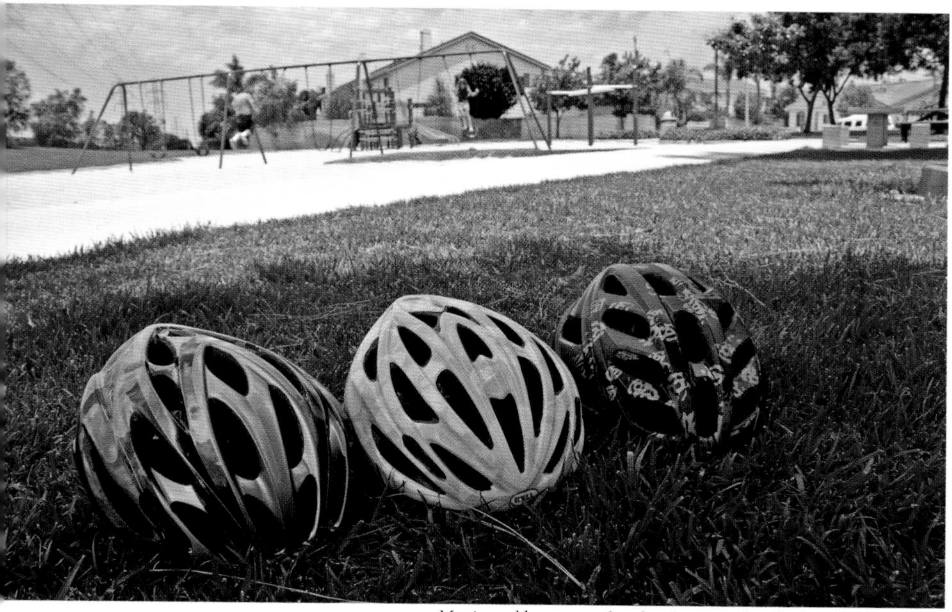

Manicured lawns, sand and a playground make for a kids' paradise.

Distance 1.16 miles

errain

Vide, cement path, through a greenbelt.

low to Get There

3y bus, OCTA route 33 passes along the Magnolia treet edge of the park.

By car, take Interstate 405 and exit at Magnolia treet, southbound. At 2.5 miles turn right onto Garield Street and after about a quarter mile, turn left.

menities and Things to Do

'laygrounds and a vast green space to frolic.

bout

'his L-shaped park is named after Vernon E. Langeneck who served as Huntington Beach mayor from 950-1952. An extra wide cement path runs the length f the park and can accommodate joggers, walkers and dogs. If you're also a runner, consider jogging while your kids pace you on their bikes. Along the path are picnic tables and plenty of shady trees to lounge under. Halfway along the ride is an excellent playground. Street side parking is available on Magnolia or Garfield.

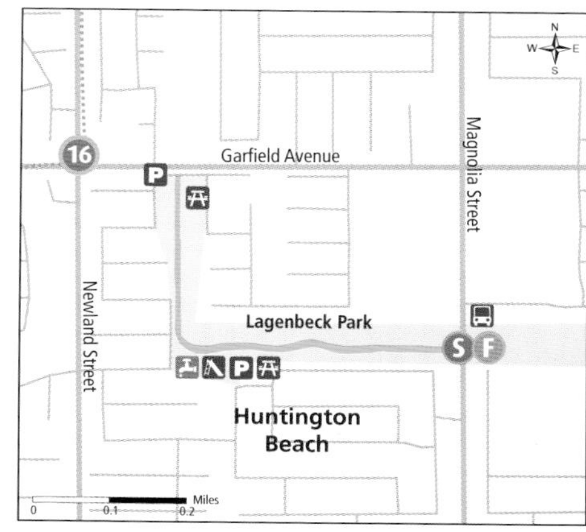

North Coast
Kids' Rides

Ride K13 - Huntington Central Park, Huntington Beach

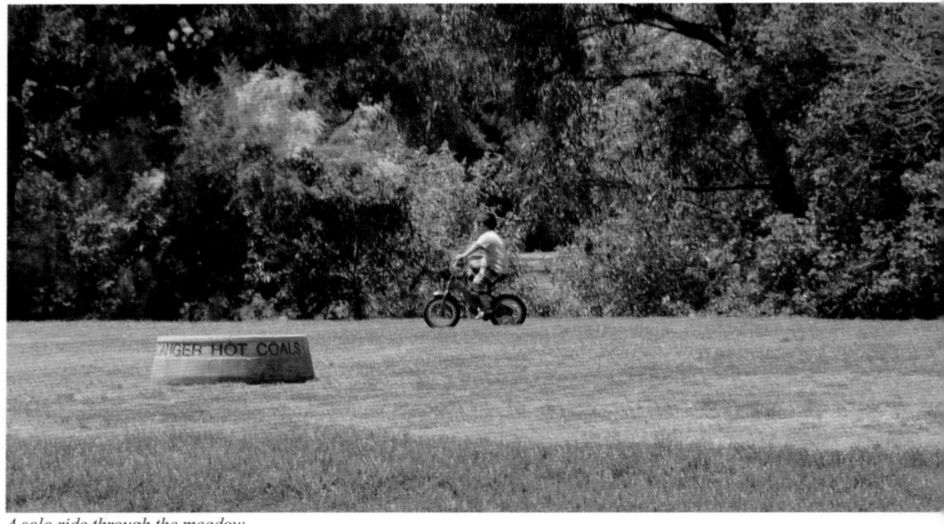

A solo ride through the meadow.

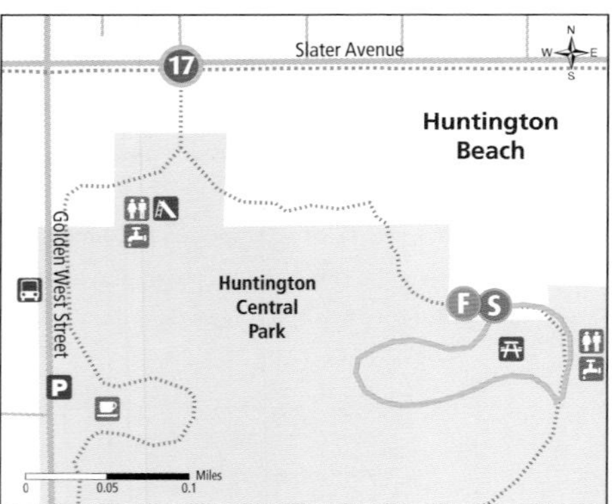

Distance 0.35 miles

Terrain

Mostly flat bike paths through meadows.

How to Get There

By bus, take OCTA route 25.

By car, take Interstate 405 to Goldenwest Street and exit southbound. Travel for three miles until you reach Central Park and turn left into parking lot.

Amenities and Things to Do

This is a large park with a full day's worth of activitie that include playgrounds, an adventure playground dog park, nature center, a library, an equestrian cente fitness course, sports complex, disc golf course and wonderful little restaurant.

About

This peaceful park is crisscrossed by a number of bik paths. The route shown here is a paved loop through meadow in the northeast section of the park. Enjoy picnic lunch or read a book as your children do loo after loop along the undulating path. Nearby is a playground as well as the Park Bench Café nestled besid Talbert Lake. This outdoor café serves excellent breakfast and lunch fare in an amazingly beautiful setting On weekends, expect a long wait.

The Central Library is a beautiful building perche upon a hilltop overlooking Talbert Lake and is wel worth a visit for story time or just to enjoy the view On the other side of Goldenwest, the park is equall beautiful with plenty to do. Here you will find the dis golf course, equestrian center and Huntington Lake.

Ride K14 - Riverdale Park, Anaheim

Distance 0.3 miles

Terrain

Mostly flat with a slight rise at the end.

How to Get There

By car, take exit 33 Tustin Avenue, southbound, off of the 91 Freeway. Take the first left onto Riverdale Avenue and travel for one mile, the park will be on your left.

Amenities and Things to Do

Riverdale Park is a small but well-appointed space with picnic tables and shelters, restrooms, barbecues, basketball courts, baseball diamond and a playground.

About

This ride is a short there and back affair which will allow younger kids a lot of safe bicycling practice. This park's greatest attribute however, is the fact that it is located adjacent to the Santa Ana River Trail and makes for a perfect place to start and end a longer family ride.

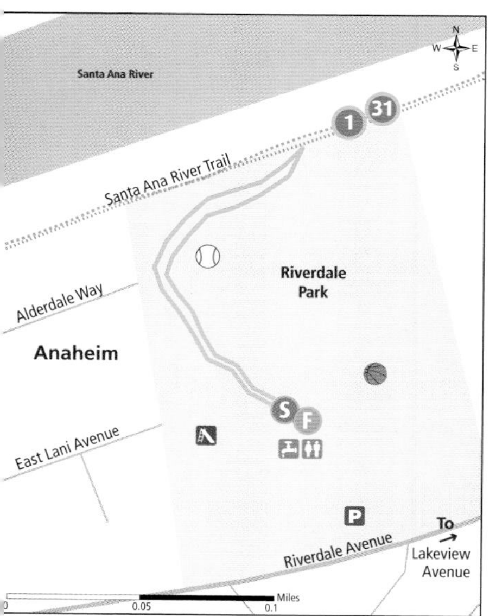

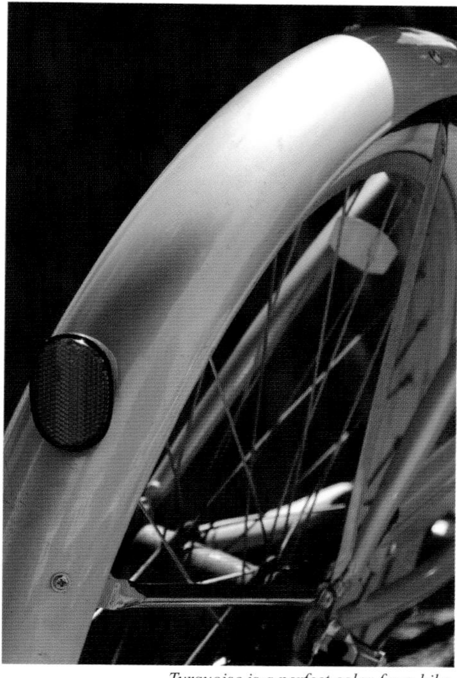

Turquoise is a perfect color for a bike.

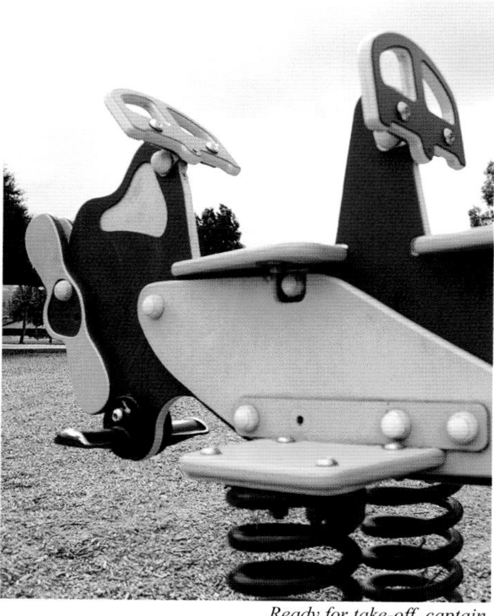

Ready for take-off, captain.

Central Inland
Kids' Rides

Ride K15 - Northwood Community Park, Irvine

Distance 0.49 miles

Terrain

This is a completely flat ride over a wide, smooth bike path.

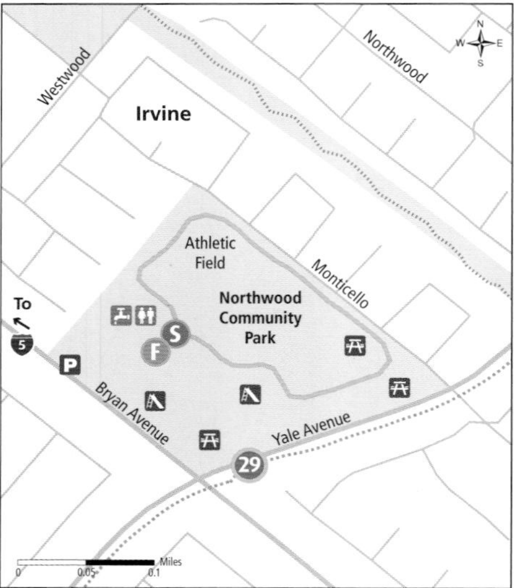

How to Get There

By bus, OCTA bus 79 stops at Bryan Avenue alon Yale Avenue.

By car, take exit 99, Culver Drive, northbound o of Interstate 5 and travel 0.6 miles before turning righ onto Bryan Avenue. The park will be on your left afte 0.5 miles.

Amenities and Things to Do

This wonderful park has basketball, racquet ball an tennis courts along with barbecues, picnic tables an a large green space. But, as your kids will tell you, th best part of the park is Castle Northwood.

About

Oh to be a child again! This well designed park ha many amenities but its playground will certainly be th highlight. Complete with walls and banners and play ground equipment resembling castle towers, you wi wish for the days you played at knights and dragon and princesses. The ride starts between the playgroun and the basketball courts and loops around the ope green space and baseball diamond.

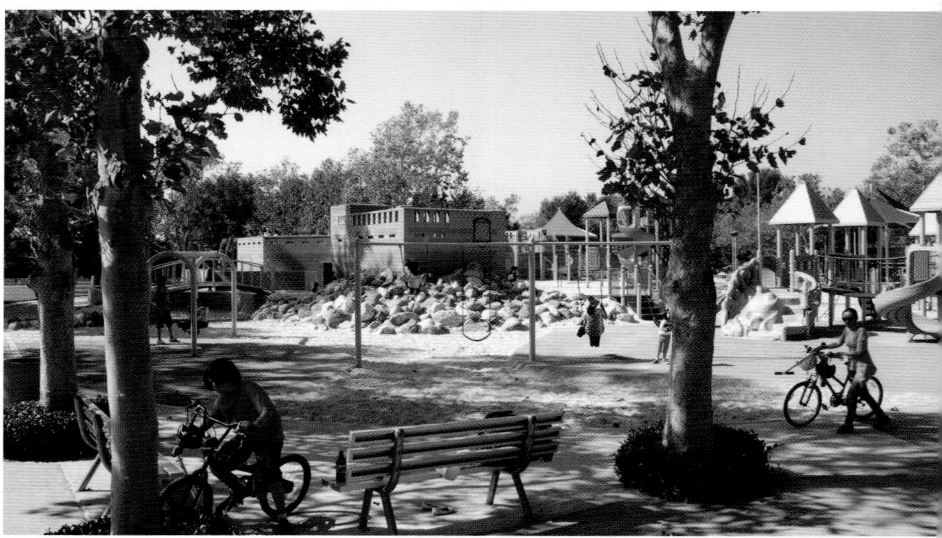

Knights and princesses will enjoy riding their steeds through this park.

Ride K16 - Cedar Grove, Tustin

istance 0.32 miles

errain

nis ride is flat, with half of the route on cement paths, e other half on packed dirt.

ow to Get There

y car, take exit 101, Tustin Ranch Road, northbound f Interstate 5. After 2.7 miles turn left onto Pioneer 'ay, and then left onto Pioneer Drive after 0.1 miles. ne park will be on your left.

menities and Things to Do

nis park has sheltered picnic tables, basketball courts, ree playgrounds, grass fields and a nature trail.

bout

edar Grove Park is located at the bottom tip of Peters anyon. This green space is a pleasant combination of wn, playground and woods. The woods are courtesy f the Irvine Company who planted 14 Coast Red-oods and 321 Deodor Cedars in the early 1900s to e if they could be grown commercially. This mature ove is now a peaceful nature walk. On the opposite de of the grove is Peters Canyon Trail, part of Ride 25 nd a great opportunity for a family ride.

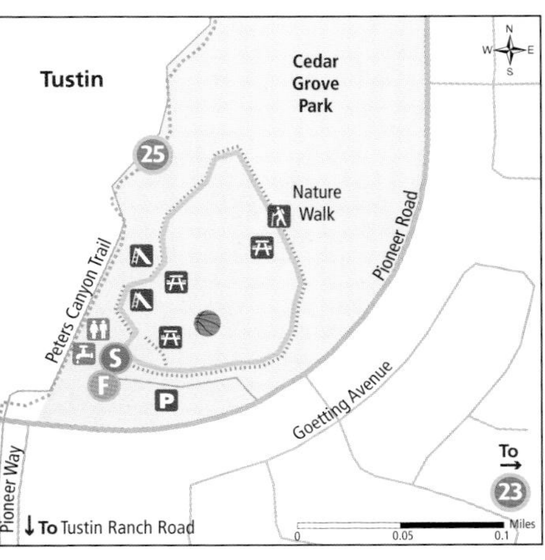

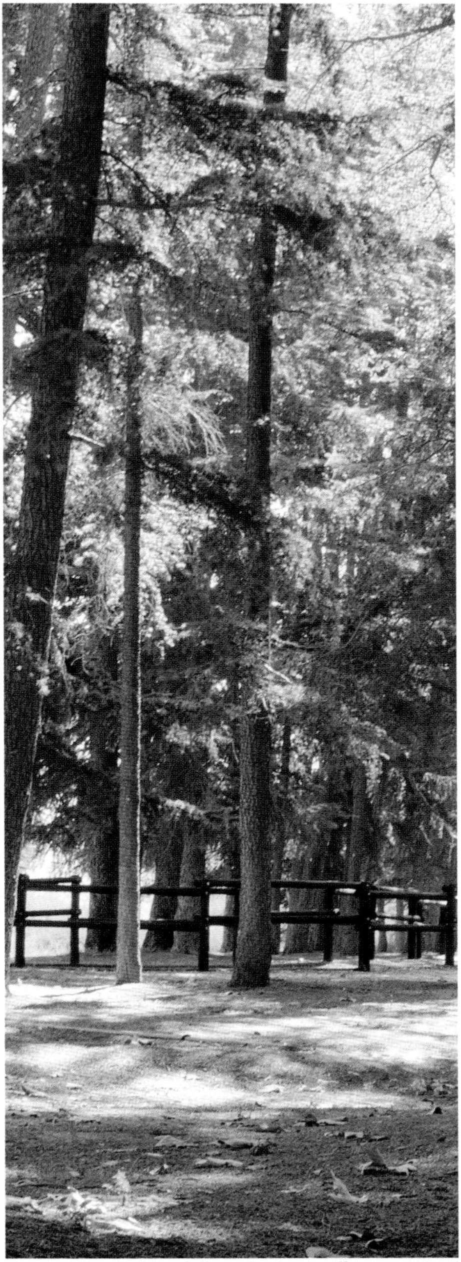

A walk through the cedar grove will transport you!

Central Inland
Kids' Rides

Ride K17 - Grijalva Community Park, Orange

Distance 0.37 miles

Terrain

Completely flat, this ride travels over cement as well as hard-packed gravel paths.

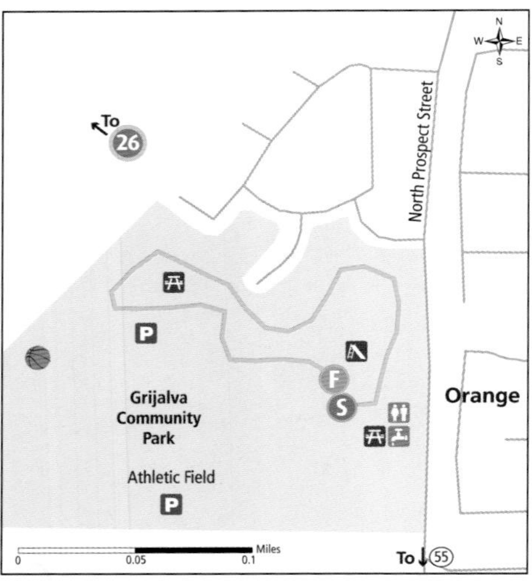

How to Get There

By car, take exit 14, Chapman Avenue, off Californ Highway 55. Travel east on Chapman for 0.6mil then turn left onto Prospect Street. Grijalva Comm nity Park will be on your left, park near the Santiag Creek Trail.

Amenities and Things to Do

This attractive, 26 acre park is filled with a sand vo leyball court, soccer fields, basketball courts, tw playgrounds and a sports center. You will also fin barbecues, restrooms, picnic tables and meanderin walkways.

About

Grijalva is a newer, well-designed park that young kids especially will enjoy. The route loops around th playground, always in sight of the shaded picnic table For older kids, there are trails that explore other par of the park. Situated alongside Santiago Creek Trai this park is the jumping off point for family friendl Ride 26.

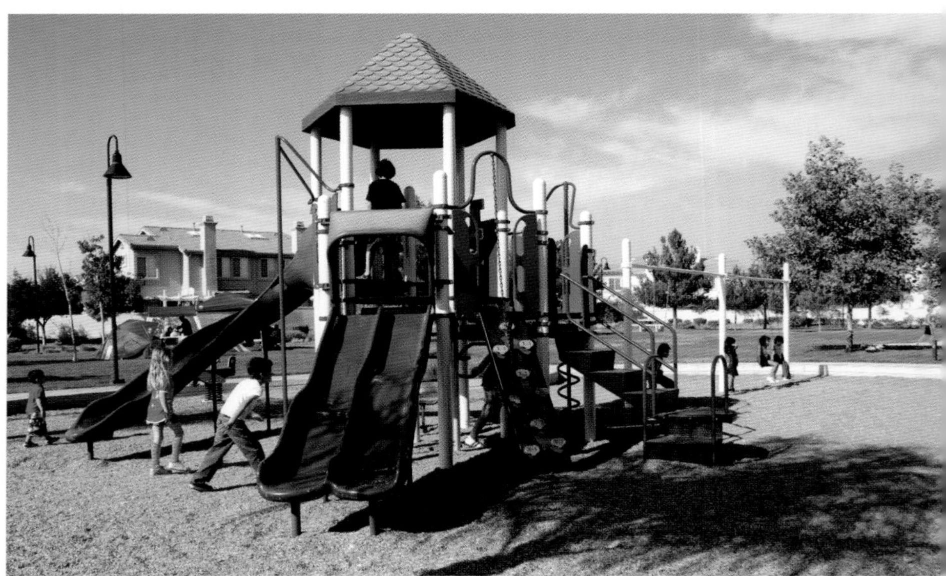

They will never want to leave this park.

Ride K18 - Tustin Centennial Park, Tustin

istance 0.67 miles

errain

lat, paved paths.

low to Get There

y car, take exit 101 Red Hill Road, southbound, off f Interstate 5. After 0.5 miles turn left onto Walnut venue, followed by a right onto Oxford Avenue at 0.3 iiles. Turn left onto Roanoke Avenue, the Centennial ark parking lot will be on your right.

menities and Things to Do

his large park has a vast green lawn, a tree shaded icnic area with barbecues and four playgrounds. Also vailable are basketball courts, horseshoe pits, a fitness ourse and a sand volleyball court.

bout

his is a quiet neighborhood park that is an excellent ace for kids who are learning to ride their bikes. The ute is long and mostly straight except at each end id obstacles are few. The ride loops around the large een space and there are fun playgrounds available.

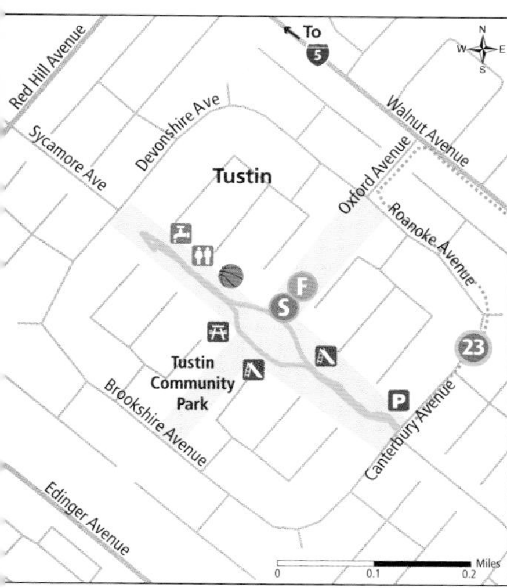

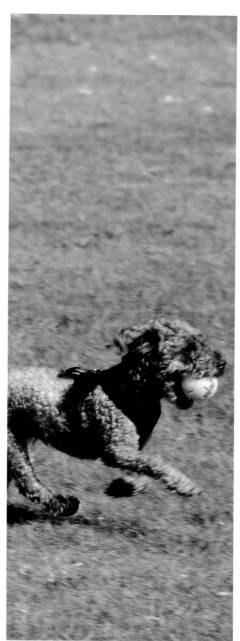

Bring a freind along and enjoy the wide open space.

Ride K19 - Hart Park, Orange

Distance 0.71 miles

Terrain

Mostly flat with one modest hill to climb.

How to Get There

By bus, OCTA number 59 makes a stop at the park along Glassell Street.

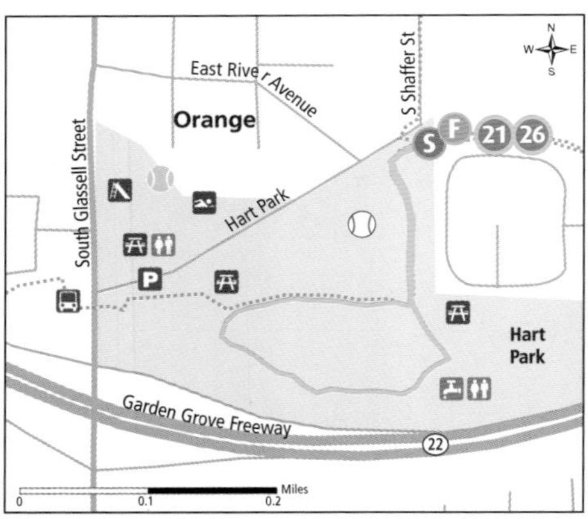

By car, take CA-22 to exit 16, Glassell/Grand. Tu north onto Glassell Street and travel for 0.1 miles b fore turning onto Fairway Drive which will take yo directly into the park.

Amenities and Things to Do

Along with baseball fields, playgrounds and a swir ming pool open during the summer, Santiago Cre Trail passes through this park making a longer fami ride a great option.

About

Evidence of Santiago Creek can be seen by the cany that bisects this park and once flowed freely throu here. On the northern half of this 40 acre park is t pool and playgrounds. The southern half is where t looping ride takes place. Start the ride where Santia Creek Trail enters the park near the parking lot a travel along this well maintained path until you clin the small hill up to the restrooms. Continue along t park's edge until you rejoin the trail and head back the start.

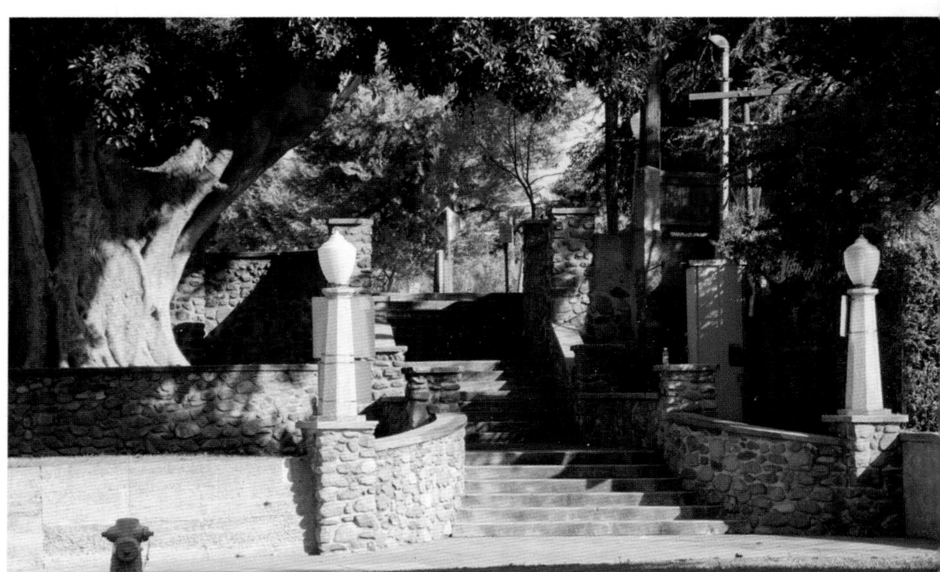

This is an old-fashioned park with mature trees and lots of stonework.

Ride K20 - Woodbridge Community Park, Irvine

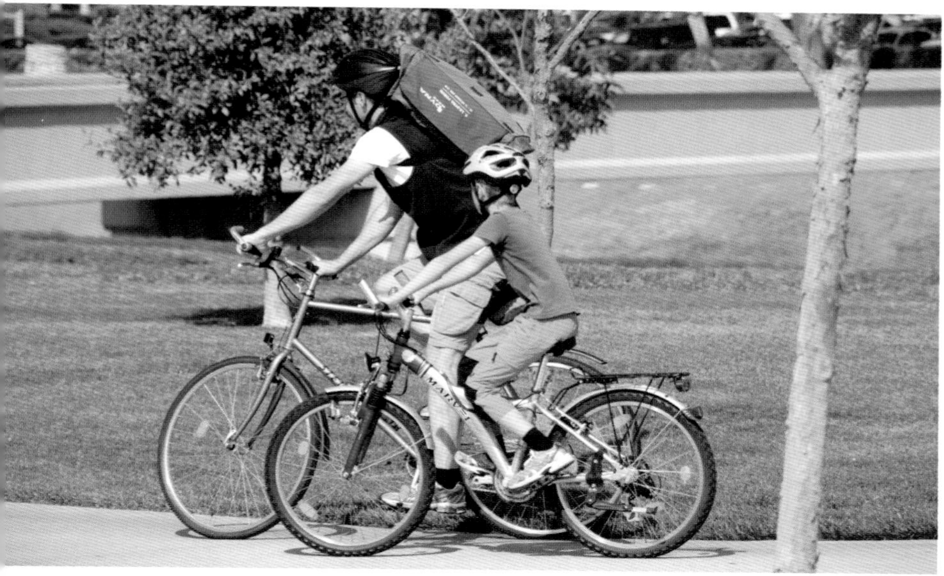

These two youngsters are off on an adventure.

istance 0.44 miles

errain

his is a flat ride on wide, pristine sidewalks.

low to Get There

y bus, OCTA bus 175 makes a stop beside the park.

By car, take exit 5, Culver Drive, off of Interstate 05 head north for 1.1 miles. Turn right onto Alton arkway and after half a mile turn left onto Lake Road. ark will be on your right.

menities and Things to Do

his park features basketball, volleyball and racquetall courts, wide green spaces as well as barbecues and icnic tables.

bout

Voodbridge Community Park, with its wide, smooth aths is an excellent place for youngsters to learn to de their bikes. The park is connected to the San Diego Creek Trail as well as being connected to a bike thoroughfare that runs car-free through the nearby Woodbridge Village shopping center. All of which makes longer family rides safe and easy.

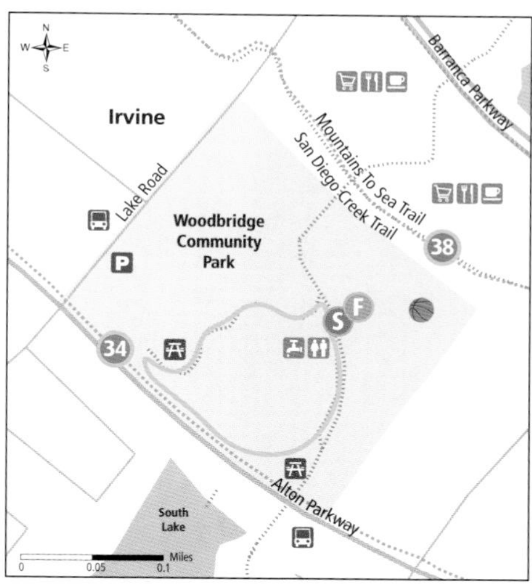

Ride K21 - Buffalo Hills Park, Newport

Distance 0.98 miles

Terrain

This is a flat ride traveling smooth sidewalk paths.

How to Get There

By car, from Pacific Coast Highway, turn onto MacArthur Boulevard heading northbound. Take second right onto San Miguel Drive and travel for 0.9 miles before making a left turn onto Port Sutton Drive. Turn right onto Newport Hills Drive and then left on Port Seabourne Place, the park entrance will be on your left.

Amenities and Things to Do

Buffalo Hills Park has basketball courts, picnic table, soccer fields, restrooms and a pleasant playground set.

About

This is a long, narrow park with a bike path running through it and is an excellent ride for young riders. At the turnaround point, the path crosses Newport Hil Drive and will take you into Harbor View Nature Par which is a very attractive park with a ravine and creek passing through. Some of the paths here can b quite steep, keep an eye on younger riders.

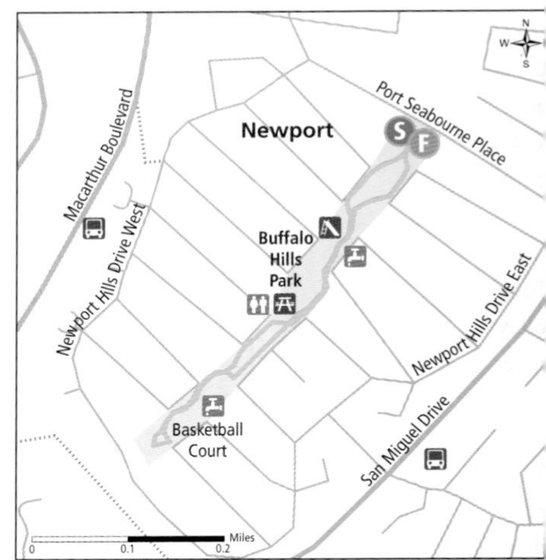

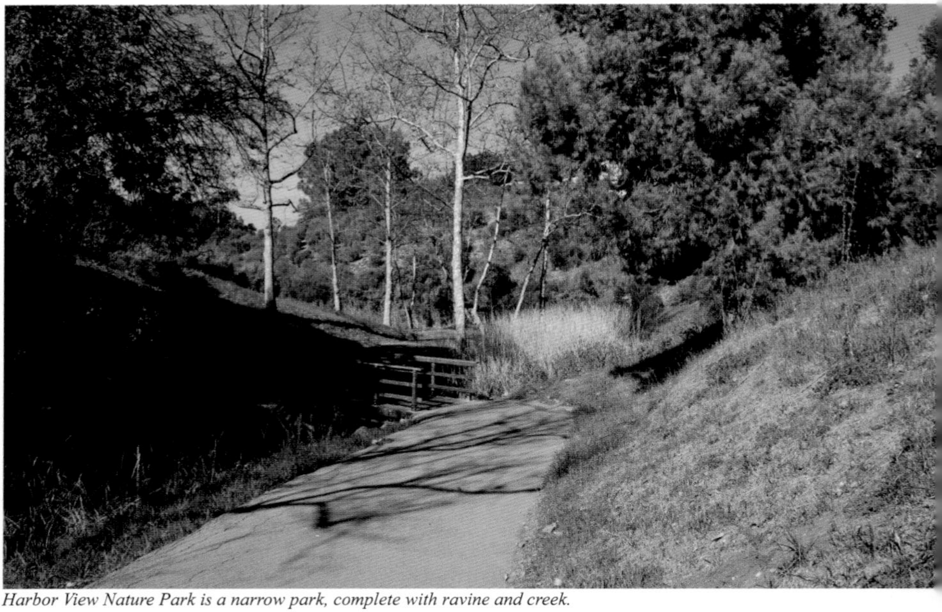

Harbor View Nature Park is a narrow park, complete with ravine and creek.

Ride K22 - Turtle Rock Community Park, Turtle Rock

)istance 0.51 miles

'errain

'wo slight inclines are part of this otherwise flat ride.

low to Get There

3y car, take Exit 4 University Drive off of Interstate 405 and head south. After 0.7 miles turn left onto Ridgeline Drive, 1.4 miles later make a left onto Turtle Rock Drive. Turn left onto Sunnyhill, park will be on our right.

\menities and Things to Do

'his park features restrooms, playgrounds, tennis and olleyball courts, large green space, a creek and a na-ure center.

\bout

'his attractive park is nestled in the San Joaquin Hills nd features a creek flowing through a wooded area vhich makes for an excellent place to search for frogs nd watch the ducks. The ride passes through the play-round before running parallel to the creek. On the op-osite end of the park is the Turtle Rock Nature Center, ve acres of trails and an interpretive center full of in-ormation on local flora and fauna.

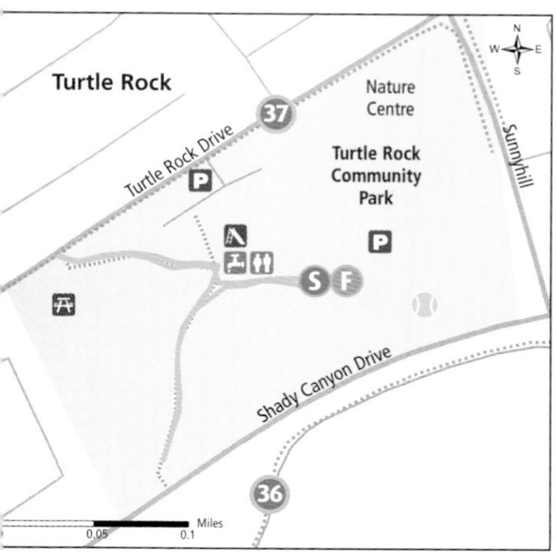

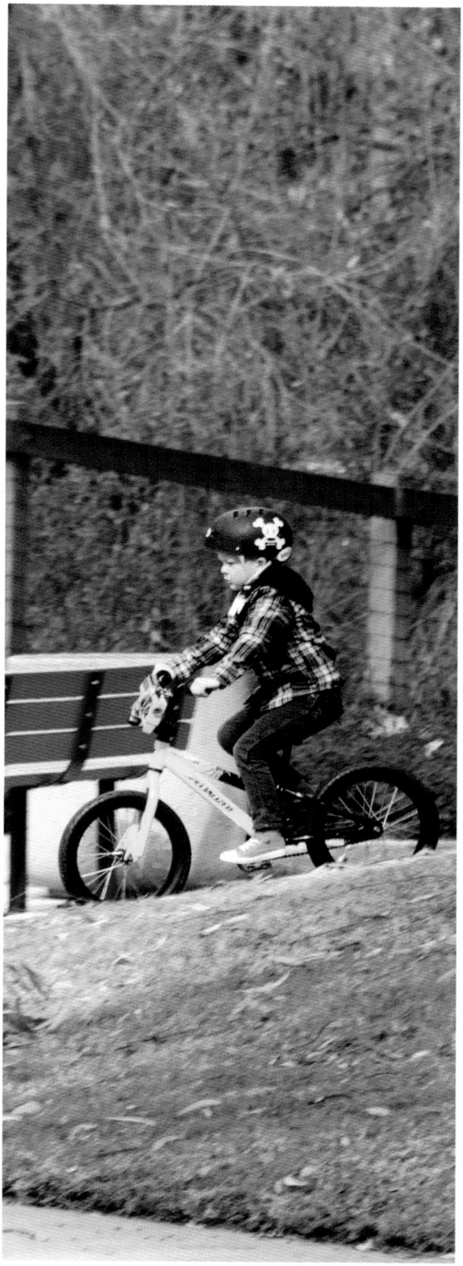

Whoa! That's a big hill!

Central Coast
Kids' Rides

Ride K23 - Civic Center Park, Irvine

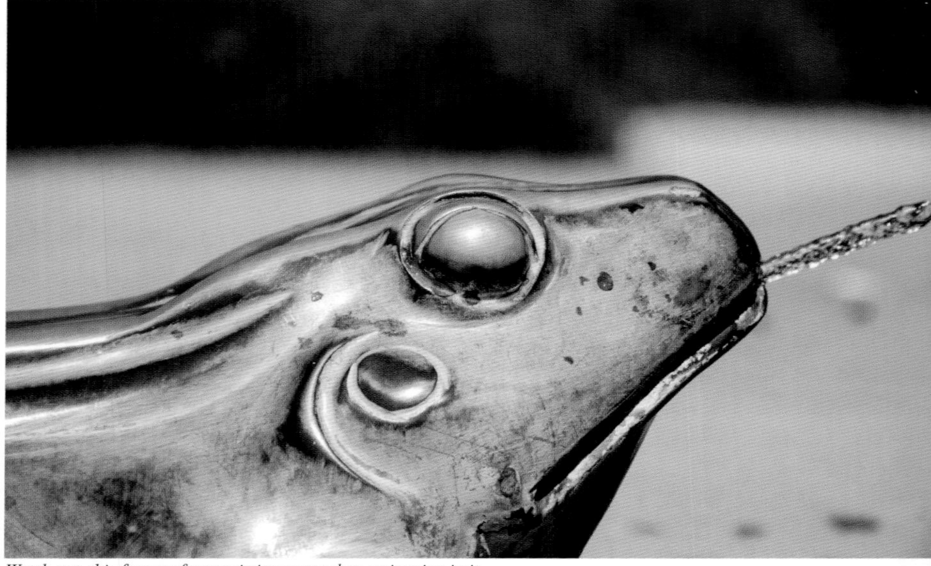

Watch out, this frog prefers squirting water than swimming in it.

Distance 0.28 miles

Terrain

A mostly flat ride on broad, well-maintained paths.

How to Get There

By bus, OCTA number 473 stops at the park.

By car, take exit 7, Jamboree Road, off Interstate 405 and head north for 0.4 miles. Turn left at Main Street and after 0.5 miles turn left onto Harvard Avenue. At San Juan turn left into parking lot.

Amenities and Things to Do

Softball diamonds, soccer fields, tennis courts, barbecues, picnic shelters and an amphitheater are all available here. Kids will be thrilled with the giant tot lot.

About

With walkways shaded by colorful bougainvillea and lined with roses, a fountain featuring spouting frogs and vast swathes of green, this delightful park has a little something for everyone. Bike paths meand throughout the park and seemingly all trails lead to t multi-leveled, gigantic playground.

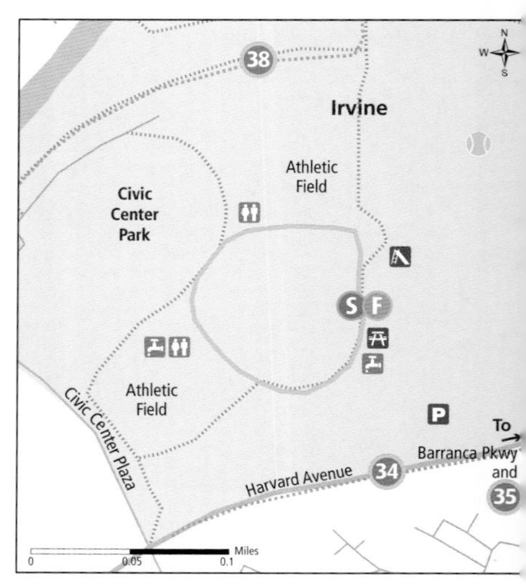

Ride K24 - Culverdale Wilderness Park, Irvine

stance 0.42 miles

:rrain

is is a flat ride over well-maintained sidewalks.

ow to Get There

/ **bus**, OCTA route 79 stops along Culver Drive out 0.25 miles away.

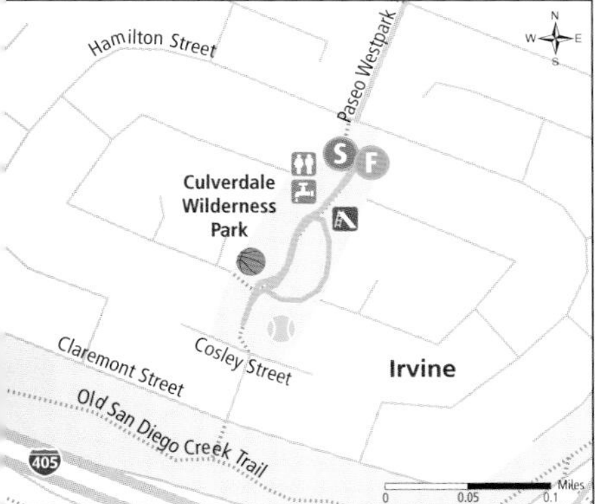

By car, take exit 5 northbound, Culver Drive, off the 405 Freeway. After 0.4 miles, turn left onto San Leandro, followed by a left onto PaseoWestpark after 0.3 miles which dead ends at the park parking lot.

Amenities and Things to Do

Culverdale is an attractive park featuring basketball and tennis courts, a swimming pool, playground and shaded picnic tables. Nearby is the Old San Diego Creek Trail which allows for a longer family ride.

About

This ride takes place in a pocket of green surrounded by attractive homes. The park is a quiet, safe place for young riders to gain experience. Although the ride is short, Old San Diego Creek Trail passes right by this park. This trail is beautifully maintained and virtually untraveled, even on weekends. Once on this trail families can build up miles in a safe environment, eventually connecting to the larger network of trails covered in the Central Coast section.

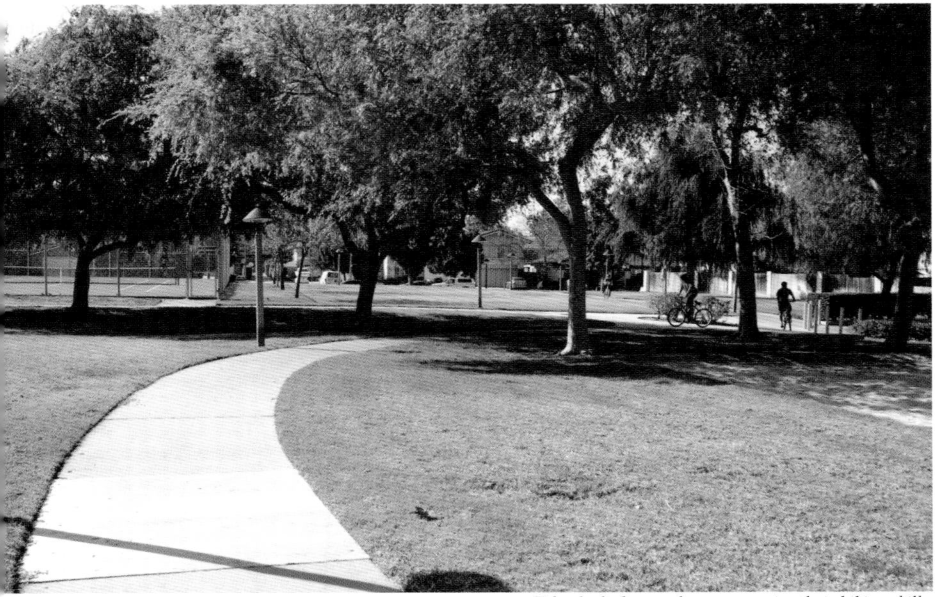

Take the little ones here to practice their biking skills.

Ride K25 - Fairview Park, Costa Mesa

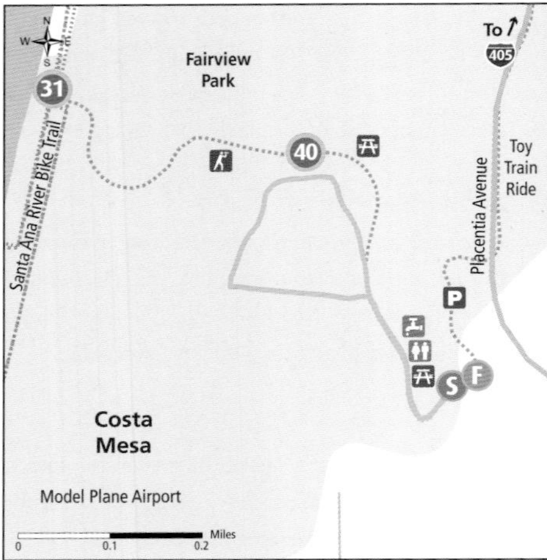

Distance 0.89 miles

Terrain

A flat ride across paved paths as well as hard-packed gravel trails.

How to Get There

By car, take exit 11, Harbor Boulevard, off of Inte state 405. Travel south on Harbor for 0.5 miles, tu right onto Baker Street, followed by a right onto Me Verde Drive. Mesa Verde turns into Placentia Aven and after 2.2 miles the park will be on your right.

Amenities and Things to Do

Fairview Park is crisscrossed with trails, plenty rustic open space, a miniature model train ride, picn tables and restrooms. There is also a model airplar airport.

About

This park sits atop a plateau overlooking the Santa Ar River and the communities that grew beside it. Mea der through tall grasses and wildflowers as bees bu about and butterflies loft lazily by. Below is Talbe Nature Preserve and a stroll through here will give yc a feel for what coastal Southern California looked lik before all the people arrived.

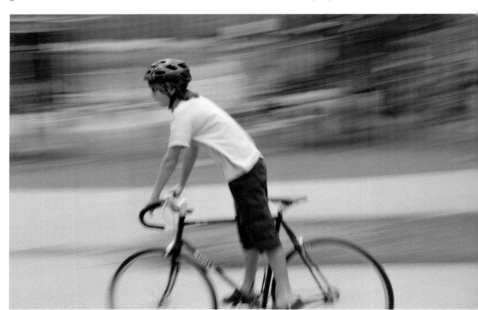

Full speed ahead!

Ride K26 - Altisima Park, Rancho Santa Margarita

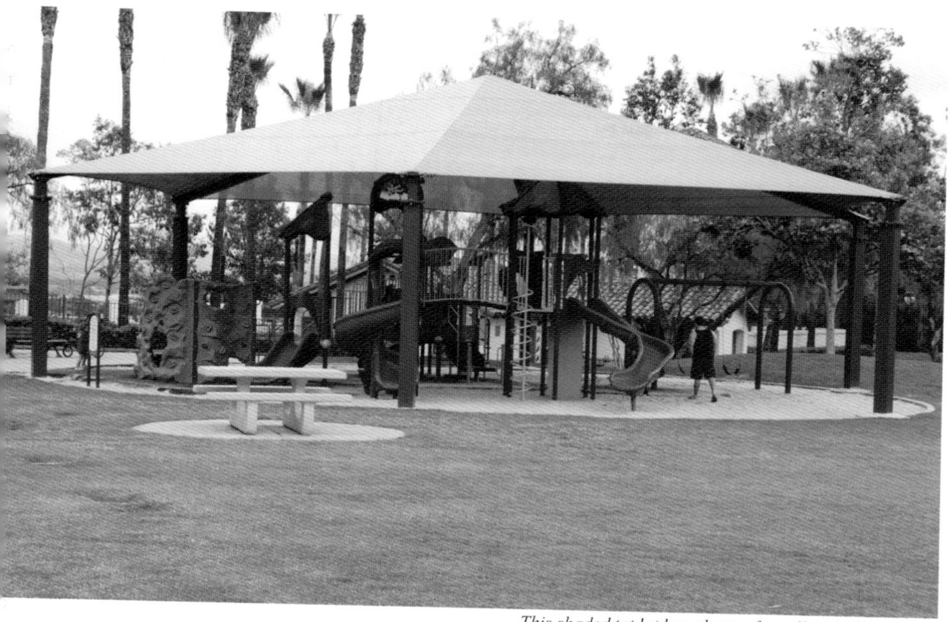

This shaded tot lot has plenty of excellent hiding places.

istance 0.39 miles

errain

his is a flat ride along park paths.

ow to Get There

y car, take exit 20, Los Alisos Boulevard, off Califor-ia Highway 241 and head north. After 0.6 miles turn eft into Altisima Park parking lot.

menities and Things to Do

his attractive park has a giant tot lot, baseball fields, ennis courts, picnic tables, barbecues and restrooms. here is also a swimming pool reserved for residents f Rancho Santa Maragrita.

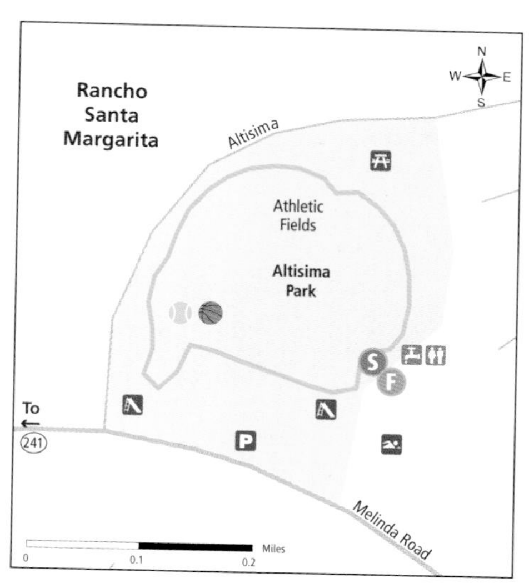

bout

erched above Upper Oso Reservoir, this park boasts pectacular views of the hillsides above and valleys elow. The bike path travels through sculpted green lawns, looping around large fields and baseball diamonds. The playground is shaded and large, complete with slides, climbing walls and plenty of places to hide.

Ride K27 - Serrano Creek Park, Lake Forest

Distance 0.99 miles

Terrain

This ride is mostly flat with a couple of mild inclines across wide, well-maintained paths.

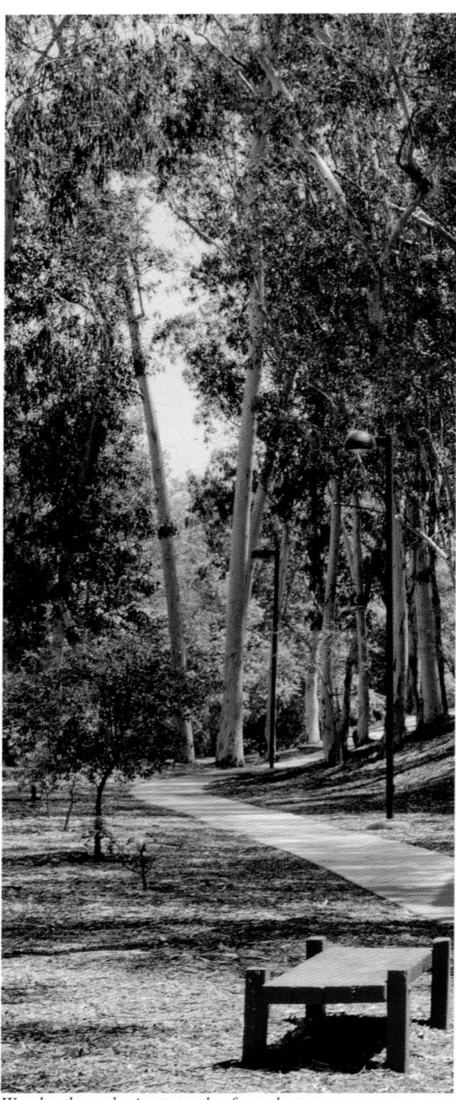

Wander through giant stands of eucalyptus.

How to Get There

By bus, OCTA route 177 makes a stop at the intersection of Lake Forest Drive and Serrano Road. The park is about a quarter mile walk along Serrano.

By car, exit 92, Lake Forest Drive, off Interstate 5 heading northeast bound. After 2.1 miles turn left onto Serrano Road, park is on your right, parking is on the street.

Amenities and Things to Do

At Serrano Creek Park you will find a playground, picnic tables, restrooms, barbecues and a walking/nature trail.

About

Groves of stately eucalyptus run the length of this peaceful park. The ride starts at the small but well equipped tot lot and from there along wide sidewalks through corridors of trees. At the turnaround point the path splits and continues but is not suited to kids riding alone. For a longer family outing these trails eventually connect to Serrano Creek Trail which runs all the way to Whiting Ranch Wilderness Park, 4.5 miles away over dirt trails.

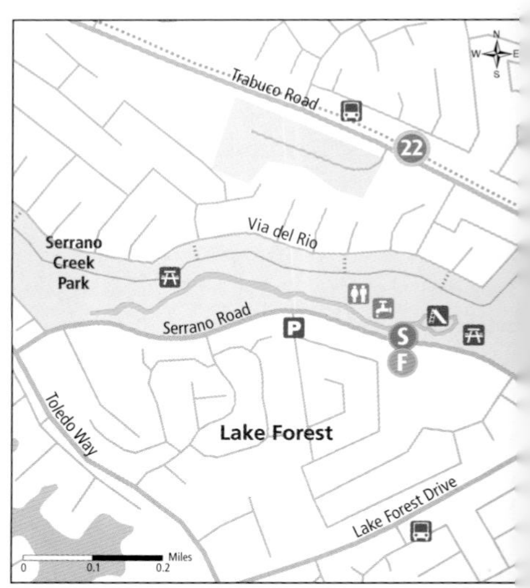

Ride K28 - Sheep Hill Park, Laguna Hills

Distance 0.42 miles

Terrain

This is a flat looping ride.

How to Get There

By bus, OCTA route 188 makes a stop near Sheep Hill Park.

By car, take exit 90, Alicia Parkway, off of Interstate 5, and head south for 1.7 miles. Turn right onto Moulton Parkway and after 0.6 miles turn right on Laguna Hills Drive. Park on street next to Sheep Hill Park.

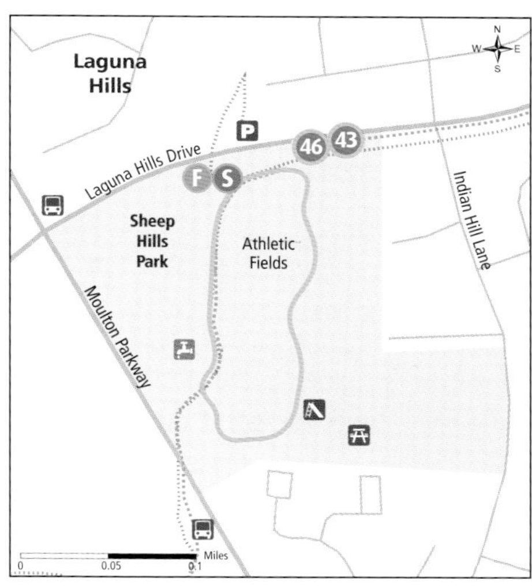

Amenities and Things to Do

You will find playing fields, baseball diamonds, picnic tables, and a tot lot at Sheep Hill Park. Also, Aliso Creek Trail runs through the park connecting to longer family rides. Oddly, there are no restrooms, only temporary port-a-potties.

About

Traveling wide, fat walkways this ride loops around the park's expansive field. An ideal park for youngsters just starting out. Once they are ready for longer rides consider trips on Aliso Creek Trail which overlaps this ride near the start and on the opposite end leaves the park. Also worthy of exploration is the Sheep Hill Park path that starts behind the playground and heads uphill, eventually turning into a graveled trail. Follow the path for 1.3 miles to reach El Conejo Park, Kids' Ride 32.

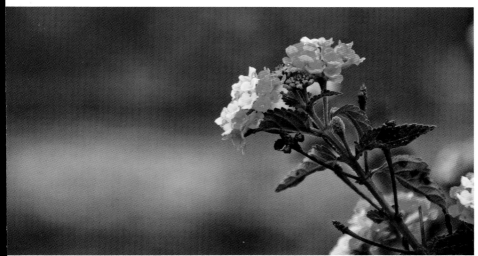

Along the Sheep Hill Trail, stop and enjoy the flowers.

Ride K29 - Yosemite Park, Laguna Niguel

Distance 0.34 miles

Terrain

This ride loops around the park along wide walkways. There is one modest rise in this otherwise flat ride.

How to Get There

By car, take exit 3, La Paz Road, off of CA-73 toward Moulton Parkway, then turn right onto Moulton. After 0.9 miles turn right onto Aliso Creek Road, then turn right onto Yosemite Road after 0.1 miles. The park will be on your right, parking is available on the street.

Amenities and Things to Do

This park has over five acres of turf with a playground, volleyball nets, drinking fountains and picnic tables.

About

Surrounded by mature pine trees, Yosemite Park is an excellent park for youngsters to practice their bike skills. Once the kids are ready for a longer ride, head downhill alongside Yosemite Road to the tunnel that will take you under La Paz Road and into Laguna Niguel Regional Park, site of Ride 47.

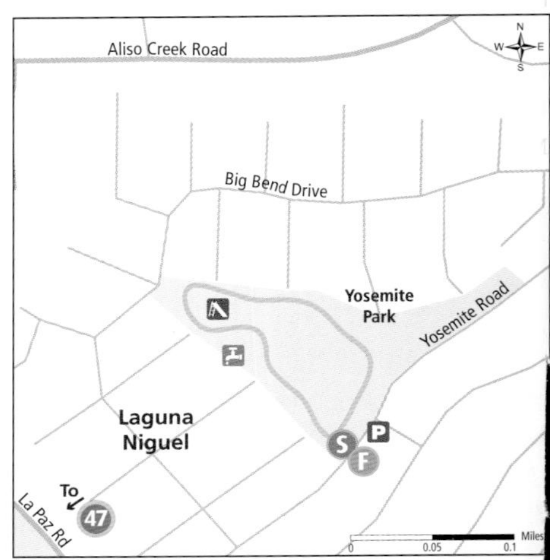

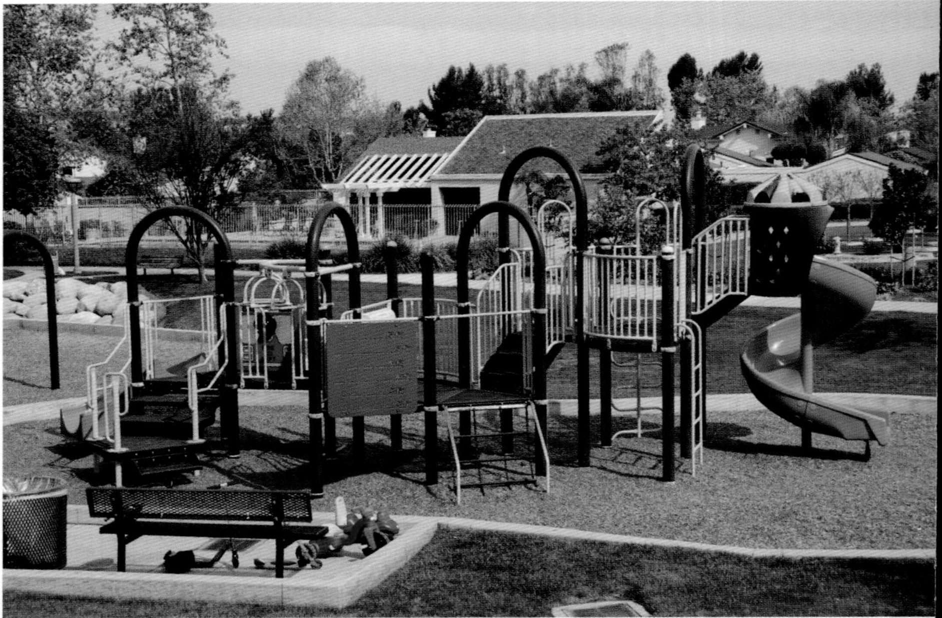

After a few loops on the bike path, relax and let the kids work off that extra energy on the tot lot.

Ride K30 - El Toro Park, Lake Forest

Distance 0.70 miles

Terrain

This ride travels gently uphill for the length of the park before returning downhill to its start.

How to Get There

By bus, take OCTA route 177 to the intersection of Muirland and Los Alisos boulevards.

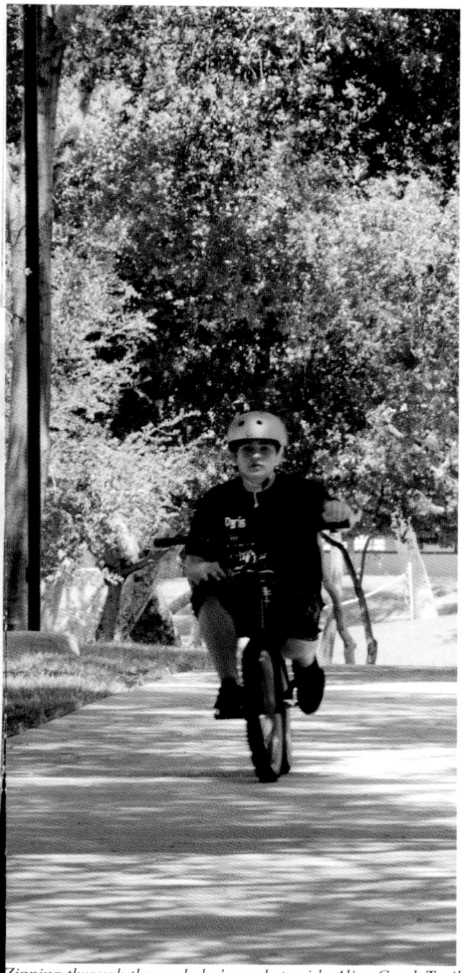

Zipping through the park, he's ready to ride Aliso Creek Trail.

By car, take exit 90, Alicia Parkway, off of Interstate 5, and head north one mile before turning left on Muirlands Boulevard. Turn left onto Aliso Parkway and after 0.4 miles, turn right onto Rockfield Boulevard. Take the first right onto Larkwood Lane, you will find parking on the street.

Amenities and Things to Do

This park boasts barbecues, restrooms, tennis courts, shelters, picnic tables, a large playground and outdoor fitness equipment. Aliso Creek Trail also passes along one edge of this park.

About

The bike path runs and loops the length of this tree-shaded park. Not for novice riders with its slight incline and fast descent, this is a ride for kids who have a firm understanding of cornering and brakes. Aliso Creek Trail, Ride 43, offers the opportunity for a longer family ride. Keep in mind the entrances to the trail are quick downhills and often damp.

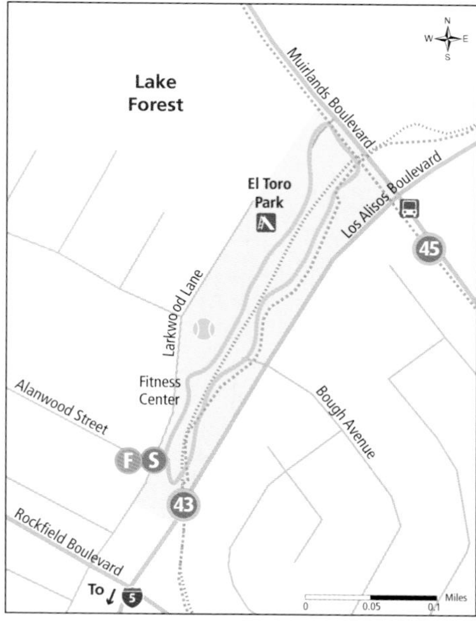

Ride K31 - Sea Terrace Park, Dana Point

Distance 0.67 miles

Terrain

This ride is mostly flat with one modest rise.

How to Get There

By bus, OCTA routes 1 and 85 make stops beside the park.

By car, take exit 79, Pacific Coast Highway, off of Interstate 5 and head northbound. After 3.5 miles turn left onto Ritz Carlton Drive then take the first right into the parking lot. To reach the park, pass through pedestrian tunnel under Pacific Coast Highway.

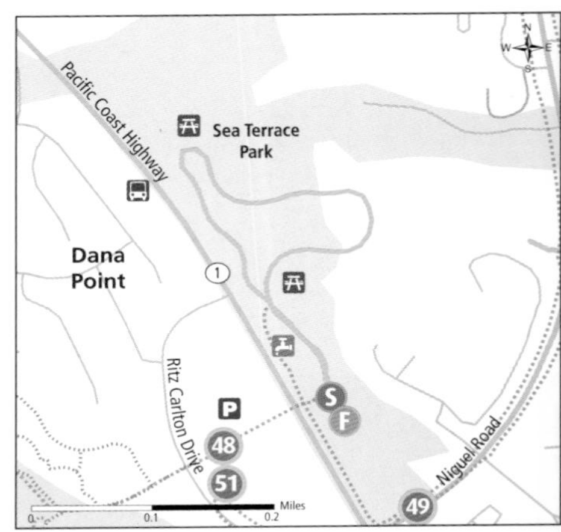

Amenities and Things to Do

Barbecues, picnic tables and benches under a gazebo, ocean views, dog runs and large stretches of green space.

About

Although not typical of most other kid rides, this park is so beautifully landscaped and the paths so smooth and well-maintained that this park just begs to be explored by bike. These 22 acres are covered in rolling fields lined with Mediterranean plants flowering nearly all year round. Kick the soccer ball around, enjoy a picnic. At the start, pause to enjoy the beautiful circle rose garden. Best of all, when the kids get hot and sweaty, head downhill to Salt Creek Beach to play in the surf.

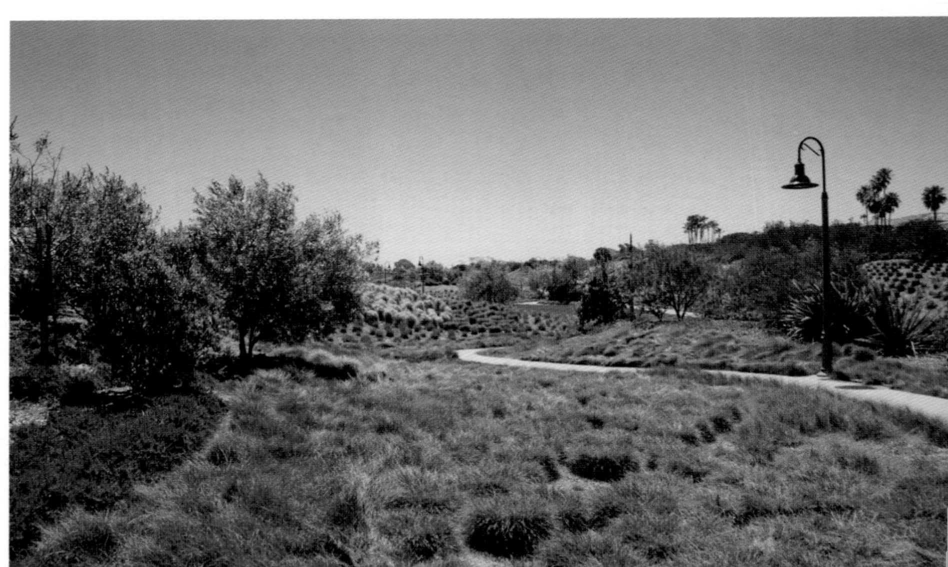

Follow the paths as they meander through this unusual park.

Ride K32 - El Conejo Park, Laguna Hills

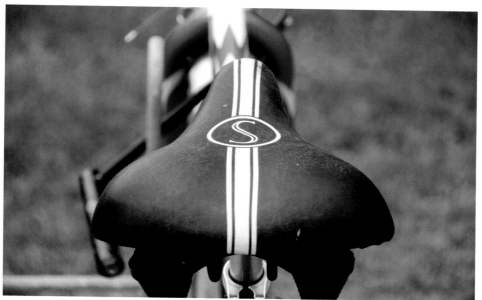

The comfort of your saddle will often dictate how enjoyable your ride is.

Distance 0.22 miles

Terrain

This a flat looping ride at the base of a hill.

How to Get There

By car, take exit 90, Alicia Parkway, south bound off of Interstate 5. After 1.3 miles turn left onto Paseo De Valencia. Take the first right onto Sunburst Avenue, followed by a left onto Largo Drive. Turn left on Linda Vista, then a right on El Conejo Lane which ends at park. Parking is on the street.

Amenities and Things to Do

This park's amenities include a tot lot, basketball court, picnic tables, benches and a sports field.

About

This charming little park features a looping ride ideal for youngsters starting out on the bike. Nestled between homes, hillsides and trees, this is an excellent place for a ride and a picnic. On the far side of the park is a hiking trail that traverses the hilltop as it carries you to Sheep Hill Park, site of Kids' Ride 28, 1.3 miles away.

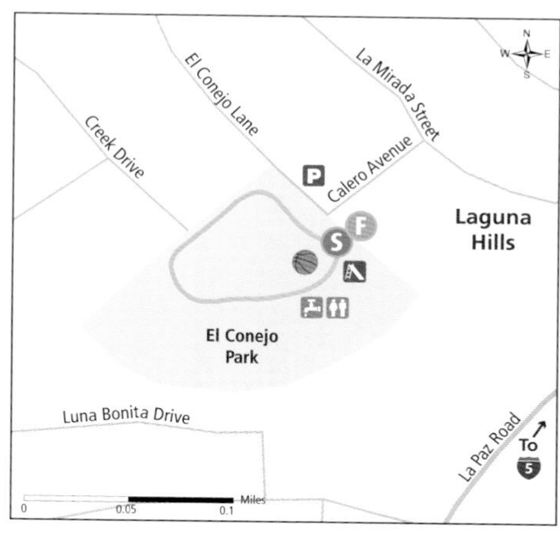

Notes

Notes

Notes

Notes

B R Bike Shops & Rentals in and around Orange County

B1 Adrenaline Bike Shop - Anaheim
1035 North Armando Street, Suite Q
ANAHEIM
Tel: 714 630 8233
www.adrenalinebikes.com

B2 Anaheim Bike Shop
5675 E La Palma, ANAHEIM
Tel: 714 779 7521
www.ahbikes.com

B3 Rock n Road Cyclery
5701 Santa Ana Canyon Road, Anaheim Hills
Tel: 714 998 2453
www.rocknroadcyclery.net

B4 2 Wheeler Dealer
1039 East Imperial Highway , BREA
Tel: 714 671 1730
www.twdcycling.com

B5 Professional Bike Parts
615 North Berry Street, Suite F , BREA
Tel: 714 255 9172

B6 Buena Park Bicycles
6042 Beach Boulevard , BUENA PARK
Tel: 714 521 8120
www.fullertonbicycle.com

B7 Volume Bike Corp
7342 Melrose St , BUENA PARK
Tel: 714 690 6454

B8 E Bike Tology
357 16th Place , COSTA MESA
Tel: 714 278 2148

B9 Erowheels
426 East 19th Street , COSTA MESA
Tel: 949 722 6342

B10 Two Wheels One Planet
420 East 17th Street , COSTA MESA
Tel: 949 646 7706
www.twowheelsoneplanet.com

B11 Bike Land of Cypress
5530 Lincoln Avenue , CYPRESS
Tel: 714 995 6541
www.ocbikeland.com

B12 Wheel Fun Rentals - Dana Point *(Rentals)*
25300 Dana Point Harbour Drive , DANA POINT
Tel: 949 496 7433
www.wheelfunrentals.com

B13 EZ Green Bikes *(Rentals available)*
34193 Golden Lantern Street, DANA POINT
Tel: 949 661 2761

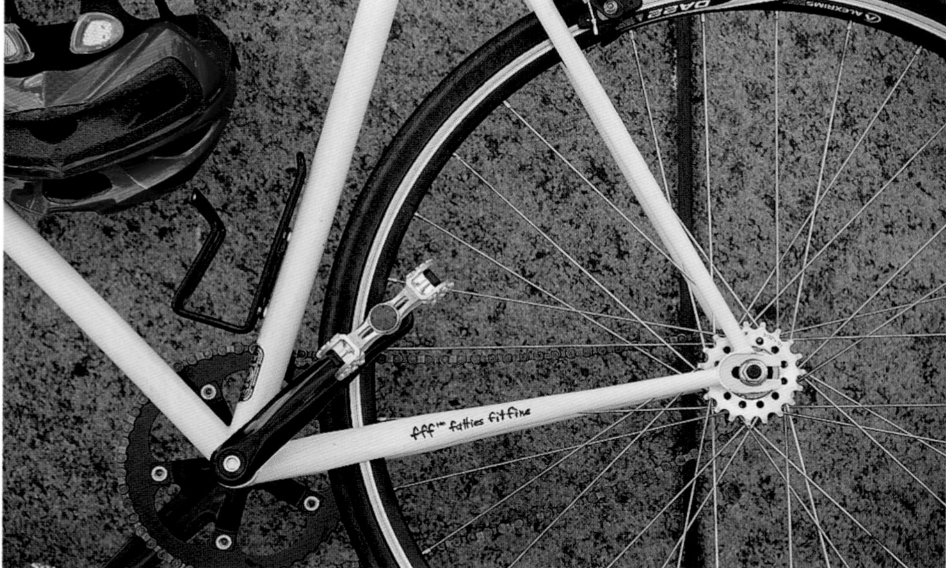

Bike Shops & Rentals in and around Orange County

B14 Performance Bikes
8850 Warner Bikes, Fountain Valley
Tel: 714 842 3480
www.performancebike.com

B15 Bicycle Discovery - Fountain Valley
8800 Warner Avenue , Fountain Valley
Tel: 714 841 1366
www.bicycle-discovery.com

B16 Bike & Source
18474 Amistad , Fountain Valley
Tel: 714 593 8171

B17 Jax Bicycle Center - Fullerton
2520 E. Chapman Avenue , FULLERTON
Tel: 714 441 1100

B18 Fullerton Bicycles and Buena Park Bicycles
424 East Commonwealth Avenue , FULLERTON
Tel: 714 879 8310
www.fullertonbicycle.com

B19 East West Bikes
(formerly Bannings Bikes)
206 North Harbor Boulevard, FULLERTON
Tel: 714 525 2200
www.ewbikes.com

B20 Wheelcare
12691 Monarch Street , GARDEN GROVE
Tel: 714 891 6222

B21 Garden Grove Bicycle Shop
8602 Garden Grove Boulevard , GARDEN GROVE
Tel: 714 537 6695

B22 Richards Cyclery
11943 Valley View Street , GARDEN GROVE
Tel: 714 379 2717
www.richardscyclery.com

B23 Team Bike Works
8464 Indianapolis Ave , HUNTINGTON BEACH
Tel: 714 969 5480

B24 Jax Bicycle Center - Huntington Beach
401 Main Street , HUNTINGTON BEACH
Tel: 714 969 8684
www.jaxbicycles.com

B25 Wheel Fun Rentals - Huntington Beach
(Rentals)
21351 Pacific Coast Highway , HUNTINGTON BEACH
Tel: 714 374 5533
www.wheelfunrentals.com

B26 Out-Spoke-N *(Rentals available)*
16400 Pacific Coast Highway,
Suite #100-101, HUNTINGTON BEACH
Tel: 562 592 6000
www.rideoutspoken.com

B27 Jax Bicycle Center - Irvine
14280-A Culver Drive , IRVINE
Tel: 949 733 1212
www.jaxbicycles.com

B28 The Bike Source
17777 Main Street, Suite E , IRVINE
Tel: 949 622 8103

B29 Irvine Bikes
6616 Irvine Center Drive, IRVINE
Tel: 949 453 9999
www.irvinebicycles.com

B30 Rock n Road Cyclery
6282 Irvine Blvd, IRVINE
Tel: 949 733 2453
www.rocknroadcyclery.net

B31 Ladera Cyclery
25662 Crown Valley Parkway, LADERA RANCH
Tel: 949 429 7784

B32 Laguna Beach Cyclery *(Rentals available)*
240 Thalia , LAGUNA BEACH
Tel: 949 494 1522
www.lagunacyclery.net

B33 Bicisport Bicycles
26538 Moulton Parkway, Suite A , LAGUNA HILLS
Tel: 949 643 1620

B34 Bicycle Retailer & Industry News
25431 Cabot Rd, Suite 204, LAGUNA HILLS
Tel: 949 206 1677

B35 Supergo Bike Shops
24721 Alicia Parkway, LAGUNA HILLS
Tel: 949 707 0344

B36 Rock n Road Cyclery - Laguna Niguel
27281 La Paz Road. Suite N, LAGUNA NIGUEL
Tel: 949 360 8045
www.rocknroadcyclery.net

B37 Two Wheels One Planet
24844 Muirlands Blvd, LAKE FOREST
Tel: 949 581 8900
www.twowheelsoneplanet.com

B R Bike Shops & Rentals in and around Orange County

B38 Bike Company
21098 Bake Parkway, Suite 112, LAKE FOREST
Tel: 949 470 1099
www.bikeco.com

B39 Pacific Cycle
21076 Bake Parkway, Suite 100, LAKE FOREST
Tel: 949 461 5944

B40 Cycle Werks - Mission Viejo
27672 Crown Valley Parkway, MISSION VIEJO
Tel: 949 364 5771
www.cyclewerks.net

B41 Rock n Road Cyclery
27825 Santa Margarita Parkway, MISSION VIEJO
Tel: 949 859 5076
www.rocknroadcyclery.net

B42 Easy Ride Tricycle Rentals
107 Palm Street , NEWPORT BEACH
Tel: 949 566 9850

B43 Bike Doctor
3415 Newport Boulevarde, NEWPORT BEACH
Tel: 949 673 3884

B44 Bikes & More
2823 Newport Boulevarde, NEWPORT BEACH
Tel: 949 675 2727

B45 Chicago Bike *(Rentals available)*
4525 West Coast Highway, NEWPORT BEACH
Tel: 949 650 4203

B46 Let it Roll Bike Shop *(Rentals available)*
3305 Newport Boulevarde, NEWPORT BEACH
Tel: 949 723 5681
www.letitroll1.com

B47 Newport Beach Bike Skate Rental
(Rentals)
2200 West Oceanfront, NEWPORT BEACH
Tel: 949 675 1065

B48 Newport Bike & Beach Rental
(Rentals)
106 22nd Street , NEWPORT BEACH
Tel: 949 673 2618

B49 Adrenaline Bike Shop - Orange
366 South Tustin Street, ORANGE
Tel: 714 288 2012
www.adrenalinebikes.com

B50 Orange Cycle
210 South Glassell Street, ORANGE
Tel: 714 532 6838
www.orangecycle.com

B51 American Flyer Bicycle Company
987 North Enterprise Street, ORANGE
Tel: 714 633 5334

B52 Bike Alley
2823 East Chapman Avenue, ORANGE
Tel: 714 997 3980
www.bikealleybmx.com

B53 Switchback Cyclery
3436 East Chapman Avenue, ORANGE
Tel: 714 628 3913
www.switchbackcyclery.com

B54 Cycle Werks - San Clemente
1421 North El Camino Real, SAN CLEMENTE
Tel: 949 492 5911
www.cyclewerks.net

B55 Orange County Bicycle Coalition
2400 Calle Monte Carlo, SAN CLEMENTE
Tel: 949 492 5737

B56 San Clemente Cyclery
2801 South El Camino Real, SAN CLEMENTE
Tel: 949 492 8890

B57 Buy My Bikes
32302 Camino Capistrano, SAN JUAN CAPISTRANO
Tel: 949 493 5611
www.buymybikes.com

B58 Janets Bike Shop
221 North Broadway, SANTA ANA
Tel: 714 953 6748

B59 S & M Bikes
1300 South Lyon Street, SANTA ANA
Tel: 714 835 3400
www.sandmbikes.com

B60 Sta-Tru Wheels
201 West Dyer Road, SANTA ANA
Tel: 714 432 0248
www.statruwheels.com

B61 Main Street Cyclery
135 Main Street, SEAL BEACH
Tel: 562 430 3903
www.mainstreetcyclery.com

B R Bike Shops & Rentals in and around Orange County

B62 Sandpiper Bike Repair
231 Seal Beach Boulevarde, Suite 3, SEAL BEACH
Tel: 562 594 6130

B63 King's Bicycles Store
1190 Pacific Coast Highway # D, SEAL BEACH
Tel: 562 598 9322
www.kingsbikestore.com

B64 Dons Schwinn Cyclery
121 North Prospect Avenue, TUSTIN
Tel: 714 544 5910
www.donsbikes.com

B65 Santiago Cycling
115 North Prospect Avenue, TUSTIN
Tel: 714 544 6091
www.santiagocycling.com

B66 The Path Bike Shop
215 W. 1st Street, Suite 102, TUSTIN
Tel: 714 669 0784
www.thepathbikeshop.com

B67 Performance Bicycle
2745 El Camino Real, TUSTIN
Tel: 714 838 0641
www.performancebike.com

B68 Santiago Cyclery
115 N Porspect Avenue, TUSTIN
Tel: 714 544 6091
www.cyclingpros.com

B69 A-1 Cycle
13752 Goldenwest Street, WESTMINSTER
Tel: 714 893 3706
www.a-1cycle.com

B70 Epic Rideshop
16483 Magnolia Street, WESTMINSTER
Tel: 714 848 0888
www.epicbmx.com

B71 G's Cylcery and Wheels
6713 Greenleaf Avenue, WHITTIER
Tel: 562 698 9426

B72 Jax Bicycle Center - Yorba Linda
17593 Yorba Linda Boulevard, YORBA LINDA
Tel: 714 996 9093
www.jaxbicycles.com

B73 Bicycles San Clemente *(Rentals available)*
1900 N El Camino Real, SAN CLEMENTE
Tel: 949 492 5737
www.bicyclessanclemente.com

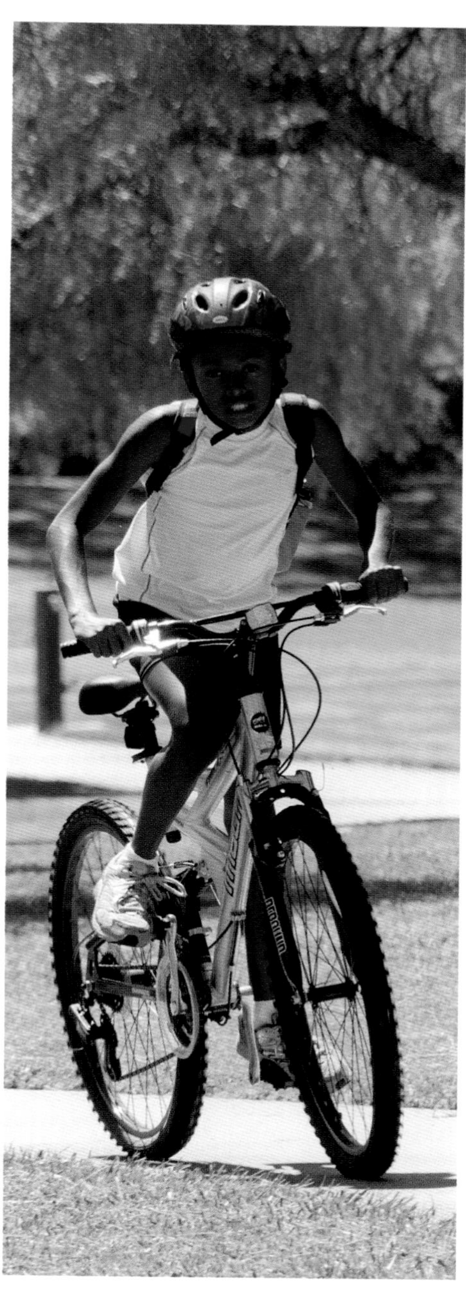

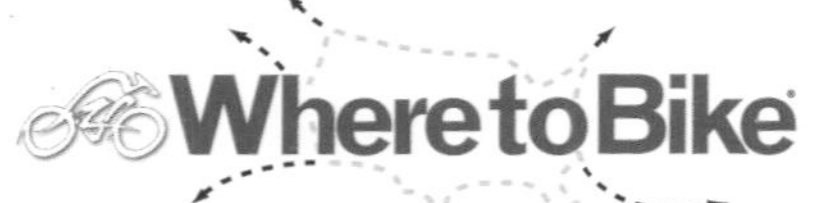

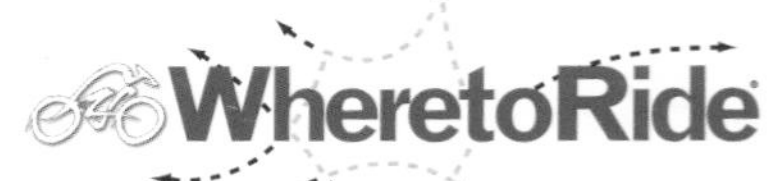

Also in this Series!

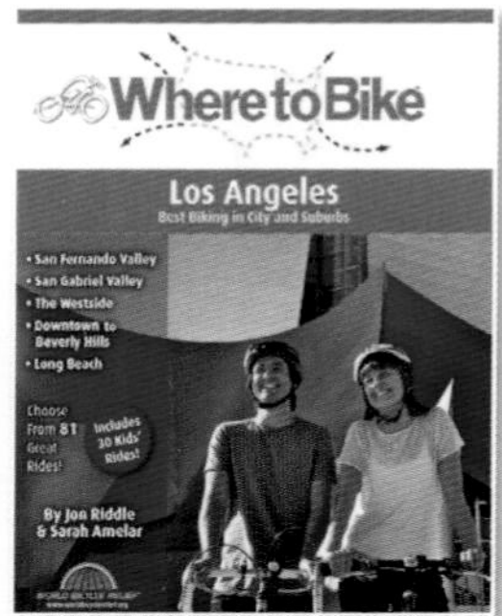

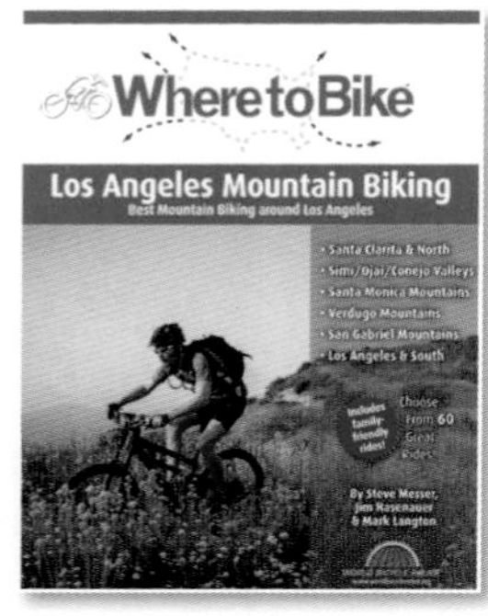

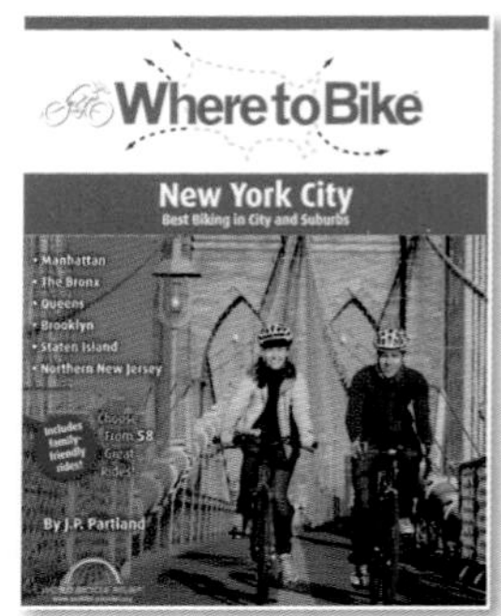

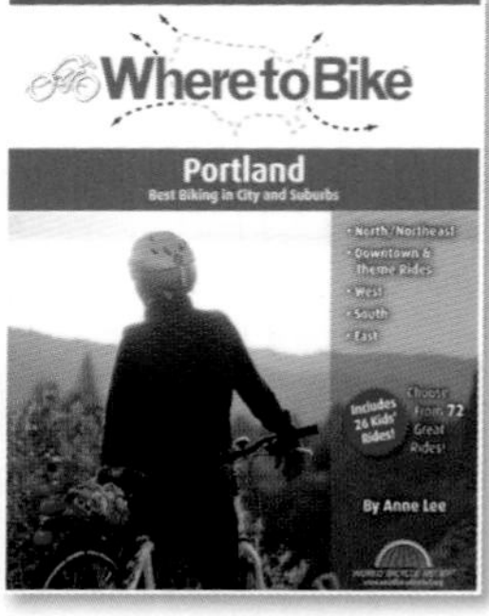

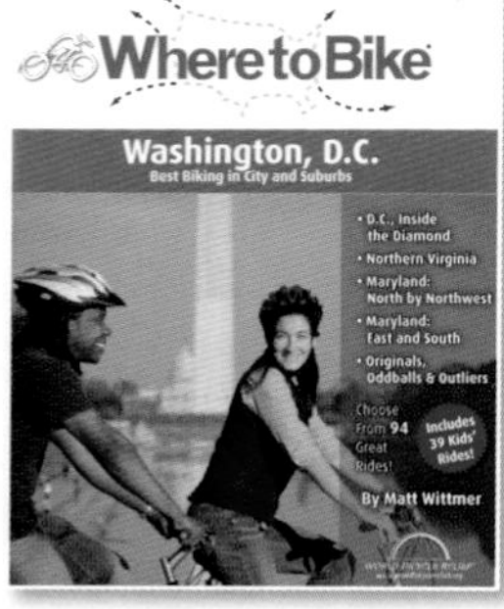

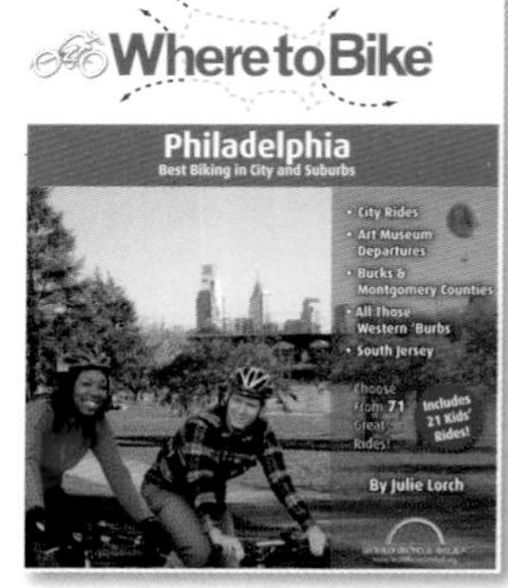

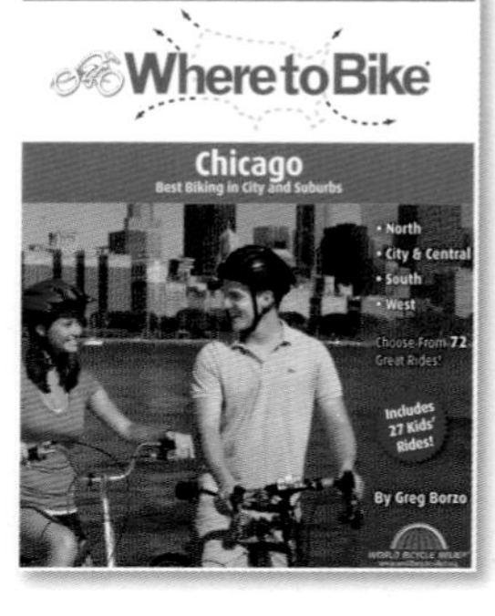

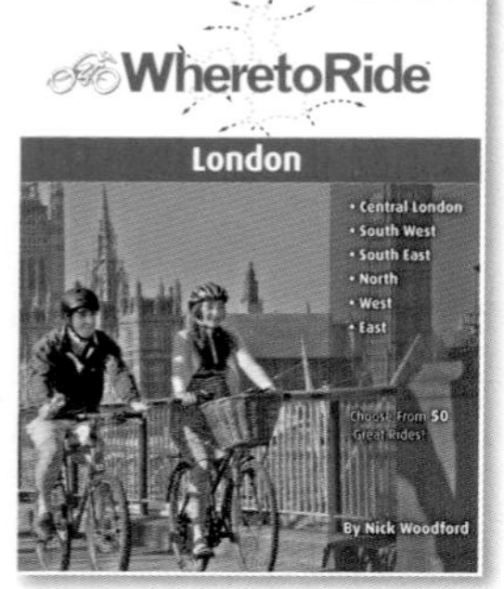

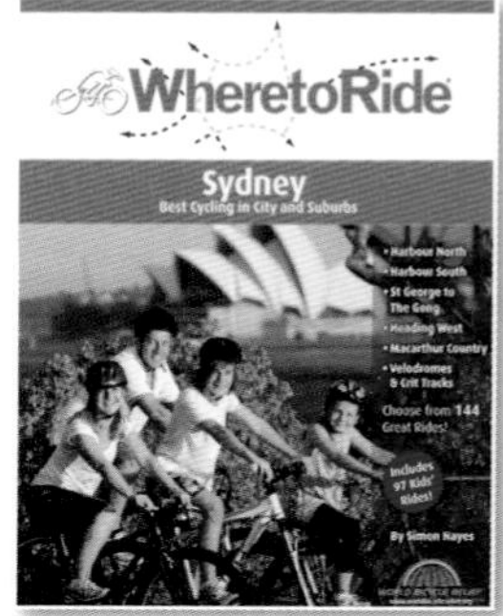

www.**WheretoBikeGuides**.com

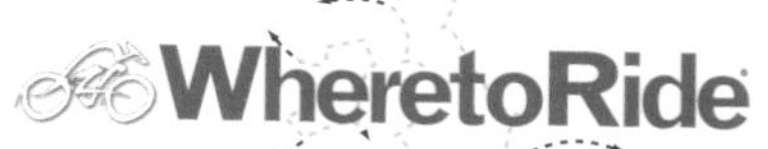

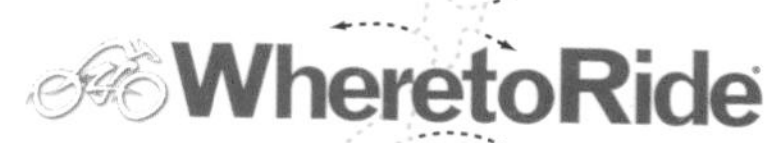

Also in this Series!

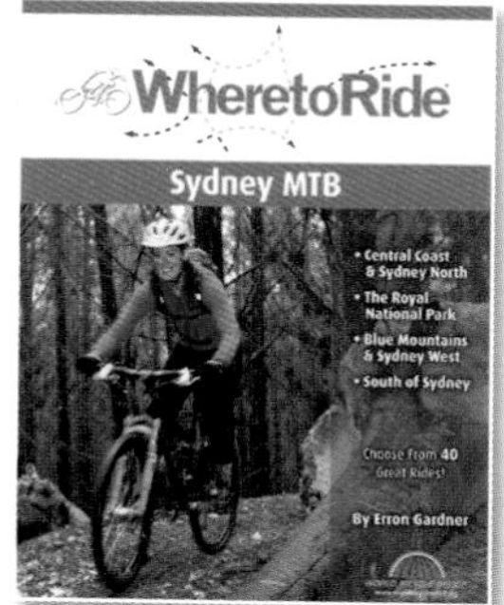

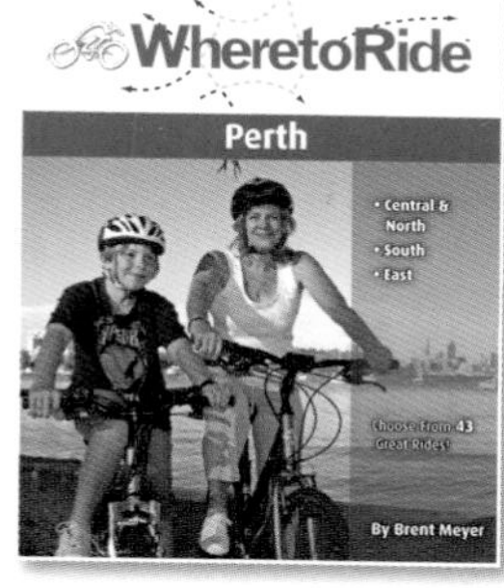

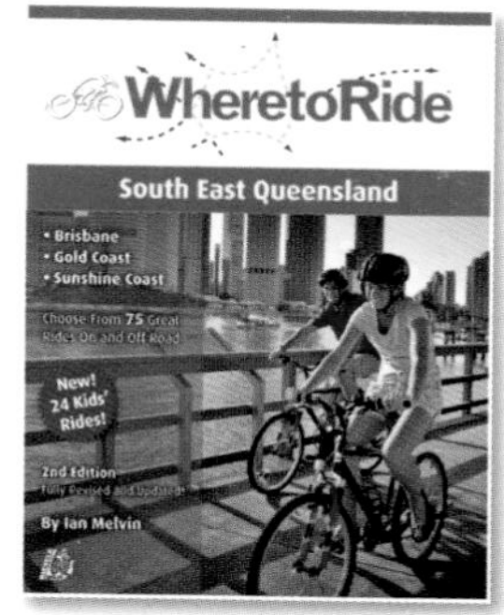

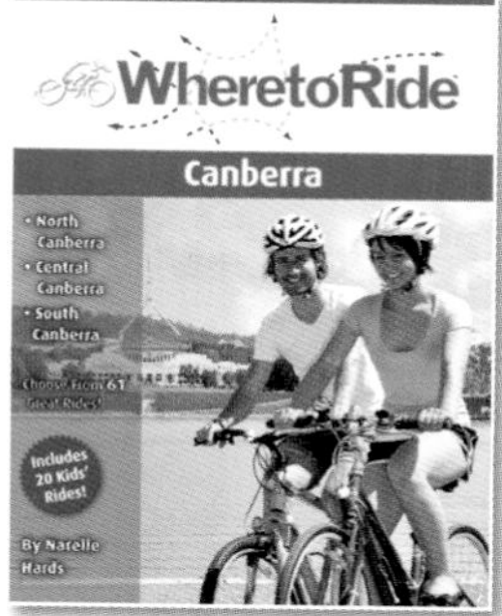

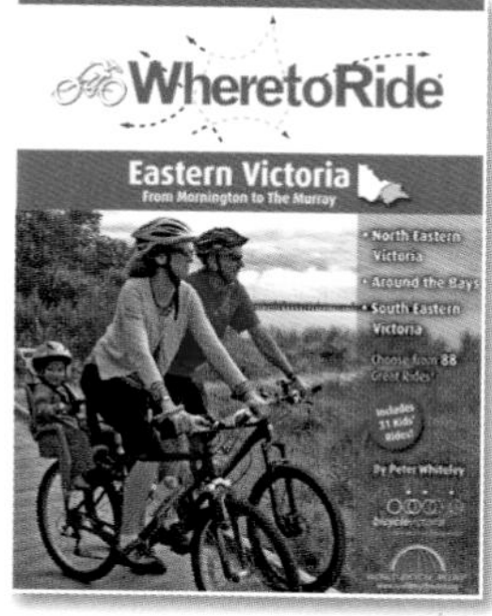

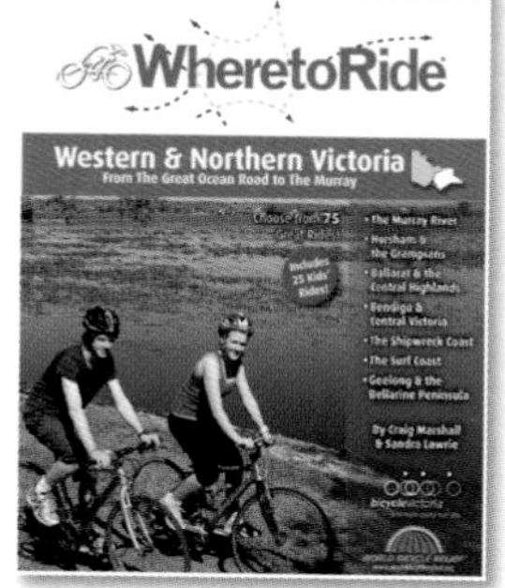

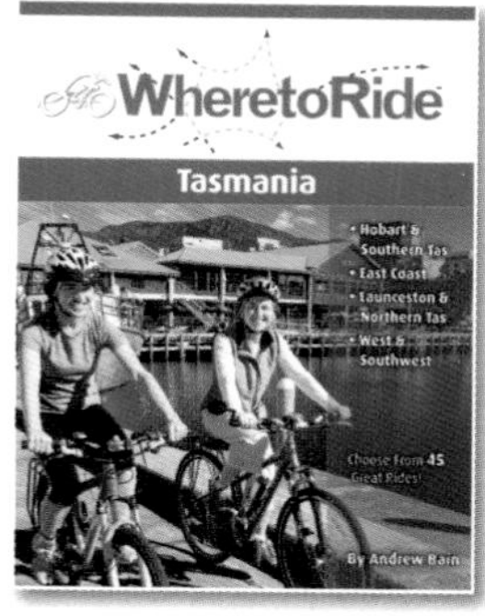

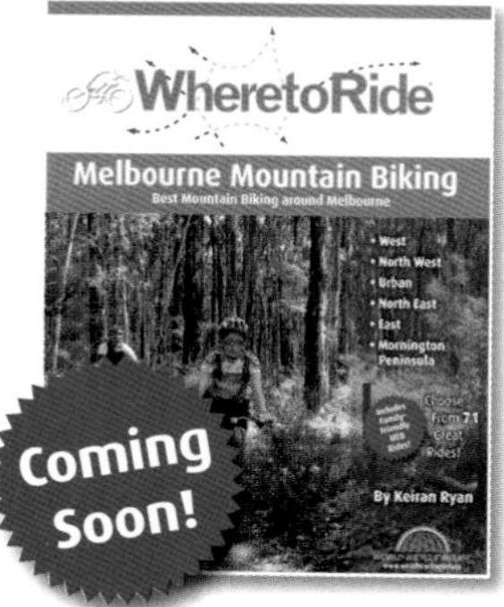

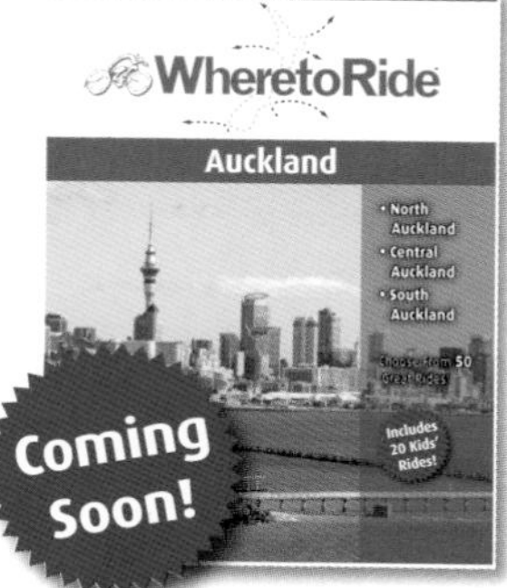

www.**WheretoBikeGuides**.com

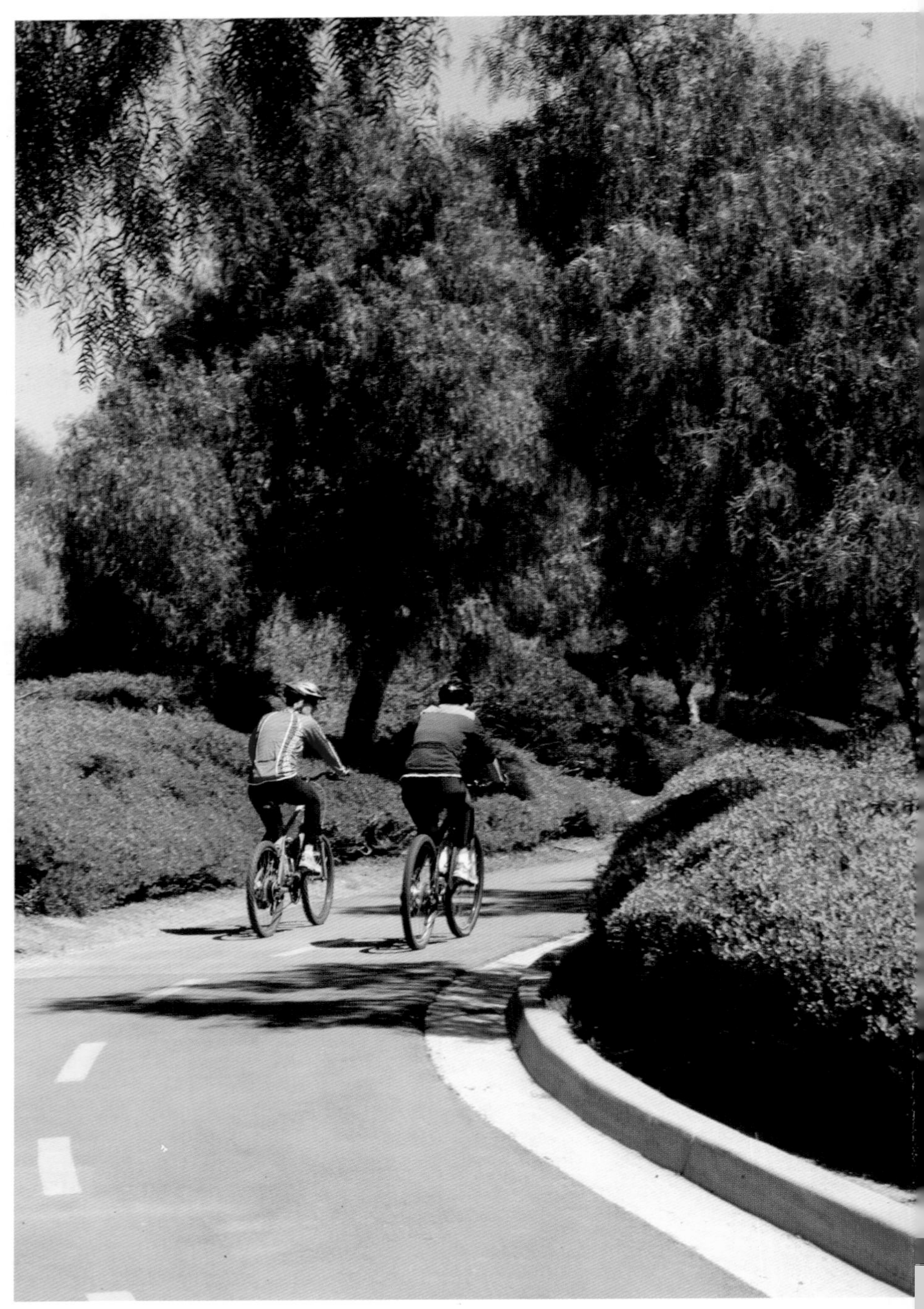